Surgical Exposure of the Spine: An Extensile Approach

Edited by
Edward C. Benzel, MD
Illustrated by
Michael Norviel

The American Association of Neurological Surgeons
Park Ridge, Illinois

ISBN: 1-879284-25-1

Printed in U.S.A.

Daniel L. Barrow, MD, Chairman
AANS Publications Committee

Joanne B. Needham, AANS Staff Editor

AANS1M995

Dedication

To Nancy Segall Bashook,
whose knowledge, insight, energy, and enthusiam
have furthered the education of so many.

Acknowledgment

We thank Jeffrey Gibson for his assistance with the illustrations.

Many of the illustrations in this book are modifications of drawings from other sources.

Contents

List of Contributors

Joseph T. Alexander, MD
Major, United States Army Medical Corps
Assistant Chief, Neurosurgery Service
Brooke Army Medical Center
Fort Sam Houston, Texas

John A. Anson, MD
Assistant Professor of Neurosurgery
University of New Mexico
School of Medicine
Division of Neurosurgery
Albuquerque, New Mexico

Nevan G. Baldwin, MD
Assistant Professor of Neurosurgery
University of New Mexico
School of Medicine
Division of Neurosurgery
Albuquerque, New Mexico

Edward C. Benzel, MD, FACS
Professor and Chief of Neurosurgery
University of New Mexico
School of Medicine
Division of Neurosurgery
Albuquerque, New Mexico

Charles L. Branch Jr, MD
Associate Professor of Neurosurgery
Division of Surgical Sciences
Bowman Gray School of Medicine
Wake Forest University
Winston-Salem, North Carolina

Arnold H. Menezes, MD, FACS, FAAP
Professor and Vice Chairman
Division of Neurosurgery
University of Iowa Hospitals and Clinics
University of Iowa College of Medicine
Iowa City, Iowa

Stephen M. Papadopoulos, MD
Department of Neurosurgery
University of Michigan Medical Center
Ann Arbor, Michigan

Richard L. Saunders, MD
Professor and Chairman, Neurological Surgery
Dartmouth Medical School
Dartmouth-Hitchcock Medical Center
Lebanon, New Hampshire

Eric J. Woodard, MD
Staff Neurosurgeon
Neurosurgery and Spinal Surgery Associates
Rapid City, South Dakota

AANS Publications Committee

Preface

Surgical Exposure of the Spine: An Extensile Approach is intended to serve as a surgical anatomical reference. Its content is descriptive and pictoral. Chapter architecture is repetitive so that data and anatomical concept acquisition is facilitated.

The inclusion of the word "extensile" in the title of the book is by design. It is taken from the work of Henry (Henry AK: *Extensile Exposure, ed 2.* Baltimore: Williams & Wilkins, 1957). It implies, as its inclusion in the title of Henry's book *Extensile Exposure,* the intent of creating an avenue through which an anatomical and safe surgical exposure is gained.

The following is an excerpt from the preface to the first edition of Henry's book (Henry AK: *Extensile Exposure Applied to Limb Surgery.* Edinburgh, Scotland: Livingstone, 1946):

> Exposures that will vie effectively with the "great arsenal of chance" must be a match for every shift, and therefore have a range, *extensile,* like the tongue of the chameleon, to reach where it requires. . . . *Bone and spine and contents* [my italics] carries our anatomy and forms its central fact, *bone and spine and contents* [my italics] wherever possible is made the core of each exposure. . . .

Thus, the surgeon's ability to expose the spine and its contents must have a range that is **extensile**. It is the intent of this book to facilitate just that.

The anatomical approach to the discipline of surgery is often intuitive. Most surgeons, however, intermittently fail to adequately consider regional anatomy during the act of surgery itself. Spine surgery is no exception.

This book is designed to first portray the surgically appropriate anatomy, and then describe the surgical approaches to the spine from a practical and anatomical point of view. Techniques of anatomical structure manipulation that enhance the surgical approach are described, discussed, and depicted.

The entire spine, from the skull base to the sacrum, is covered. A variety of approaches and surgical angles and orientations of exposure are depicted.

For the most part, black and white line drawings are used in this text. This type of illustration has been found to provide the greatest amount of useful and clinically applicable information. Surgical or cadaver photographs do not depict with clarity the anatomical points and regions of interest as well as the artist does, with his ability to emphasize the relevant and to de-emphasize the relatively irrelevant.

Edward C. Benzel, MD

Chapter 1

Cervical Spine and Skull Base Anatomy

Joseph T. Alexander, MD

Cervical Triangles

The neck has traditionally been divided into a series of triangular areas for ease of anatomical description (Figure 1). The sternocleidomastoid muscle forms the prominent border of the large anterior and posterior triangles.[11,15] Within the anterior triangle, the submandibular triangle is located above the digastric muscle. The submental triangle is bounded by the ventral belly of the digastric muscle, the hyoid bone, and the midline. The carotid triangle is caudal to the dorsal belly of the digastric muscle, ventral to the sternocleidomastoid muscle, and dorsal to the omohyoid muscle. The muscular triangle is bounded by the omohyoid and sternocleidomastoid muscles and the midline. The posterior triangle is located between the dorsal border of the sternocleidomastoid and trapezius muscles, and is subdivided by the omohyoid muscle into the occipital and the subclavian triangles. Dorsally, the suboccipital triangle is defined by the obliquus capitis superior and inferior and the rectus capitis muscles[2] (Figure 2).

Palpable Landmarks

Some palpable features aid in preoperative localization of cervical levels. Ventrally, the hyoid bone is at the level of the C3 vertebra. The thyroid cartilage is at the level of the C4 vertebra, while the cricoid cartilage is at the C6 level. The sternal notch of the manubrium is not a reliable guide, due to the considerable variation between individuals in the angulation of the thoracic inlet.[18] The prominent transverse process of the atlas can be palpated between the mastoid process and the dorsal border of the mandible. Dorsally, the large spinous process of the axis can be located in the midline of the suboccipital region. The spinous process of the C7 vertebra is prominent in the lower cervical midline. In the anesthesized patient, the anterior arch of the atlas can be palpated in the midline of the upper pharynx.[7]

Fascial Planes

Knowledge of the cervical fascial planes is critical in the ventral and lateral approaches to the spine. Exploitation of the natural planes between these layers simplifies the

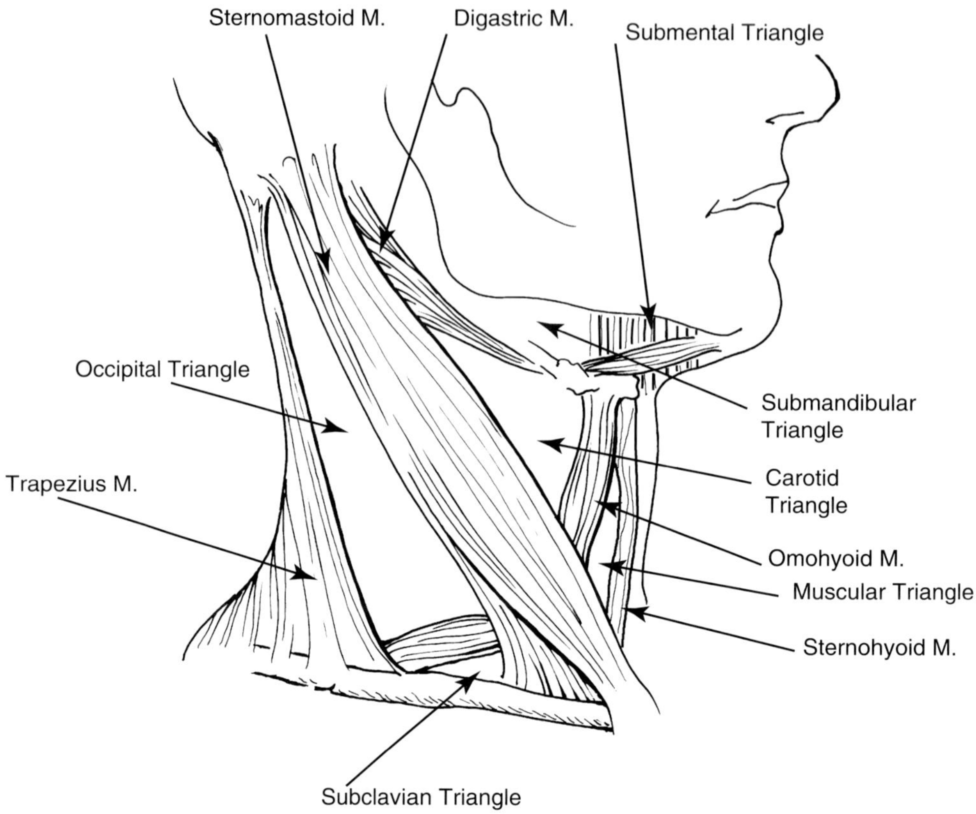

Figure 1. The triangles of the ventral neck region.

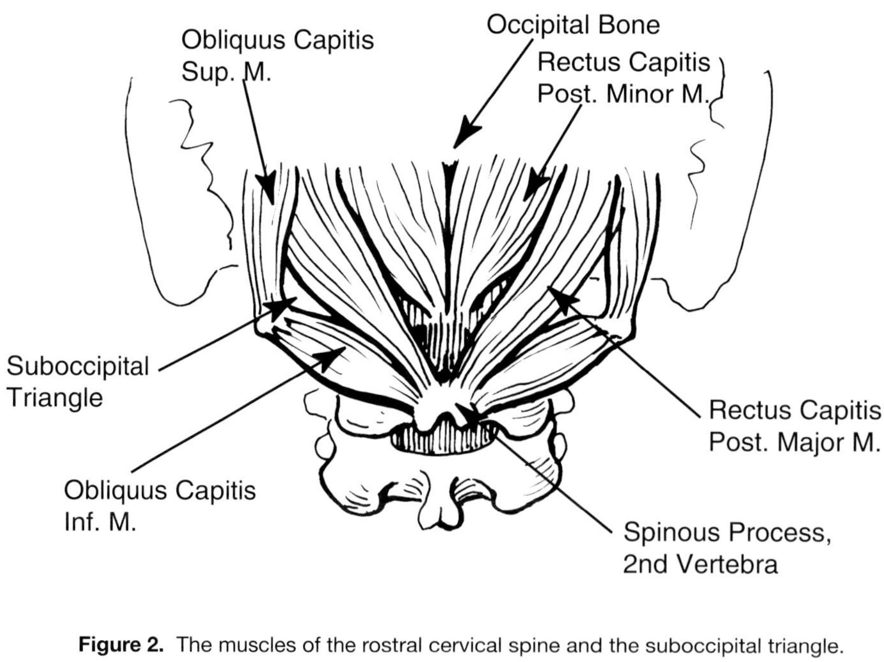

Figure 2. The muscles of the rostral cervical spine and the suboccipital triangle.

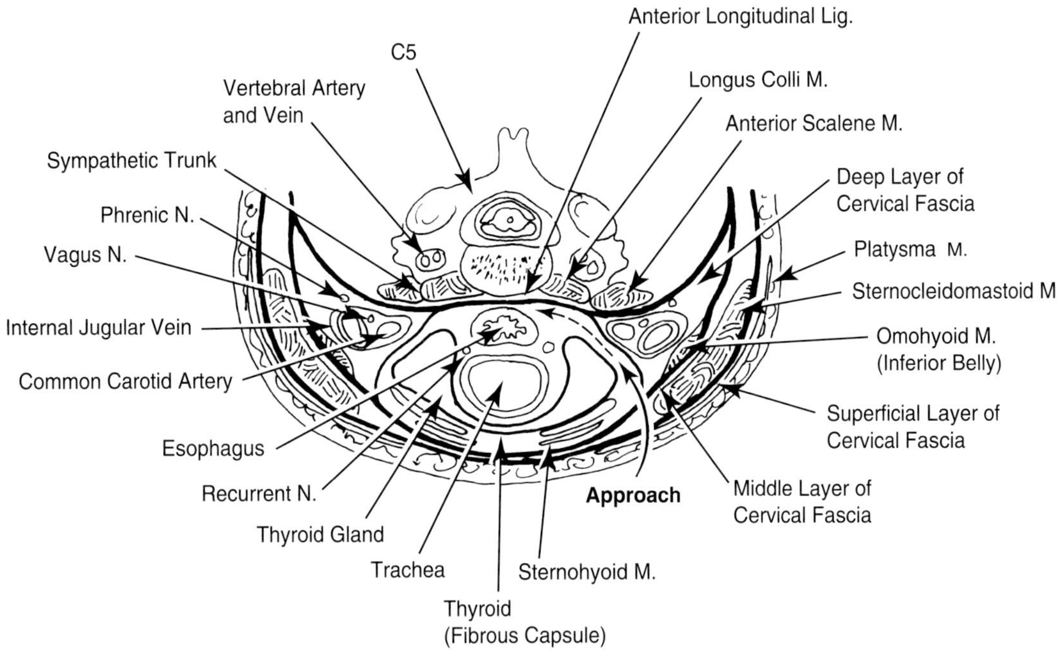

Figure 3. Fascial planes of the ventral neck region. The fascial planes are depicted by dense lines. "Approach" depicts the common approach for the exposure of the ventral cervical spine.

surgical dissection, and the fascia itself provides some additional protection for the visceral and neurovascular structures that it encloses. The fascia is commonly divided into one superficial and three or four deep layers[11,21] (Figure 3). The superficial layer is located in the subcutaneous tissue and encloses the platysma muscle. The superficial layer of the deep fascia surrounds the neck and contains the sternocleidomastoid and trapezius muscles. The middle layer can be subdivided into the visceral fascia (containing the trachea, esophagus, thyroid gland, and recurrent laryngeal nerve) and the alar fascia (which forms the carotid sheaths bilaterally). The deep layer, also called the prevertebral fascia, encloses the vertebral bodies, the ventral and dorsal paraspinal muscles, and the cervical and brachial plexuses. Sibson's fascia forms the floor of the subclavian triangle and covers the pleura at the apex of the lung.

Bony Anatomy

The pertinent bony anatomy of the cervical region includes the base of the skull.[7] Beginning at the foramen magnum, the paired occipital condyles are located in the ventrolateral quadrants and are convex caudally (Figure 4). The long axes of the occipital condyles project ventromedially and are situated at approximately 90° to each other. The styloid process and the exit of the eustachian tube from the skull are found on a line between the mastoid process and the pterygoid tubercle at the base of the medial pterygoid plate. The pterygoid tubercle buttresses the rostral aspect of the clivus, and the hard palate defines the posterior nasal aperture. The vomer fuses with the upper clivus at this aperture. The pharyngeal tubercle is located on the midline of the clivus two-thirds of the way from the vomer to the foramen magnum, and is the

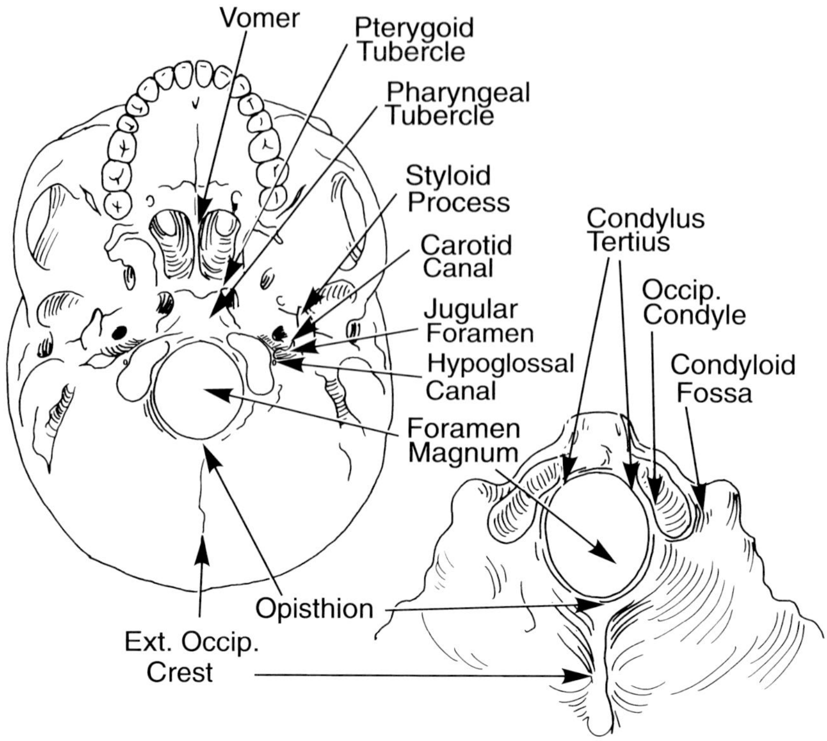

Figure 4. The base of the skull and the occipital condyles.

point of attachment for the pharynx. The hypoglossal canal is located lateral to the occipital condyle. Proceeding ventrally and medially, the jugular foramen, cranial nerves IX, X, and XI, and the carotid canal are found. The intrapetrous carotid artery remains superficial to the skull base in its ventromedial course. At the foramen lacerum, just dorsolateral to the pterygold tubercle, the carotid artery is unprotected caudally. Dorsal to the foramen magnum is the opisthion. The external occipital crest runs from the opisthion to the inion, and forms the attachment for the ligamentum nuchae.[20]

The C1 and C2 vertebrae (the atlas and the axis, respectively) are distinct in morphology, both from each other and from the remainder of the cervical vertebrae. The atlas consists of two wedge-shaped lateral masses connected by the short, thick anterior arch and a longer, thinner posterior arch. The transverse processes of the atlas are very prominent. The lateral masses are concave rostrally and receive the rounded occipital condyles, forming a ball and socket-type joint that restricts motion to primarily flexion and extension, due to the orthogonal positioning of the condyles. The inferior articular portion of the lateral masses face caudally and medially. On the medial aspect of the lateral masses are the tubercles for the attachment of the transverse ligament of the atlas. The vertebral artery passes through the transverse foramen, then turns dorsally and medially along the posterior arch before curving back ventrally to penetrate the dura mater[16] (Figure 5).

The C2 vertebra, or axis, provides a transition between the unique anatomy of the occipitocervical junction and the lower cervical spine. The rostral portion of the axis includes the odontoid process (or dens). This is derived embryologically from the

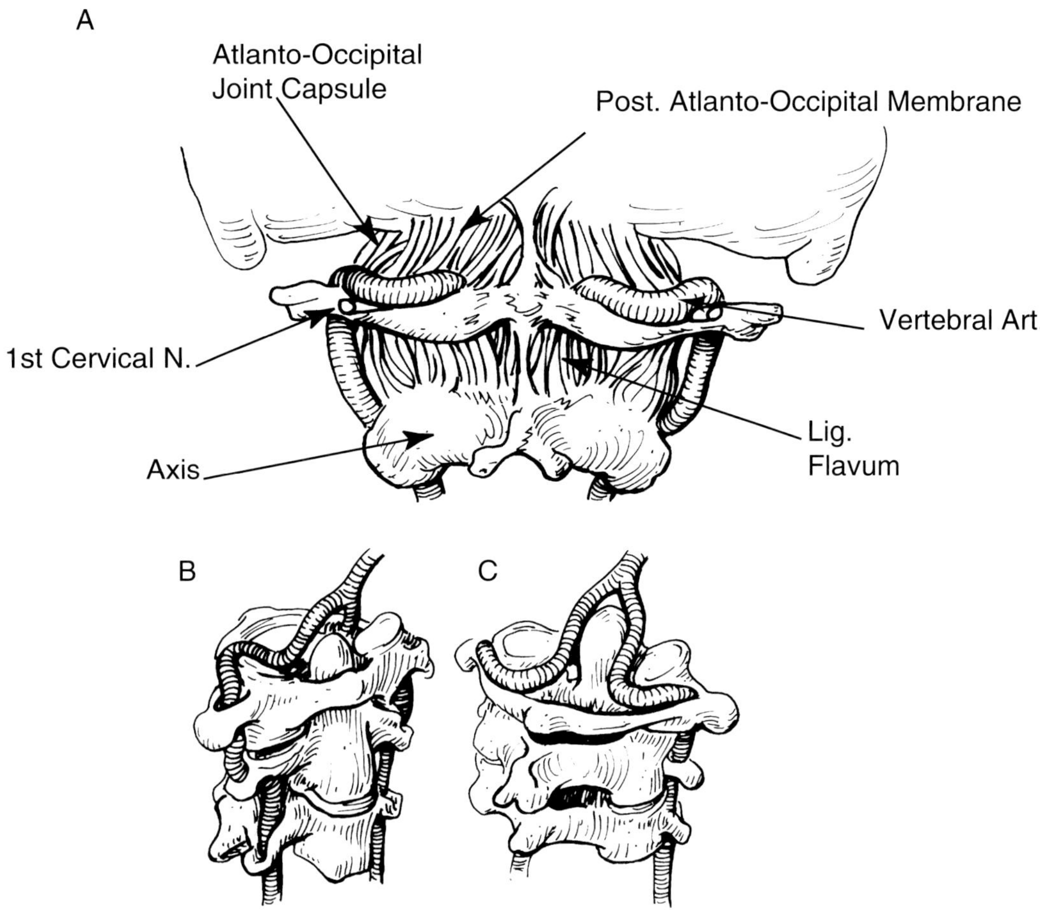

Figure 5. The course of the vertebral artery in the rostral cervical spine. The vertebral artery pierces the dura mater and the posteroatlanto-occipital membrane as depicted in **(A).** Two views depict its course through the bony rostral cervical spine and skull base **(B** and **C).**

centrum of the C1 segment. The midportion of the dens is narrowed at the level of the transverse ligament of the atlas. There is a synovial joint between the anterior aspect of the dens and the anterior arch of the atlas. The superior articular processes of the axis face upward and outward to receive the atlas. Along with lax capsular ligaments, this configuration allows for considerable rotation of the atlas on the axis, with the dens serving as the pivot point. The pars interarticularis is short and thick. From a dorsal perspective, the pars interarticularis projects 20° to 30° toward the midline and 45° rostral from the middle of the lateral masses[8] (Figure 6). The lamina are thick and the spinous process is prominent. Caudally, there is a conventional annulus and nucleus pulposus between the axis and the C3 vertebral body. The inferior articular processes of the atlas are oriented in the coronal plane.

Although the overall size of the vertebral bodies increases from the C3 to the C7 level, their general features are common. The rostral aspect of the centrum of a typical lower cervical vertebra has a bilateral rostral projection dorsolaterally (the uncus). This gives the body a rostrally concave

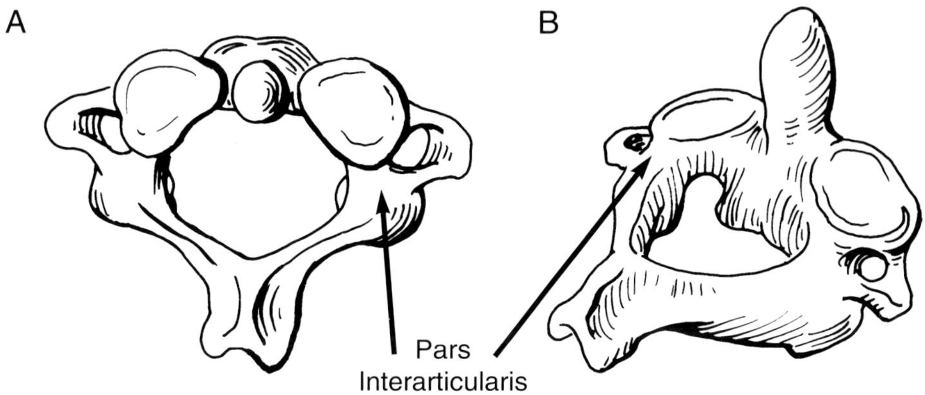

Figure 6. The C2 vertebra as viewed from a rostral orientation **(A)** and a dorsolateral orientation **(B).**

shape in the coronal plane, and enables it to receive the somewhat rounded caudal aspect of the adjacent vertebral body. The transverse process projects laterally and terminates in an anterior and a posterior tubercle (Figure 7). The anterior tubercle of the C6 vertebra is usually the most prominent, and marks the rostral turn of the vertebral artery into the foramen. At consecutive rostral levels, the vertebral artery (along with a plexus of veins) passes through the transverse foramen. On the rostral surface of each transverse process, there is a prominent groove carrying the exiting spinal nerve root.[10] The pedicles of a lower cervical vertebra are small and have a medial orientation. The lateral mass is connected both by the pedicle and by a ramus of the transverse processes. Because of the coronal orientation of the articular processes, the lateral masses have a 20° to 30° rostral orientation, as observed from a lateral perspective[9] (Figure 8). The lamina are thin and the spinous processes small and bifid in the midcervical region. The C6 spinous process is somewhat larger and that at C7 is quite prominent.

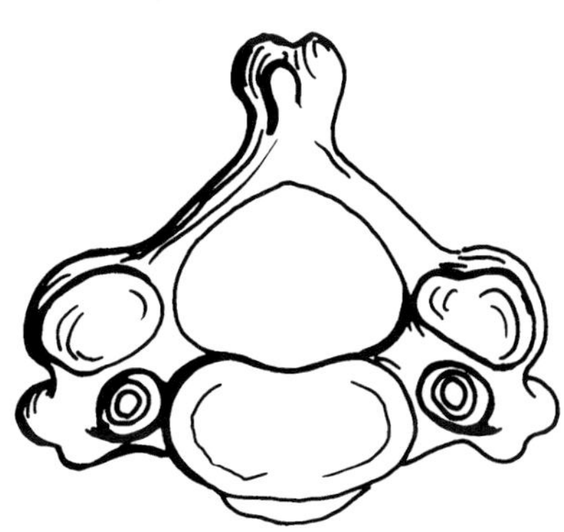

Figure 7. Mid- to low cervical vertebral body contour is depicted. Note the dorsally oriented concave shape.

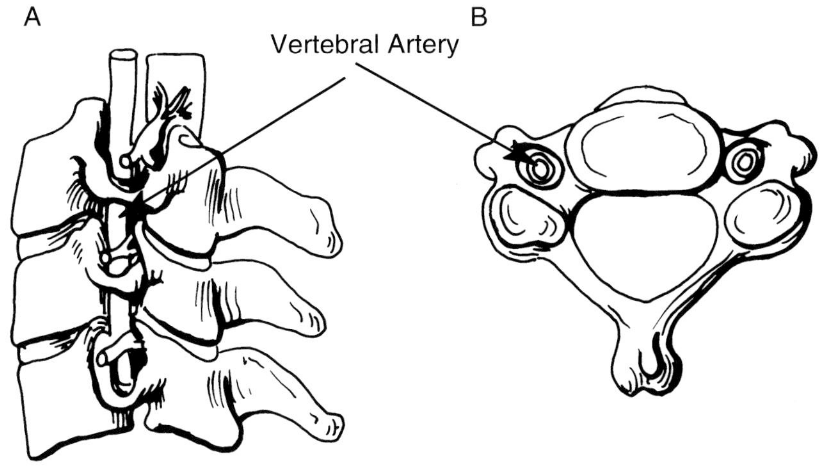

Figure 8. A lateral **(A)** and axial **(B)** view of the cervical spine. Note the orientation of the lateral masses in the parasagittal plane **(A)** and the orientation of the pedicles in the axial plane **(B).**

The cervical area is limited ventrally by the manubrium and clavicles. The thoracic inlet is composed of the first ribs bilaterally, the T1 vertebral body, and the manubrium.[1,18] A cervical rib is an anomalous structure that articulates with the C7 transverse process and the manubrium, and may at times compromise the caudal aspect of the brachial plexus at the attachment of the anterior scalene muscle.[21]

Ligaments

The ligaments of the cervical spine are crucial for the maintenance of alignment and stability.[8,22] Once again, the occipito-atlantoaxial complex has a unique configuration (Figure 9). The cruciform ligament maintains the alignment of the odontoid process with the atlas. The thick, horizontal portion of this ligament, known as the transverse ligament, attaches to the tubercles of the lateral masses of the atlas. It articulates with a synovial joint at the narrow waist of the dens. The ascending band of the cruciform ligament attaches to the inner aspect of the foramen magnum, and the descending band attaches to the body of the axis. The paired alar ligaments pass rostrally and laterally from the dens, attaching at the foramen magnum. These bands help limit lateral rotation. The apical ligament is a smaller vertical attachment from the tip of the dens. The anterior and posterior atlanto-occipital membranes attach the atlas to the skull base. The tectorial membrane is the continuation of the posterior longitudinal ligament, covers the dorsal aspect of the cruciform ligament, and attaches the axis to the skull.

The anterior longitudinal ligament spans the entire cervical spine, and helps limit extension. It is a thin structure that is firmly attached at each cervical level through dense connections to the ventral annulus fibrosus. It also is firmly attached to the anterior arch of the atlas.

The posterior longitudinal ligament is more substantial as it passes on the ventral surface of the spinal canal. It is densely attached to the fibers of the annulus fibrosus at each segmental level, but is not firmly attached to the intervening vertebral bodies. The rostral aspect is contiguous with the

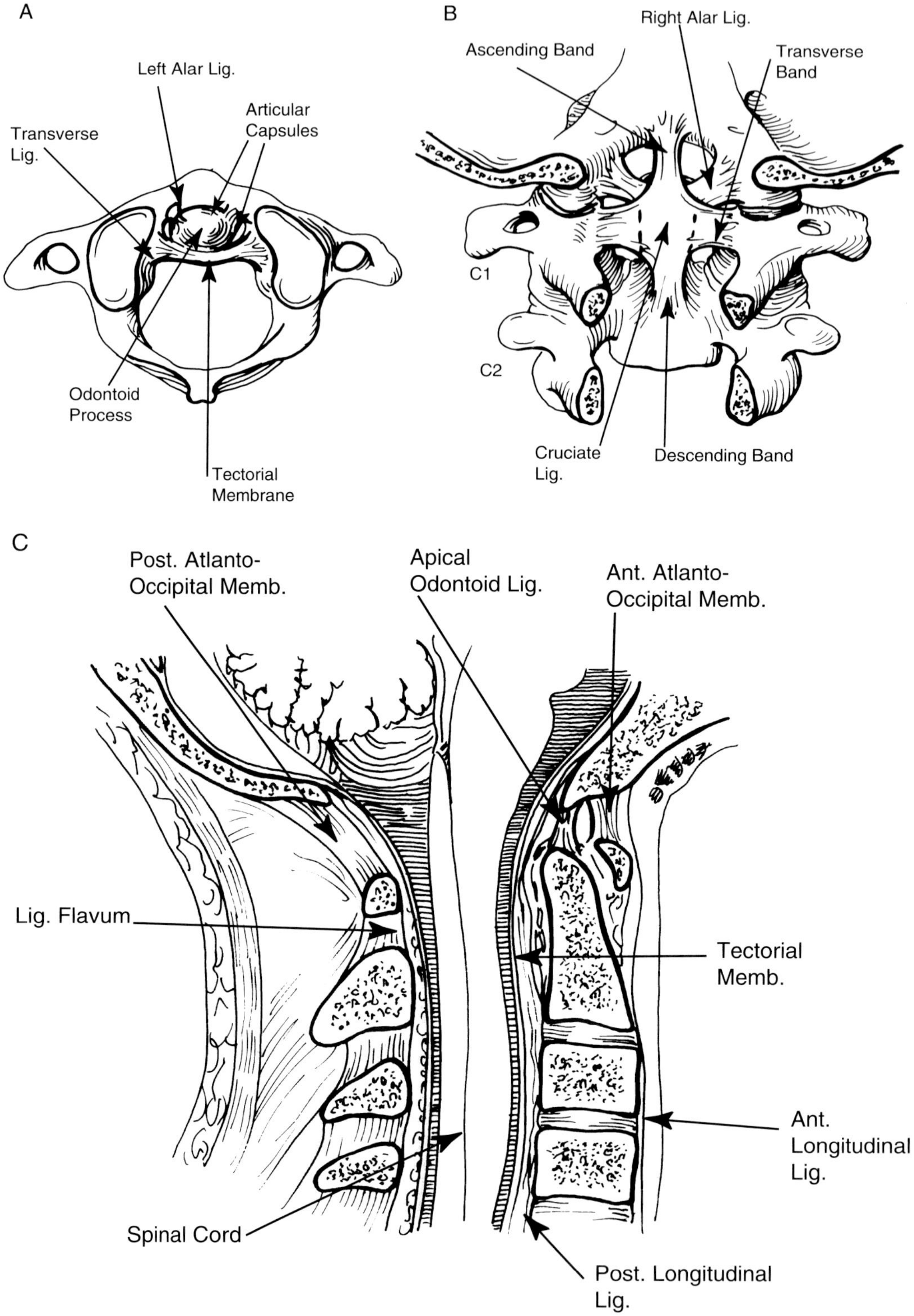

Figure 9. The ligaments of the rostral cervical spine between C1 and C2 as viewed axially **(A);** the dorsal aspect of the vertebral bodies, dens, and clivus as viewed after removing the lamina **(B)** and as viewed from a sagittal section **(C).**

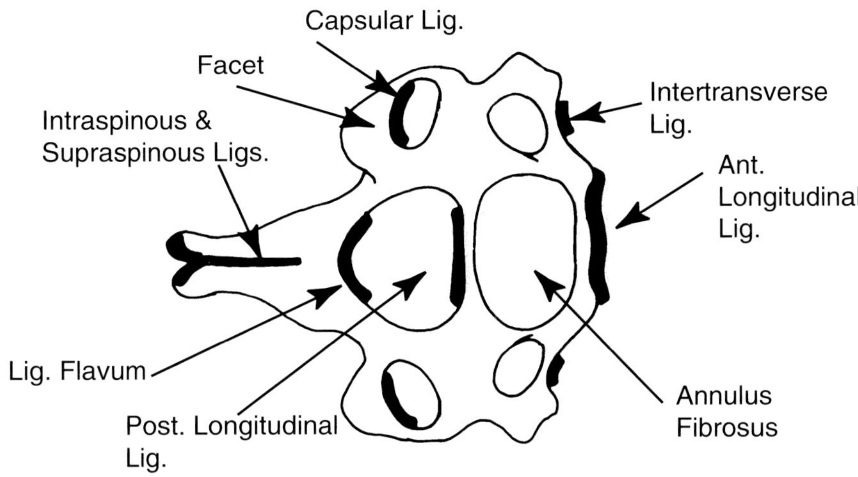

Figure 10. The ligamentous attachments of the mid- to low cervical spine.

tectorial membrane. There are a number of smaller ligaments joining the lower cervical vertebrae (Figure 10). Although the interspinous and the supraspinous ligaments are thin, they have a long lever arm with the vertebral body, and thus serve an important role in limiting flexion. The capsular ligaments are lax during normal motion, but can limit excessive flexion and rotation when under tension. The nuchal ligament consists of a band that runs from the occiput to the spinous process of C7 (the funicular portion), and a fibrous septum (the lamellar portion) that attaches to the external occipital crest, the spinous processes, and the funicular portion.[22] It appears to have only a minimal structural role in humans, but it may provide proprioceptive input to the cervical musculature.

Muscles

The muscles of the neck can be considered from the standpoint of either function (Table 1) or location.[2,6,11,14,15,20] In the ventral cervical region, the key anatomical landmark is the sternocleidomastoid muscle as it runs from the mastoid process to its dual insertion on the clavicle and the

Table 1. **Function of Cervical Muscles**

Extension	Flexion	Rotation	Lateral Flexion
Splenius capitis	Sternocleidomastoid	Sternocleidomastoid	Scalene
Splenius cervicis	Longus colli	Trapezius	Splenius capitis
Semispinalis capitis	Longus capitis	Splenius capitis	Longus colli
Semispinalis cervicis	Rectus capitis anterior	Longissimus capitis	Levator scapulae
Longissimus capitis	Stylohyoid	Obliquus capitis inferior	Iliocostalis cervicis
Longissimus cervicis	Digastric	Rectus capitis posterior major	Intertransversarii
Trapezius	Mylohyoid	Longus capitis	
Interspinal	Geniohyoid	Rotators	
Rectus capitis posterior major	Omohyoid	Multifidus	
Rectus capitis posterior minor	Sternohyoid		
Obliquus capitis superior	Sternothyroid		

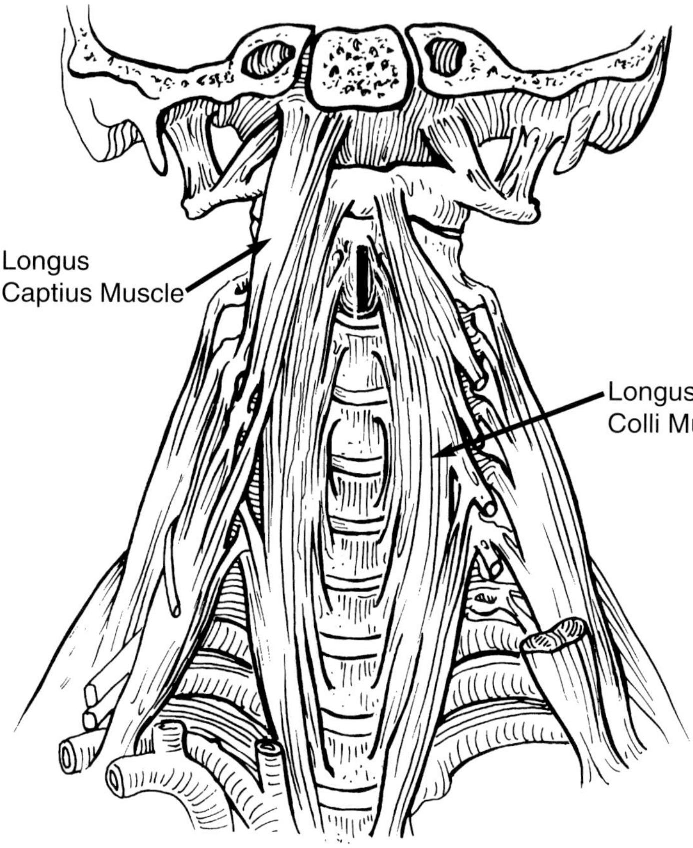

Figure 11. The prevertebral space as viewed following removal of all visceral and ventral muscular structures.

manubrium. The longus capitis and longus colli muscles define the prevertebral space, and are attached to the ventrolateral aspect of the vertebrae and the anterior tubercle of the transverse process (Figure 11). The scalene muscle group forms the floor of the occipital triangle, passing from the transverse processes to the upper ribs. The nerve roots and the brachial plexus pass between the anterior and middle scalene muscles. The strap muscles, along with the digastric muscles, stabilize the hyoid bone and larynx, and function as secondary flexors of the head and depressors of the mandible.

In the dorsal cervical region, the trapezius muscle is a prominent feature, spanning from the midline fascia to the scapula. The next layer includes the levator scapulae, the splenius capitis, and the splenius cervicis muscles. The deepest, or paraspinal, group includes the superior and inferior obliques, the semispinalis cervicis and capitis, the longissimus, and the iliocostalis muscles. Immediately adjacent to the spine are the short muscles: the rotators, the interspinal, the multifidus, and the intertransversarii muscles.

Arteries and Veins

The left common carotid artery usually originates directly from the arch of the aorta, while the right common carotid arises from the innominant artery[4,12,13,19] (Figure 12). The division of the common carotid artery into the internal and external carotid artery occurs in the carotid triangle. The small ascending pharyngeal artery arises here, and can generally be ligated, if necessary.

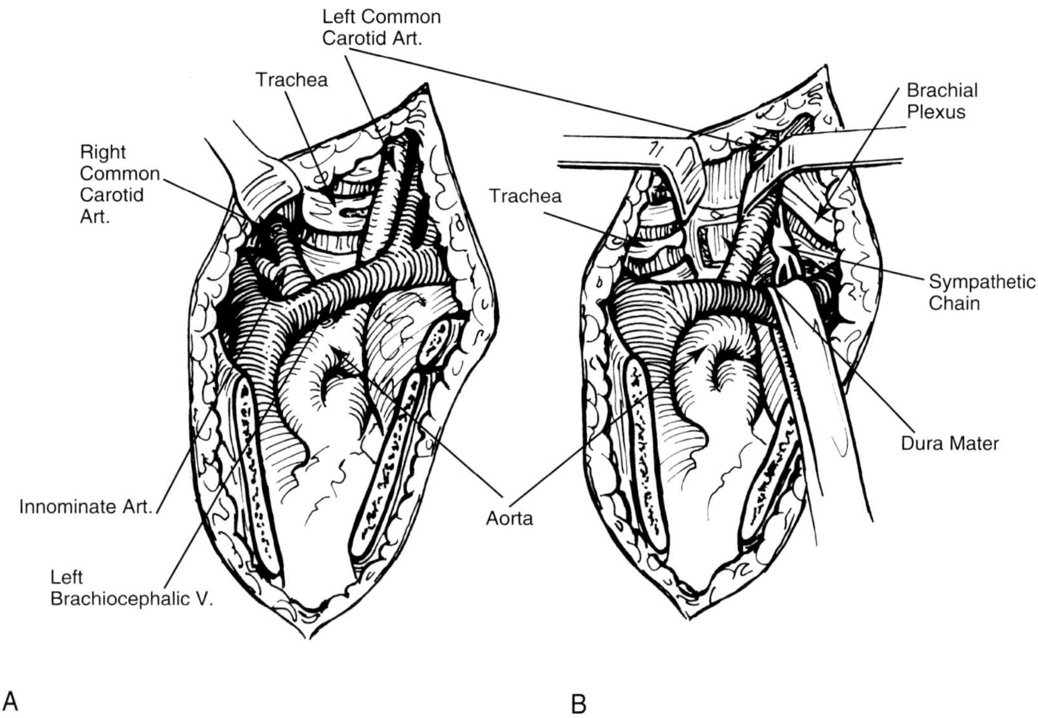

Figure 12. The vascular structures of the base of the neck **(A)** and following caudal retraction of the brachiocephalic vein **(B).**

The internal carotid artery proceeds to the skull base without further branches. The upper internal carotid artery is tethered at the skull base and is vulnerable to avulsion via excessive retraction in the rostal cervical region. The external carotid artery has several branches in the carotid triangle, including the superior thyroid, the lingual, and the facial arteries. These arteries can generally be ligated, if necessary, but care must be taken because these vessels are accompanied by nerves.

The vertebral artery generally arises as the first branch of the subclavian artery. It passes through the foramen of the C6 vertebra, and then ascends through successive foramina in the transverse processes. As noted previously, after passing through the foramina of the atlas, the vertebral artery turns medially along the posterior arch of the atlas before turning ventrally to penetrate the dura mater. The vertebral arteries unite ventral to the medulla to form the basilar artery. In most individuals, there is considerable redundancy in the vertebrobasilar system, thus allowing for unilateral occlusion of a vertebral artery. However, there are many variations of these arteries, such as one dominant vertebral artery supplying the basilar system and the other terminating in the posterior inferior cerebellar artery. If vertebral artery occlusion is planned as part of an operative approach, angiographic confirmation of collateral supply is vital.

The thyrocervical trunk is the second branch of the subclavian artery (Figure 13). It divides into the inferior thyroid artery, which courses medially, and the transverse or superficial cervical artery, which proceeds dorsolaterally.

The deep jugular veins form at the skull base and proceed in the carotid sheath to the base of the neck, where they join the brachiocephalic veins. There is a highly variable network of superficial veins located both superficially and deep to the platysma muscle. Most of the arteries of the neck have an accompanying vein. Due to the rich anas-

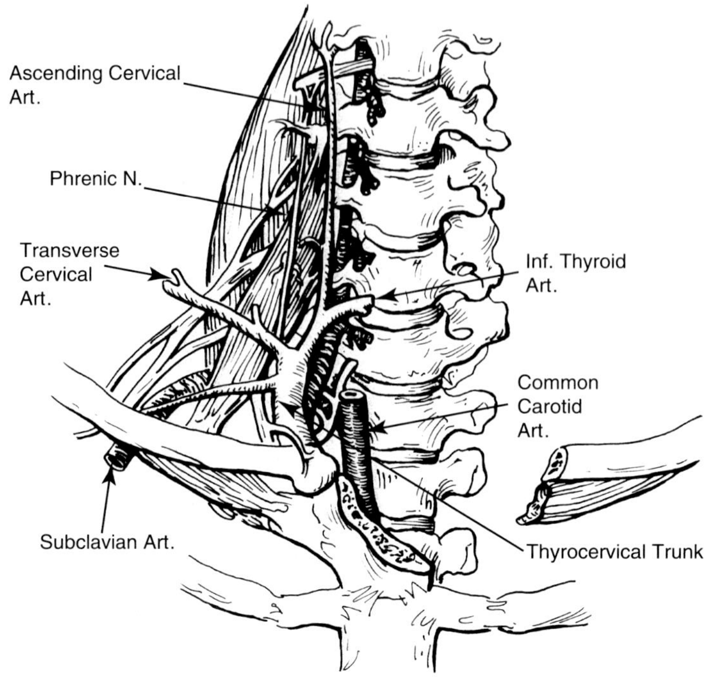

Figure 13. The thyrocervical trunk and juxtaposed structures.

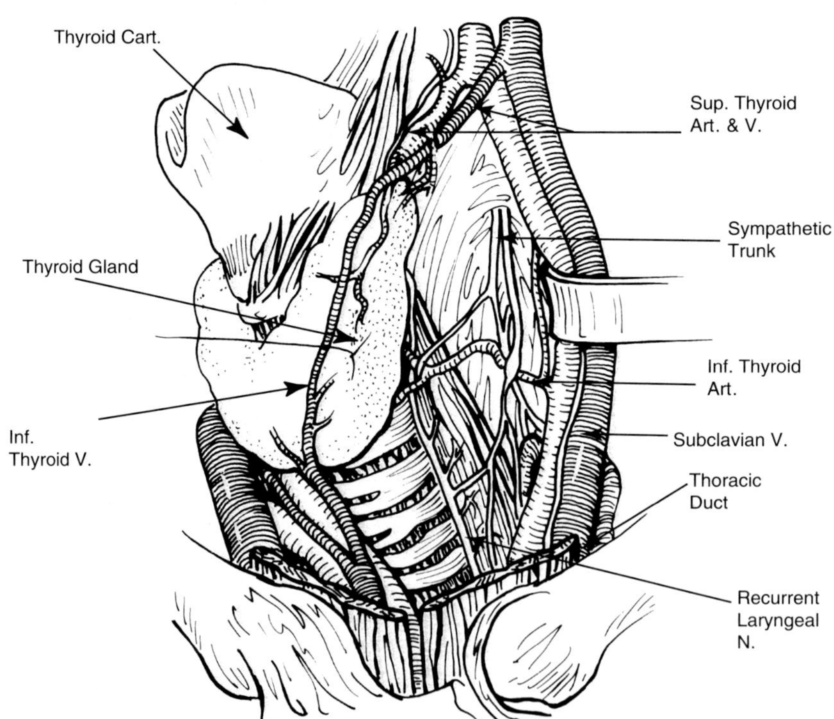

Figure 14. The deep structures of the low ventral neck region. Note the entrance of the thoracic duct into the left subclavian vein.

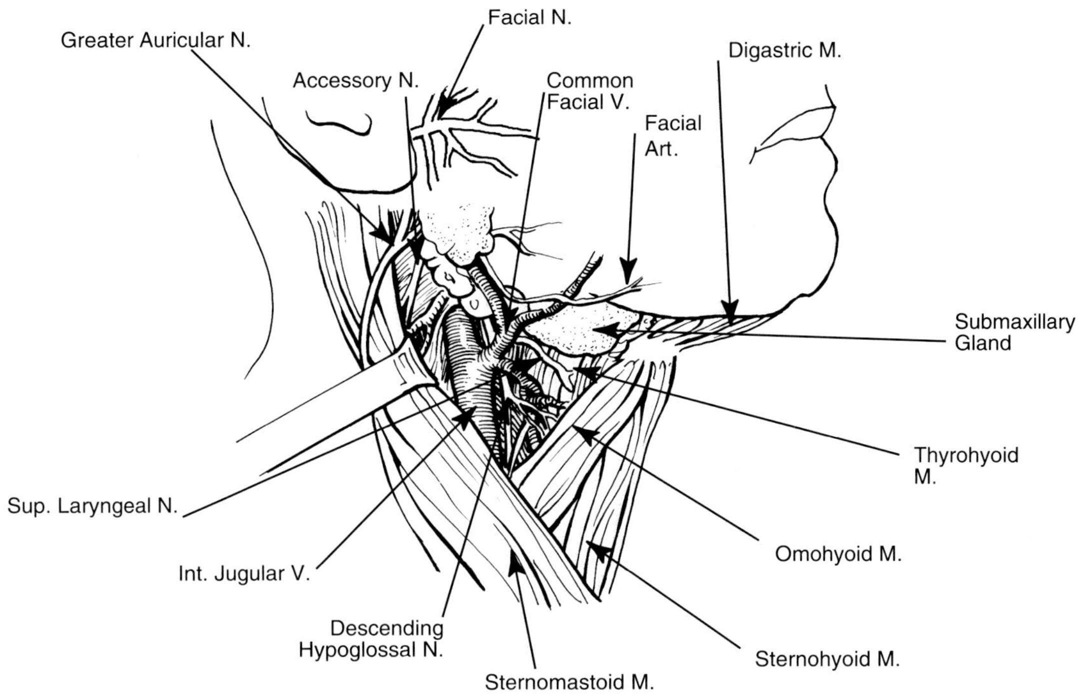

Figure 15. The submandibular region.

tomotic network comprised of the deep and superficial veins, most cervical veins can be ligated with impunity. However, in the case of certain extensive tumors, bilateral surgical approaches, or prior radiation, care must be taken to insure that adequate channels remain for venous return. The large subclavian veins can be encountered deep to the clavicle in low cervical approaches. They are thin-walled and can cause significant hemorrhage. There is a plexus of veins that accompanies the vertebral artery through the transverse foramina to the foramen magnum and that can be a troublesome source of bleeding during the dorsolateral approaches to the occipitocervical junction.

Lymphatics

The lymphatic drainage of the cervical region largely parallels that of the veins. A prominent chain of lymph nodes is found in the carotid and occipital triangles. These can generally be removed without consequence, for biopsy or convenience. The thoracic duct typically enters the left subclavian vein deep to the clavicle (Figure 14). Its course in the base of the neck can be variable, and the thoracic duct can be encountered during low cervical approaches from the left side. The thoracic duct can be ligated, if necessary, to gain exposure.

Cranial Nerves

The facial nerve exits the skull through the styloid canal and can be damaged by retraction at this level. It branches within the capsule of the parotid gland. The lowest branch of the facial nerve, the marginal mandibular nerve, runs under the mandible and can be encountered in retropharyngeal approaches (Figure 15). Damage to this branch causes drooping of the ipsilateral

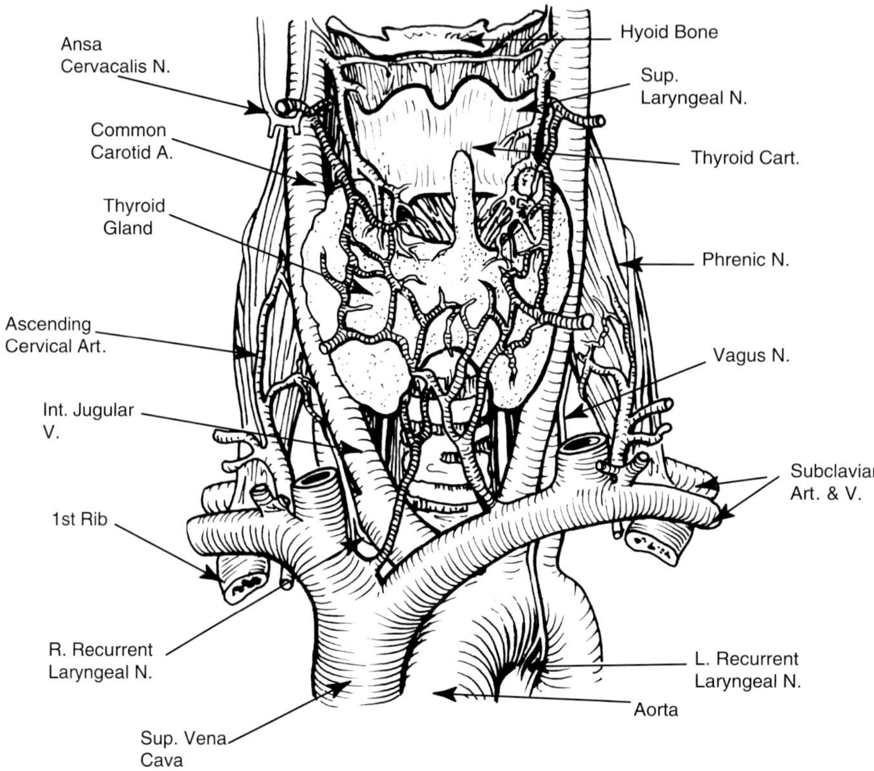

Figure 16A. The recurrent laryngeal nerves as they course about and through the vascular milieu of the low cervical spine region.

lip.[3,5,17] The glossopharyngeal and vagus nerves contribute branches to the pharyngeal plexus, supplying both motor and sensory fibers to the pharynx. An important branch of the vagus nerve is the superior laryngeal nerve, found adjacent to the superior thyroid artery. Damage to this nerve is responsible for early fatigue of the voice and difficulty producing high notes. The other important branch of the vagus nerve is the recurrent laryngeal nerve. On the left, the course of this nerve is constant, passing under the arch of the aorta and proceeding in the tracheo-esophageal groove. On the right side, the recurrent laryngeal nerve generally loops under the subclavian artery and then angles rostrally and medially to join the visceral structures (Figure 16). In some cases, the nerve is not recurrent at all on the right. The recurrent laryngeal nerve supplies most of the laryngeal muscles, and damage to this nerve causes hoarseness.

The accessory nerve crosses the carotid triangle to reach the rostral border of the sternocleidomastoid muscle one-third of the distance from the mastoid process to the clavicle. After supplying this muscle, it exits at the midportion of the sternocleidomastoid muscle and crosses the occipital triangle to supply the trapezius muscle. The hypoglossal nerve crosses the carotid canal rostral to the hyoid bone, prior to turning medially to supply the tongue. It sends an important branch, the descendens hypoglossus, to the strap muscles. The cervical sympathetic chain ascends from the thorax through the stellate, intermediate, and superior cervical ganglia (Figure 17). It is located on the ventral aspect of the longus colli and longus capitus muscles in the prevertebral space. Injury to this chain will produce an ipsilateral Horner's syndrome.

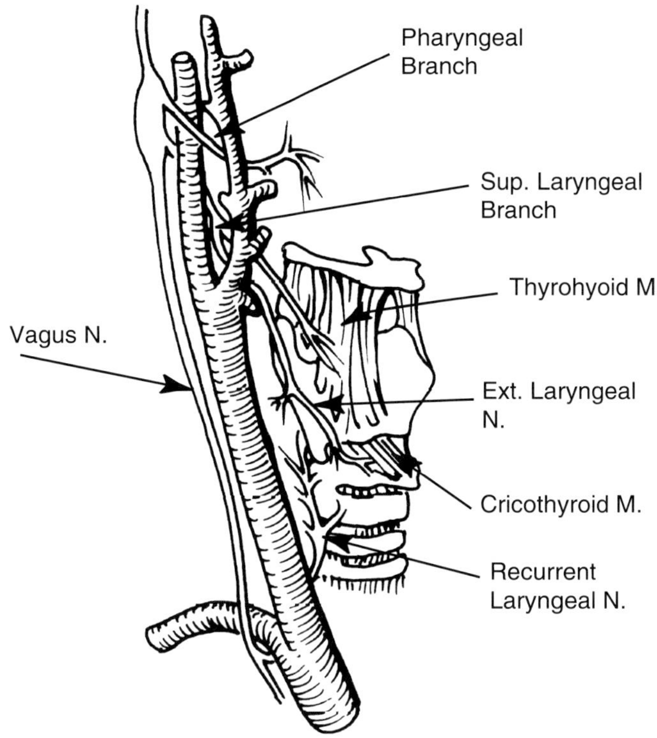

Figure 16B. The right ascending portion of the recurrent laryngeal nerve as it enters the larynx, with juxtaposed anatomical structures.

The Cervical Plexus

The cervical plexus is formed from branches of the first four cervical nerves (Figure 18). The phrenic nerve is the most important branch, also receiving a contribution from the C5 nerve root. The phrenic nerve runs on the ventral aspect of the anterior scalene muscle and must be preserved in low cervical approaches. The descendens cervicalis supplies the omohyoid muscle and joins the descendens hypoglossus through the ansa hypoglossi. Damage to this system may impair vocalization and swallowing function due to weakness of the strap muscles and consequent effects in the larynx and hyoid bone. The cervical plexus also gives off the greater auricular nerve, the small occipital nerve, and several cervical cutaneous nerves. These sensory nerves should be spared when possible; however, they may be sacrificed if necessary to provide exposure.

The Tongue and the Rostral Ventral Pharynx

The tongue can be divided, if necessary, to gain exposure in certain extended transoral procedures.[10] The midline of the tongue provides a relatively avascular plane, if this is needed. Similarly, the midline of the oropharynx is a relatively safe avenue to the upper prevertebral area (Figure 19). The pharyngeal musculature attaches in the midline at the pharyngeal tubercle of the clivus. There is modest vascular and lymphoid tissue in this portion of the pharynx. The eustachian tubes exit laterally. The retropharynx has two layers below the tubercle: a superficial mucosal layer and the deeper muscular layer. These layers should be closed separately in transoral approaches to the spine. The larynx and trachea are generally protected by the visceral fascia and the strap muscles during most cervical approaches. The parotid gland

A

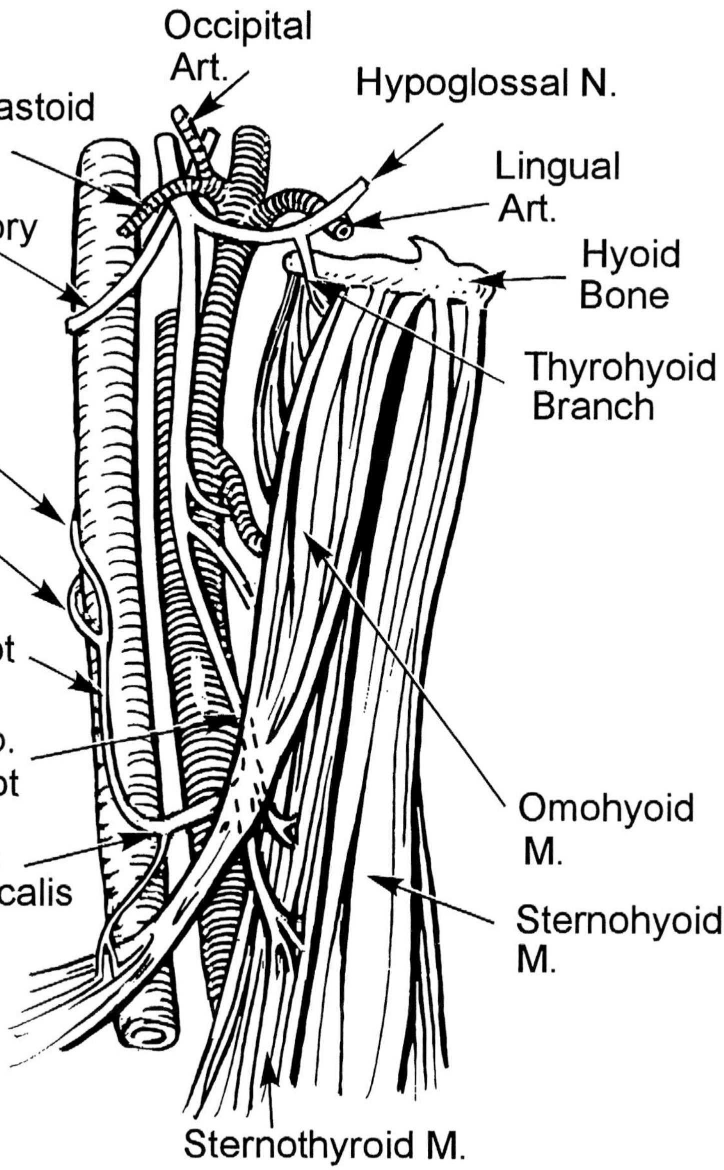

Figure 17A. The hypoglossal nerve and related structures.

B

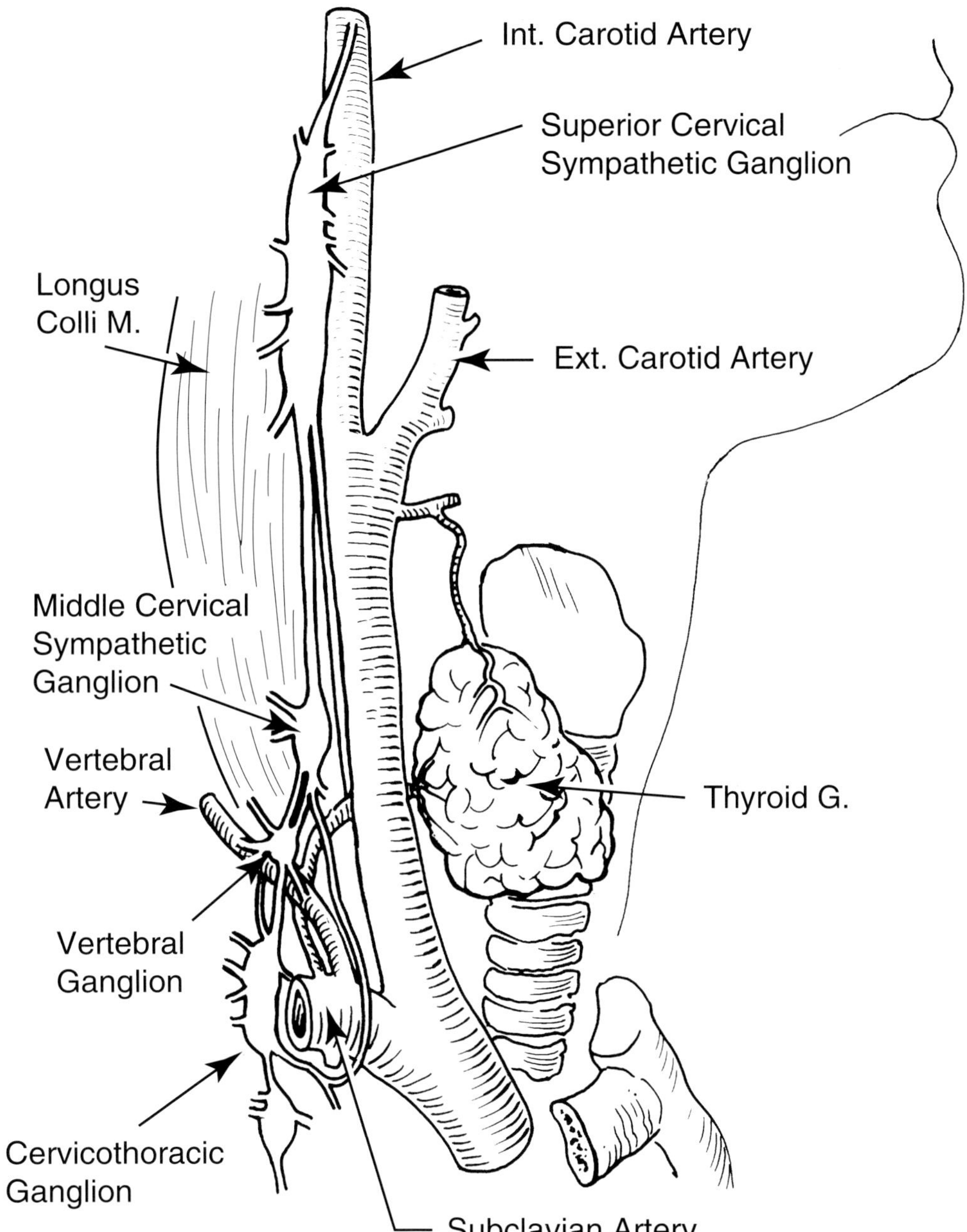

Figure 17B. The cervical sympathetic chain and related structures.

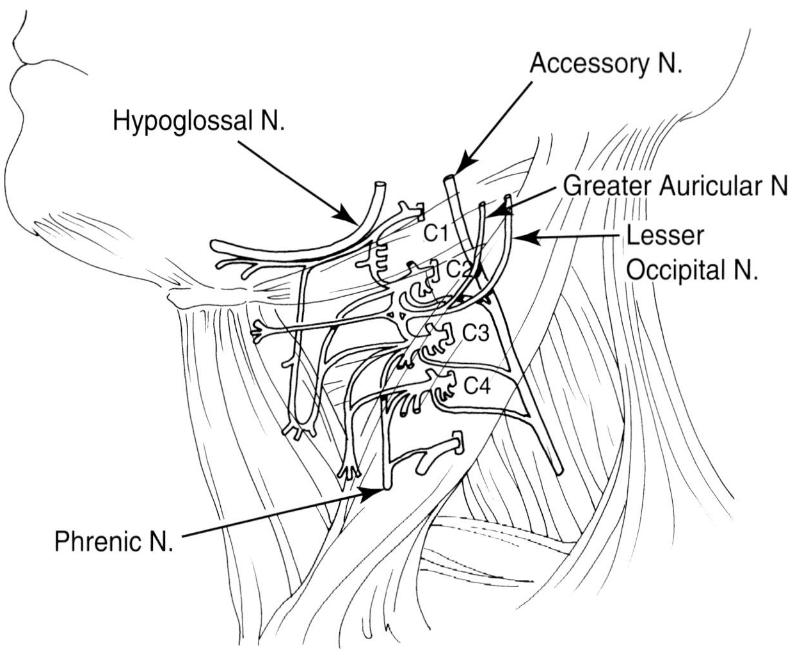

Figure 18. The cervical plexus.

must be protected during approaches through the upper cervical triangle because of the branches of the facial nerve. The submandibular salivary gland may be excised, if necessary, taking care to ligate its duct to prevent a fistula.

References

1. An HS: Surgical exposure and fusion techniques of the spine, in An HS, Cotler JM (eds): **Spinal Instrumentation.** Baltimore: Williams & Wilkins, 1992, pp 1-32
2. Anderson JE: **Grant's Atlas of Anatomy, ed 7.** Baltimore: Williams & Wilkins, 1978
3. Brazis PW, Masdeu JC, Biller J: **Localization in Clinical Neurology.** Boston: Little, Brown & Co, 1985
4. Chandler WF: **Carotid Artery Injuries.** Mount Kisco, NY: Futura Publishing, 1982
5. Chusid JG: **Correlative Neuroanatomy and Functional Neurology, ed 17.** Los Altos, CA: Lance Medical Publications, 1979
6. Clemente CD: **Anatomy, ed 2.** Baltimore: Urban & Schwartzenberg, 1981
7. Crockard HA, Johnston F: Development of transoral approaches to lesions of the skull base and craniocervical junction. **Neurosurg Q 3:**61-82, 1993
8. Dickman CA, Crawford NR, Brantley AGU, et al: In vitro cervical spine biomechanical testing. **BNI Q 9:**17-26, 1993
9. Dickman CA, Sonntag VKH, Marcotte PJ: Techniques of screw fixation of the cervical spine. **BNI Q 9:**27-38, 1993
10. Hakuba A, Komiyama M, Tsujimoto T, et al: Transuncodiscal approach to dumbbell tumors of the cervical spinal canal. **J Neurosurg 61:**1100-1106, 1984
11. Johnson RM, Murphy MJ, Southwick WO: Surgical approaches to the spine, in Rothman RH, Simeone FA (eds): **The Spine, ed 3.** Philadelphia: WB Saunders, 1992, pp 1607-1738
12. McAfee PC, Bohlman HH, Riley LH Jr, et al: The anterior retropharyngeal approach to the upper part of the cervical spine. **J Bone Joint Surg (Am) 69:**1371-1383, 1987
13. McDonnell DE: Anterolateral cervical approach to the craniovertebral junction, in Rengachary SS, Wilkins RH (eds): **Neurosurgical Operative Atlas.** Baltimore: Williams & Wilkins, 1992, pp 147-164
14. McMinn RMH, Hutchings RT, Logan BM: **Color Atlas of Head and Neck Anatomy.** Chicago: Yearbook Medical Publishers, 1981

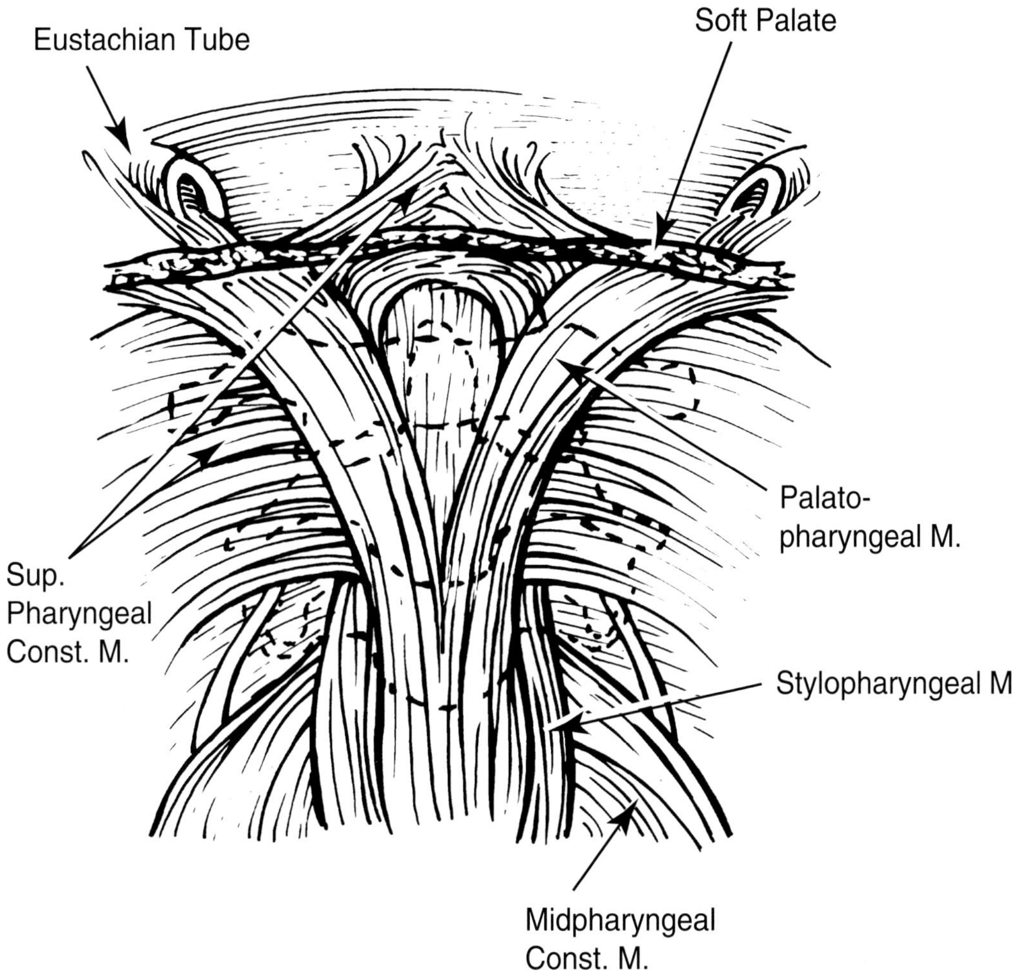

Figure 19. The midline ventral oropharynx.

15. Parke WW, Sherk HH: **The Cervical Spine, ed 2.** Philadelphia: JB Lippincott, 1989

16. Sen CN, Sekhar LN: An extreme lateral approach to intradural lesions of the cervical spine and foramen magnum. **Neurosurgery 27:**197-204, 1990

17. Shah JPI, Shana AR: Transmandibular approaches to the upper cervical spine, in Sundaresan N, Schmidek HH, Schiller AL, et al (eds): **Tumors of the Spine.** Philadelphia: WB Saunders, 1990, pp 329-335

18. Sundaresan N, DiGiacinto GV: Surgical approaches to the cervicothoracic junction, in Sundaresan N, Schmidek HH, Schiller AL, et al (eds): **Tumors of the Spine.** Philadelphia: WB Saunders, 1990, pp 358-368

19. Sundaresan N, Sachdev VP: Anterior approaches to the cervical spine, in Sundaresan N, Schmidek HH, Schiller AL, et al (eds): **Tumors of the Spine.** Philadelphia: WB Saunders, 1990, pp 344-357

20. VanGilder JC, Menezes AH, Dolan KD: **The Craniovertebral Junction and Its Abnormalities.** Mount Kisco, NY: Futura Publishing, 1987

21. von Torklus D, Nicola T: **Atlas of Orthopaedic Exposures, ed 2.** Baltimore: Urban & Schwartzenberg, 1986

22. White M, Panjabi MM: **Clinical Biomechanics of the Spine, ed 2.** Philadelphia: JB Lippincott, 1990

The opinions expressed in this chapter are those of the author and must not be construed as representing the policy of the Department of Defense or the Department of the Army.

Chapter 2

Ventral Subaxial Cervical Spine Anatomy

Richard L. Saunders, MD

Ventromedial and ventrolateral surgery of the subaxial cervical spine are performed through the retropharyngeal space.[2] The lateral extremes of this space are defined by the attachments of the prevertebral fascia to the anterior tubercles of the transverse processes (Figure 1). This fascia covers the ventral vertebral surfaces and the longus colli muscle complex. Orientation in this space is achieved by palpation of the disc spaces, the more lateral anterior tubercle, and the midline longitudinal keel on C2. The anterior tubercle is particularly prominent at C6, is not distorted by degenerative disease, and is consistently 1 cm from the uncinate process (Figure 2). The C2 keel is a characteristic bony prominence enhanced by a sharp configuration of the anterior longitudinal ligament. Accordingly, upon accessing the retropharyngeal space, the segmental level and the lateral margin of the disc space are defined readily without x-ray. A finger tip pressed just medial to the transverse process tubercle lies over the lateral aspect of the disc.

The uncinate process is the basic anatomical reference point for ventromedial surgery of the subaxial cervical spine. It marks the lateral extent of the disc space and the medial extent of the vertebral artery. Within the spinal canal, the medial aspect of the base of the uncinate process lies at or slightly medial to the base of the pedicle, and thus identifies the approximate position of the axilla of the nerve root. Because the uncinate process is often obscured by osteophytic disease, its position should be determined critically. Typically, it becomes more prominent toward the depths of the interspace and, accordingly, is best appreciated only after removal of disc material. The slope of the medial uncinate process is often subtle at the more rostral disc spaces, thus making the more lateral extent of the disc uncertain. This can be obviated by identifying the lateral "corner" of the upper vertebral body, which represents the medial surface of the unco-vertebral joint. This coincides with the opposing base of the uncinate process. From "corner-to-corner" or side-to-side, except at C2, the distance between the medial joint surfaces is 15 mm (Figure 3).

The longus colli muscles are usually symmetrically applied to the ventrolateral vertebral body surfaces. This leaves between 5 and 10 mm of the anterior longitudinal ligament exposed medially. The longus colli muscle complex covers the uncinate processes

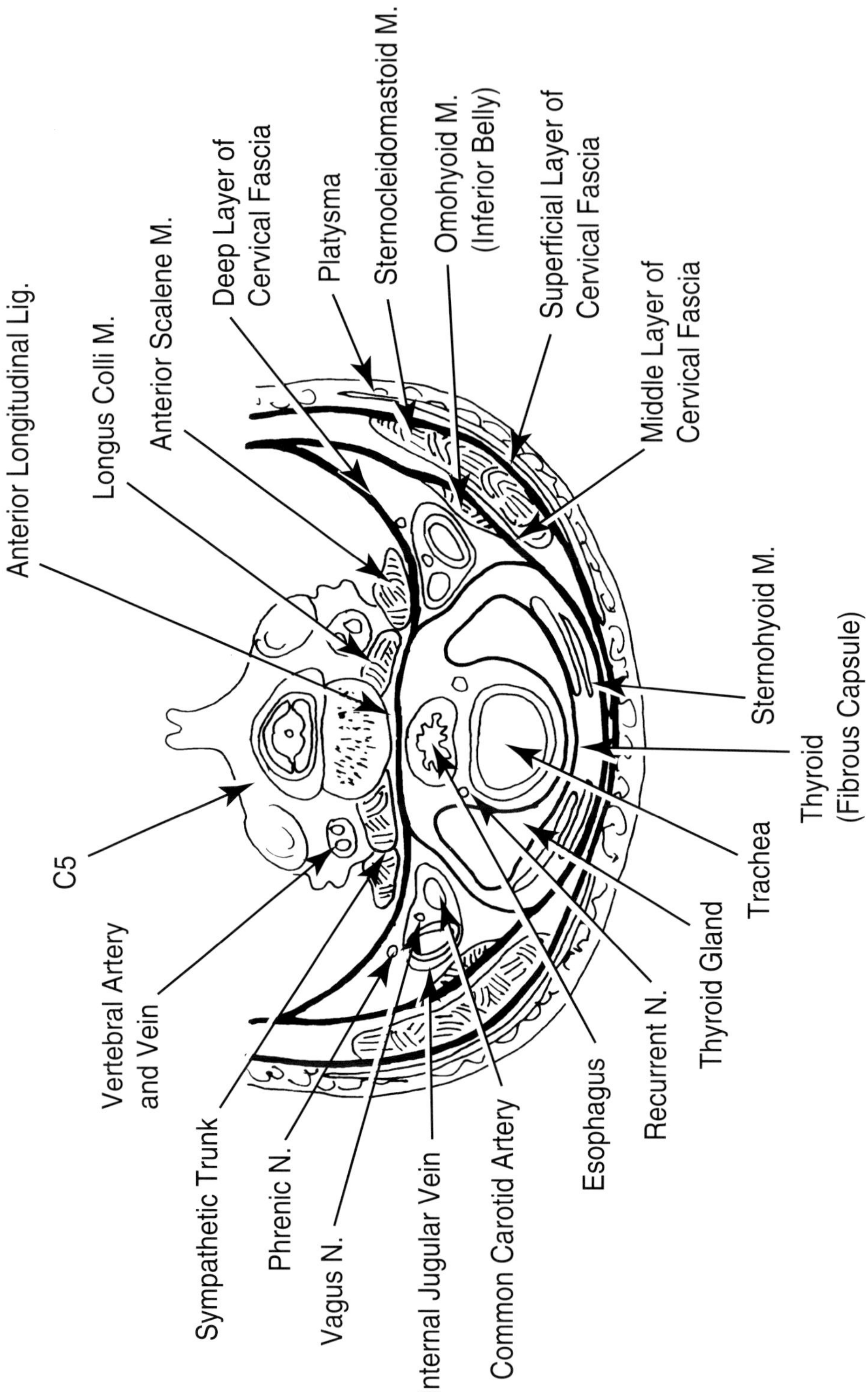

Figure 1. A depiction of the fascial planes achieved by access to the prevertebral space.

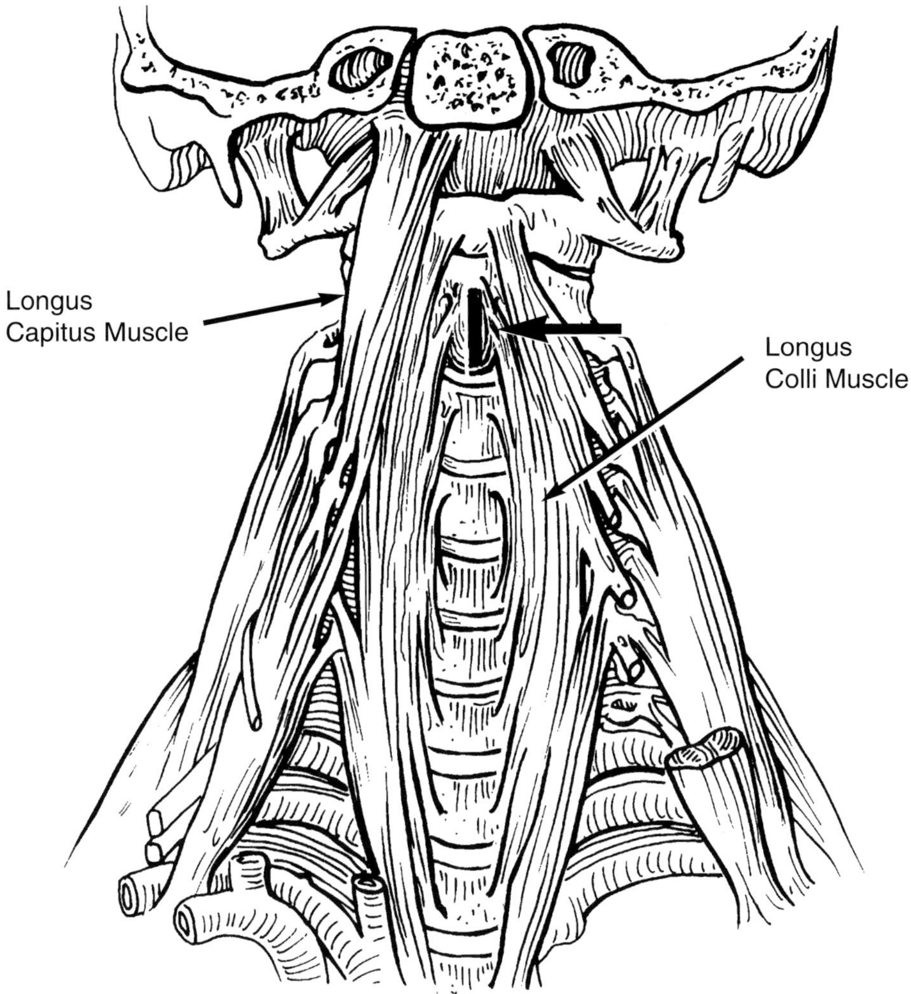

Figure 2. Prevertebral soft tissue showing a keel-like ligament marking the anterior surface of C2 *(arrow)*.

and fills the gap between the vertebral body and the anterior tubercles. (Definition of the muscle's components has no surgical importance.) The muscle can be sectioned medially, or mobilized longitudinally for lateral retraction for the definition of the uncinate processes. Usually, the contralateral longus colli muscle requires less dissection than its ipsilateral counterpart, because the obliquity of the surgical perspective allows a view under the muscle and toward the uncinate process. A large emissary vein at the caudal root of the transverse process, in line with the medial base of the uncinate process, is almost always encountered during mobilization of the longus colli muscle.

The ventral and dorsal vertebral surfaces are of equal axial height, but the ventral vertebral surface is more caudal. It overlaps slightly the ventrorostral aspect of the vertebral body below.[1] This parallelogram configuration of the vertebral body results in a

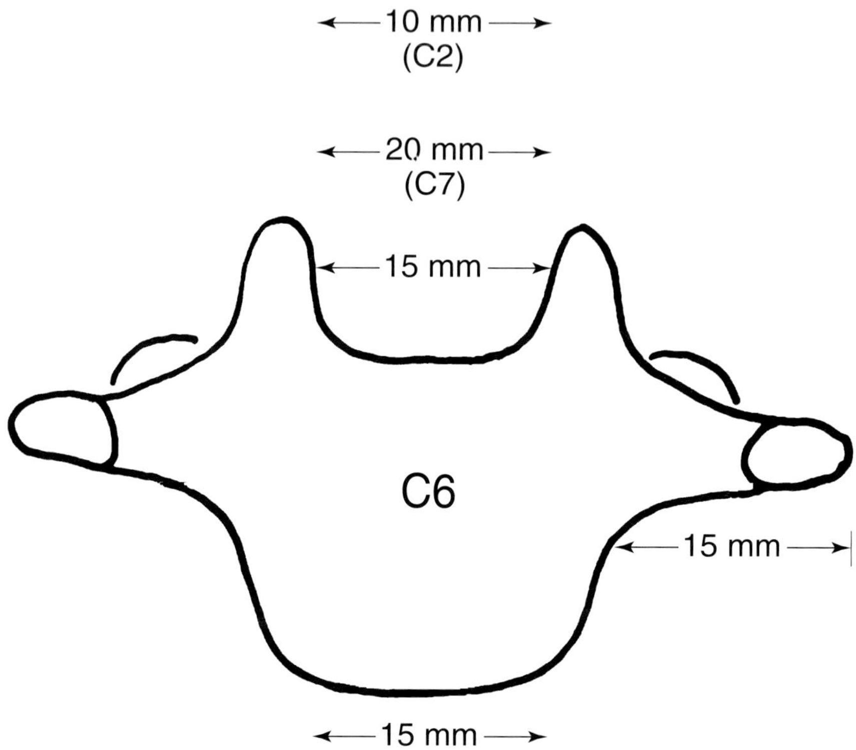

Figure 3. A depiction of the ventral cervical vertebral body, with critical surgical dimensions.

rostrocaudal angulation of the disc space from dorsal to ventral, a factor that must be considered during surgical exposure and also during mortising.

The annulus fibrosus and posterior longitudinal ligament become increasingly united as the degenerative process ensues. The posterior longitudinal ligament is identified in the midline by its longitudinal fibers, as the more amorphous annulus fibrosus is torn away. The central 5 mm of the posterior longitudinal ligament is thicker than that which extends into the lateral gutters, and may be further thickened by either the degenerative process or ossification at the level of the annulus fibrosus. Because the dorsal vertebral surface is convex, when drilling away the dorsal vertebral body cortex, the posterior longitudinal ligament is first encountered in the lateral aspects of the decompression. *The symmetry of this encounter is an indication of the degree to which a perfectly midline approach has been achieved.* Asymmetry is frequently problematic. At the center of the dorsal vertebral surface, the large vertebrobasilar vein(s) enter(s) the ligament. These are easily coagulated, but may be problematical prior to the removal of the cortical shell. Ligament excision into the lateral gutters opens a varix-like venous plexus. This is often difficult to control. Because the lateral extent of the ligament is rarely thickened, omitting lateral excision avoids needless blood loss.

The landmark for ventrolateral subaxial surgery is the anterior tubercle of the transverse process. Whereas the span of interuncinate surgery (i.e., central surgery) is 1.5 to

2 cm, the span from the tubercle to the lateral uncinate process is 1 cm or less. The ventral bony band of the foramen transversarium, referred to as the "costal process" (or costo-transverse lamelli), connects the tubercle with the uncinate base. This lamelli attaches to the vertebral body midway between the uncinate tip rostrally and the endplate caudally. It is 1 to 2 mm thick. The dorsal medial rim of the foramen transversarium is the pedicle that courses dorsolaterally from the vertebral body. Through the foramen transversarium, the upper six cervical vertebrae lend passage for the vertebral artery, encompassing veins and portions of the sympathetic plexus. The exiting nerve root lies behind the vertebral artery in a groove on the upper surface of the transverse process. To envision the region of the nerve root, the lateral uncinate process, and the vertebral artery, the longus colli muscle must be mobilized, lateral to medial with its overlying sympathetic chain, from the anterior tubercles.

References

1. Goss CM (ed): **Gray's Anatomy of the Human Body, ed 29.** Philadelphia: Lea & Febyer, 1973
2. Whitecloud TS. Anterior and posterior surgical approaches to the cervical spine, in Frymoyer JW (ed): **The Adult Spine: Principles and Practice.** New York: Revere Press, 1991, pp 987-1013

Chapter 3

Ventral Thoracic and Lumbar Spine Anatomy

Charles L. Branch Jr, MD

Surgical exposure of the thoracic and lumbar spine is often approached from a ventral or lateral route in order to facilitate decompression of the neural elements and provide ventral support of the spine. Safe and effective exposure may be accomplished at all levels by the surgeon with a thorough knowledge of the paraspinal anatomy. In this chapter, the pertinent anatomy of the structures adjacent to the ventral spine (from the upper thoracic to the lumbosacral levels) is reviewed.

Upper Thoracic Spine (T1-5)

Immediately dorsal to the upper thoracic spine are three, nearly contiguous muscle groups: the trapezius, rhomboid, and erector spinae. These muscles form the dorsal plane, ventral to which the spine is approached through the lateral extracavitary approach. The scapula is an obstruction that may be overcome with retraction after incising the fascial plane between the dorsal muscles (Figure 1). The rib attaches to the spine ventral to the corresponding transverse process at this level and then to the vertebral body at the disc space itself (e.g., the T3 rib head covers the T2-3 disc space). The autonomic chain is present just ventral to this rib articulation and remains in a relatively constant relationship to the rib articulation and vertebral body over the extent of the thoracic and lumbar spine (Figure 2).

Ventral to the vertebral body lies the concentrated collection of the tracheo-esophageal structures, surrounded ventrally by the left subclavian, left common carotid, and brachiocephalic arteries. Between these vessels and the sternum lie the vagus nerve and the jugular-subclavian venous complex. The descending thoracic aorta assumes its left paraspinous position beginning at T4 and continuing through the diaphragm at T12 (Figure 3).

Midthoracic Spine (T6-10)

In the midthoracic region, the dorsolateral plane is defined by the trapezius and longissimus muscles dorsally and the rhomboid and external intercostal muscles ventrally. Over this segment of the spine, the articulation of the rib head gradually migrates caudally so that in the lower thoracic region, its articulation is on the corresponding vertebral body

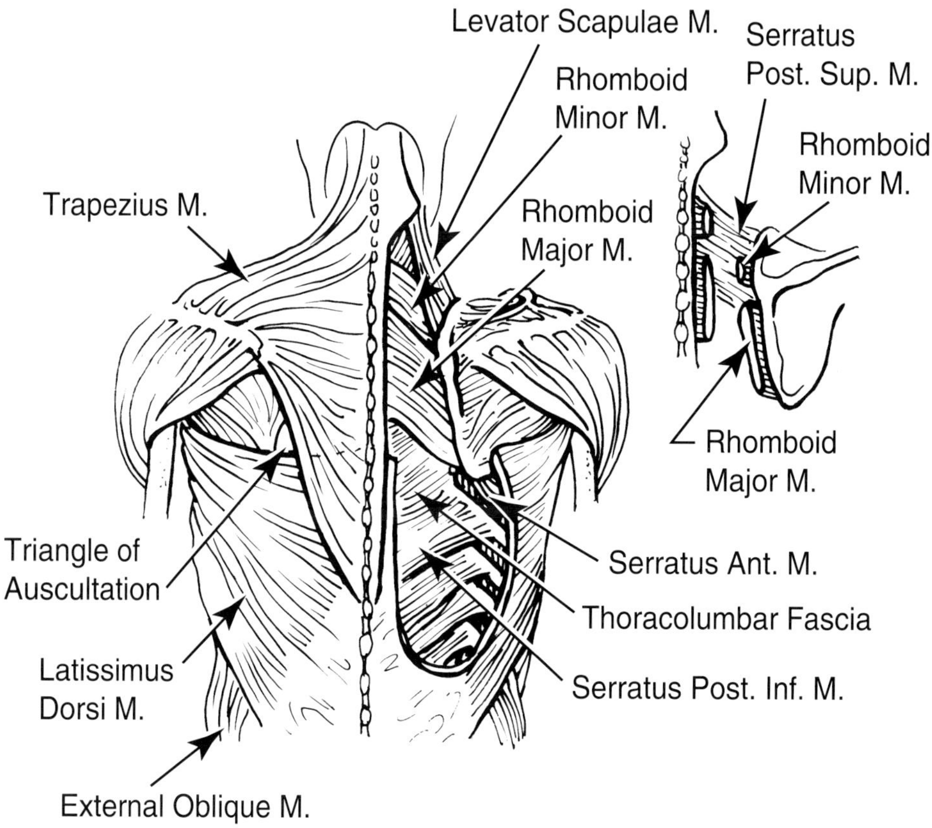

Figure 1. Dorsal view of the paravertebral muscles of the thoracic and upper lumbar spine. *Inset* depicts the incision of the rhomboid muscles to gain access to the dorsolateral thorax.

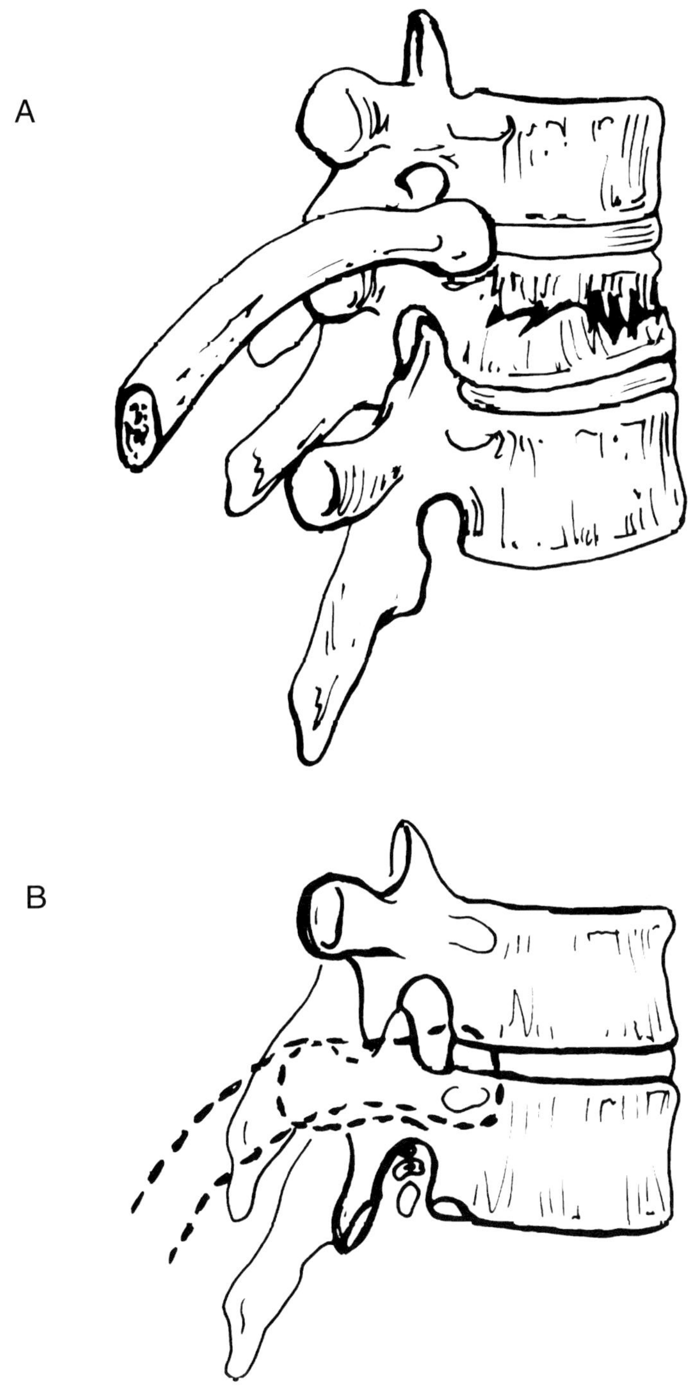

Figure 2. The relationship of the rib to the vertebral body, disc interspace, and transverse process, depicted in a case of fracture **(A)** and with the rib ghosted **(B)**.

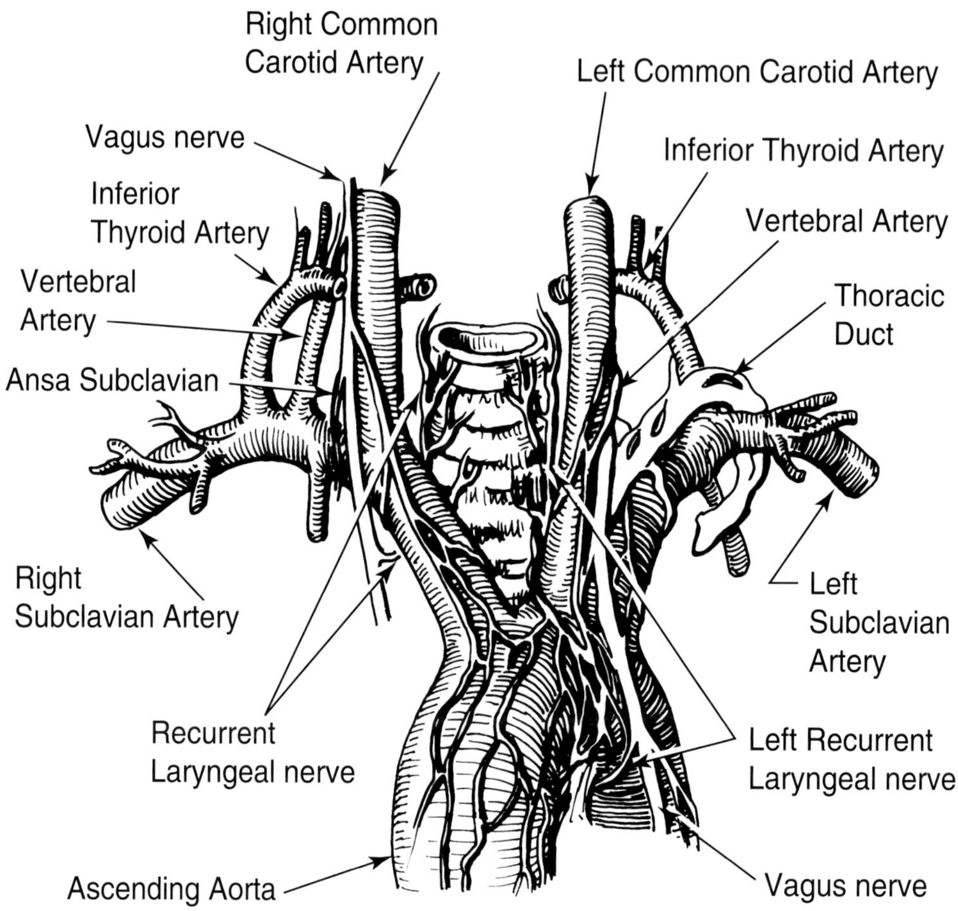

Figure 3. A depiction of the arterial structures of the upper mediastinum and their relationship to the nerves and trachea.

(as opposed to the lateral disc space in the upper lumbar spine). The aorta, esophagus, and sympathetic chains are constant throughout this segment of the spine. Above the T7 level, the superior vena cava and azygos veins are present to the right of midline; below the T7 level, the inferior vena cava is found in this same location (Figure 4).

At each midvertebral level, paired intercostal vessels are enveloped by parietal pleura. In general, the vertebral body anatomy is also relatively constant over this region, with the width and depth each ranging from 25 to 30 mm. The outer cortical diameter of the pedicles in this region is 5 mm, while the internal diameter of the cortical pedicular tube ranges from 2.5 to 3.5 mm.

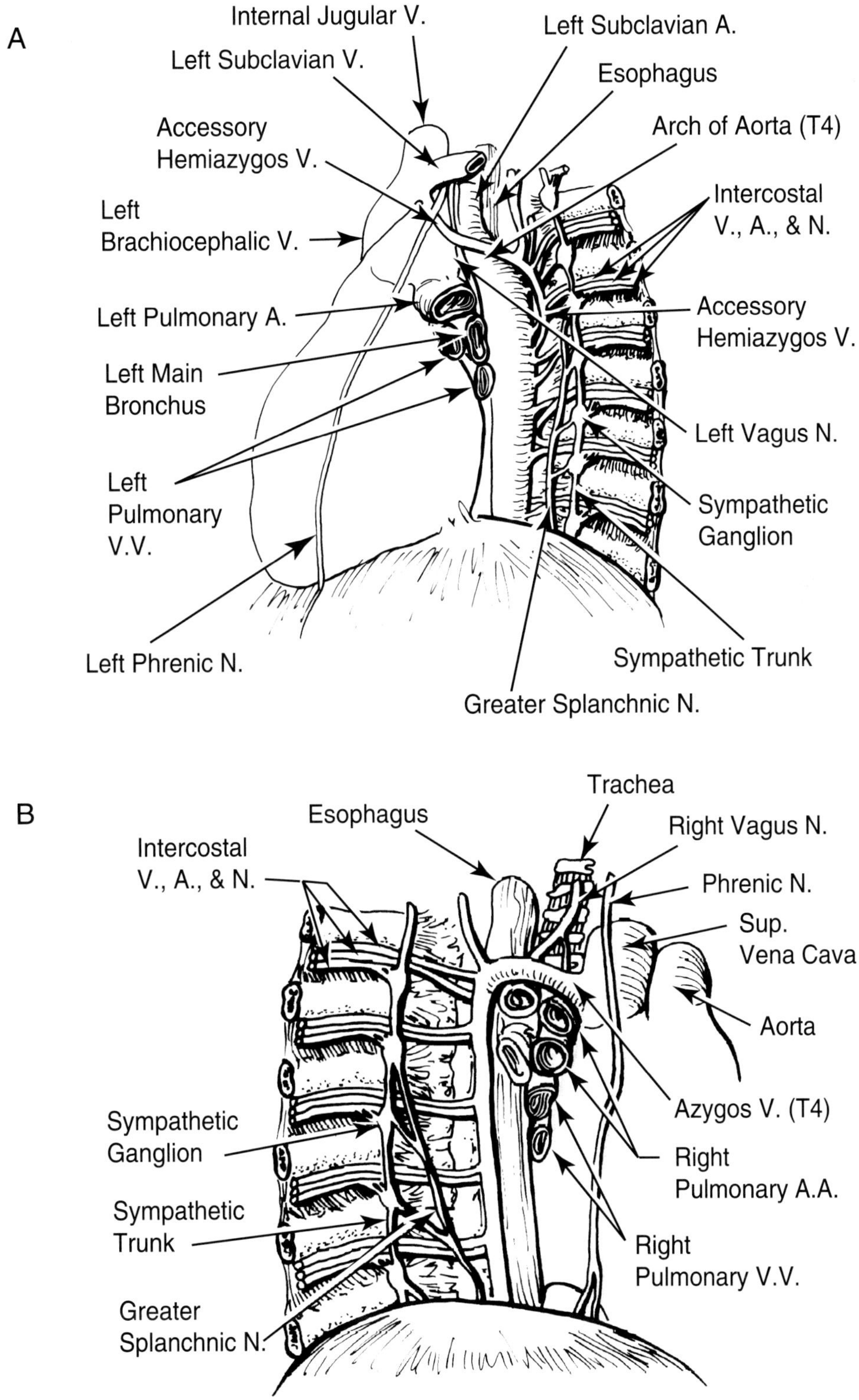

Figure 4. The left **(A)** and the right **(B)** relationships between the paravertebral vascular structures and the ribs and spine.

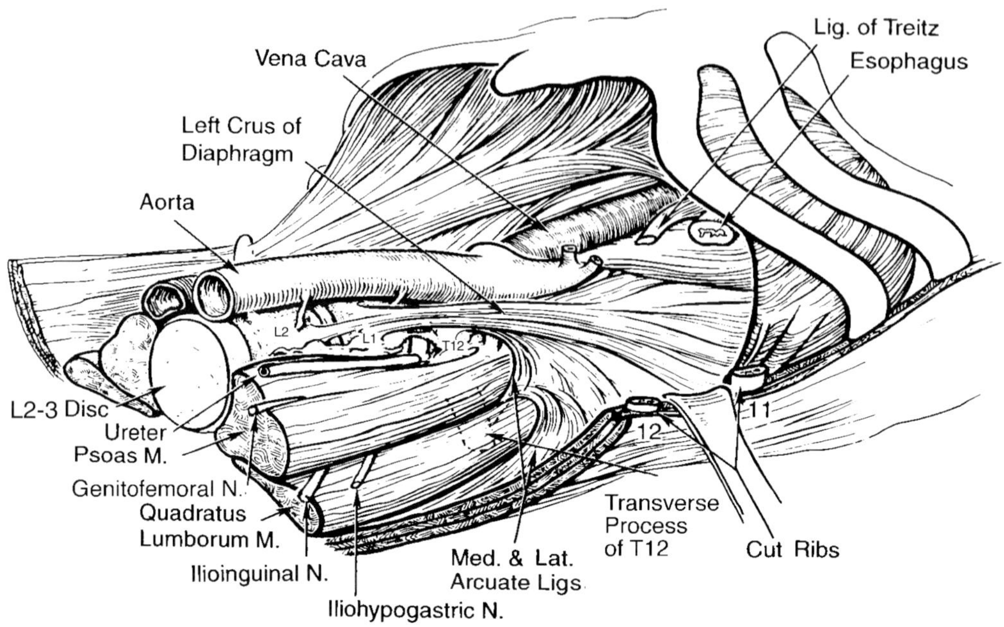

Figure 5. The rostral retroperitoneum.

Lower Thoracic Spine (T11-12)

Dorsolaterally, the erector spinae muscles remain as a discreet bundle that includes the iliocostal, transversospinal, and longissimus muscles. The ventral surface for the lateral approach is the rib and intercostal muscle plane. At this level, the rib head articulates with the pedicle and the vertebral body, with very little overlap onto the disc space.

Ventral to the spine, the diaphragm, whose dome is at the T7 or T8 level, attaches dorsally to the lower six ribs and crura of L1-4. The aorta passes through the hiatus in these crura at the T11-12 levels while the inferior vena cava and esophagus pass through the diaphragm more ventrally at the T8-10 levels. The sympathetic chains remain in the costovertebral grooves just ventral to the rib heads. The psoas muscle often originates at this level. The liver, spleen, and upper pole of the kidneys and fundus of the stomach are found intraperitoneally (Figure 5).

In the lower thoracic spine, the appearance of the vertebral body changes significantly. Whereas the ventrodorsal diameter remains about 3 cm, the lateral diameter increases to 4.5 cm. The pedicles also change toward their lumbar size, with the outer diameter approaching 8 cm and the internal diameter between 5 and 6 cm.

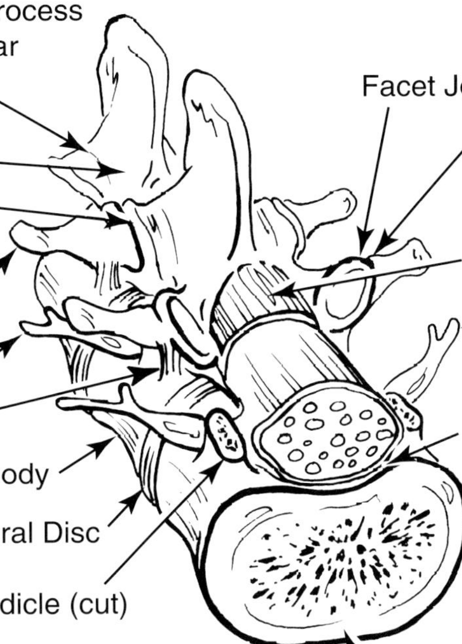

Figure 6. A depiction of the relationship of the spine to the dural sac and exiting nerve roots.

Upper Lumbar Spine (L1-2)

The dorsolateral plane in the upper lumbar spine lies between the erector spinae muscle group, dorsal to the transverse processes (transversospinal, longissimus, and iliocostal muscles) and the quadratus lumborum muscle, which is also the dorsal or retroperitoneal muscular wall. The psoas muscle, found just ventral to the transverse processes, increases in bulk as it courses caudally. The sympathetic chain remains in a consistent position on the ventrolateral vertebral body. The remnants of the crus of the diaphragm are often encountered on the ventrorostral limit of L2, between the vertebral body and the distal aorta. The renal branches of the aorta and vena cava are generally found at this level. Rarely, at this level, the aorta and vena cava bifurcate into the iliac vessels.

Pedicle and vertebral body anatomy is constant over these two levels, with inner and outer pedicle diameters of 5 mm and 7.5 mm, respectively. The ventrodorsal and lateral vertebral diameters are 3 cm and 4.5 cm, respectively.

Lower Lumbar Spine (L3-5)

Pedicle and vertebral body anatomy is less constant in the low lumbar region. However, the relationship between the dural sac and exiting nerve root is relatively constant throughout the lumbar spine (Figure 6).

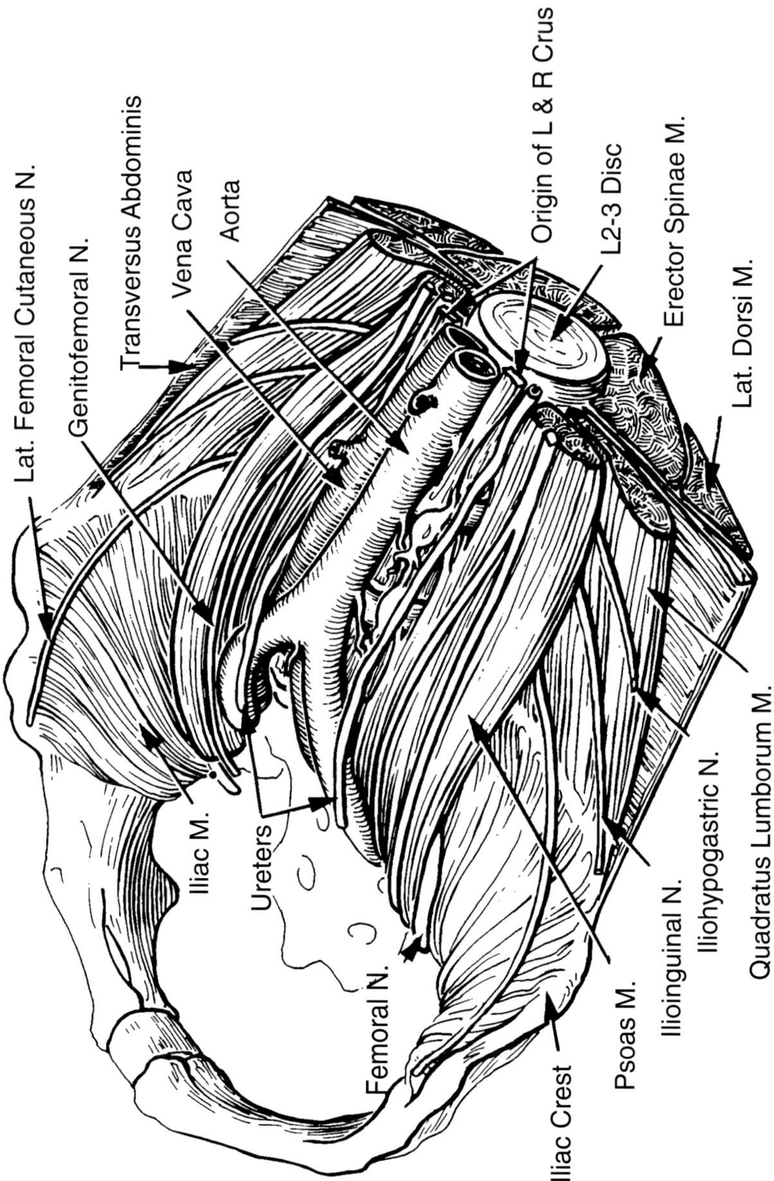

Figure 7. The caudal retroperitoneum.

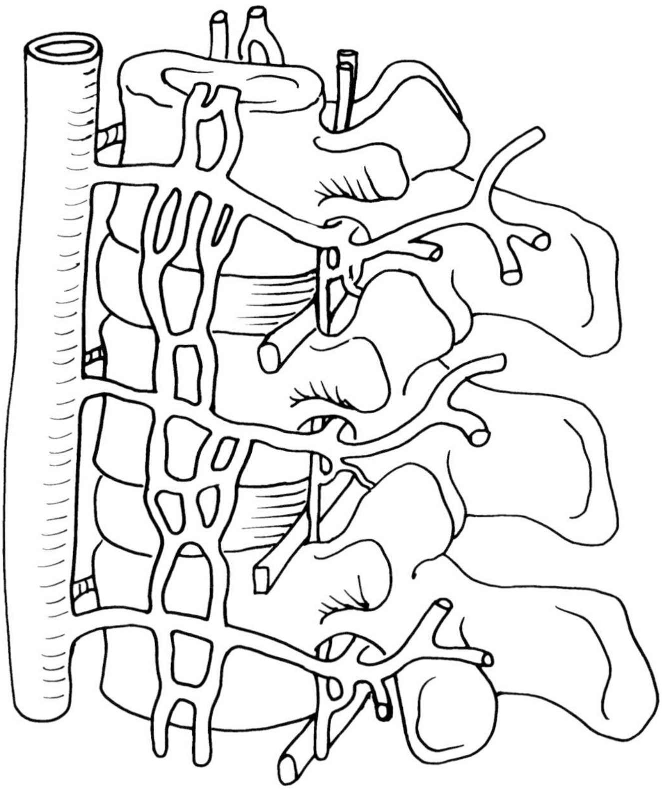

Figure 8. The lumbar paravertebral arterial anatomy.

The plane between the erector spinae muscle group and the quadratus lumborum muscle leads to the transverse process and subsequently the neural foramen. Immediately ventral is the body of the psoas major muscle. Components of the lumbar plexus (L3-5) course along the dorsomedial border of the psoas muscle, while the ureter courses along the ventral border. Also located along the medial border of the psoas muscle is the caudal extent of the sympathetic chain and the genitofemoral nerve. The vertebrae at the L4-5 levels are found ventral to the bifurcation of the abdominal aorta and vena cava. Ileocolic and mesenteric arteries and veins are often located adjacent to the aortocaval structures at this level (Figure 7). The regional lumbar arterial distribution (Figure 8) and neural network (Figure 9) are relatively consistent from level to level in the thoracic and lumbar regions.

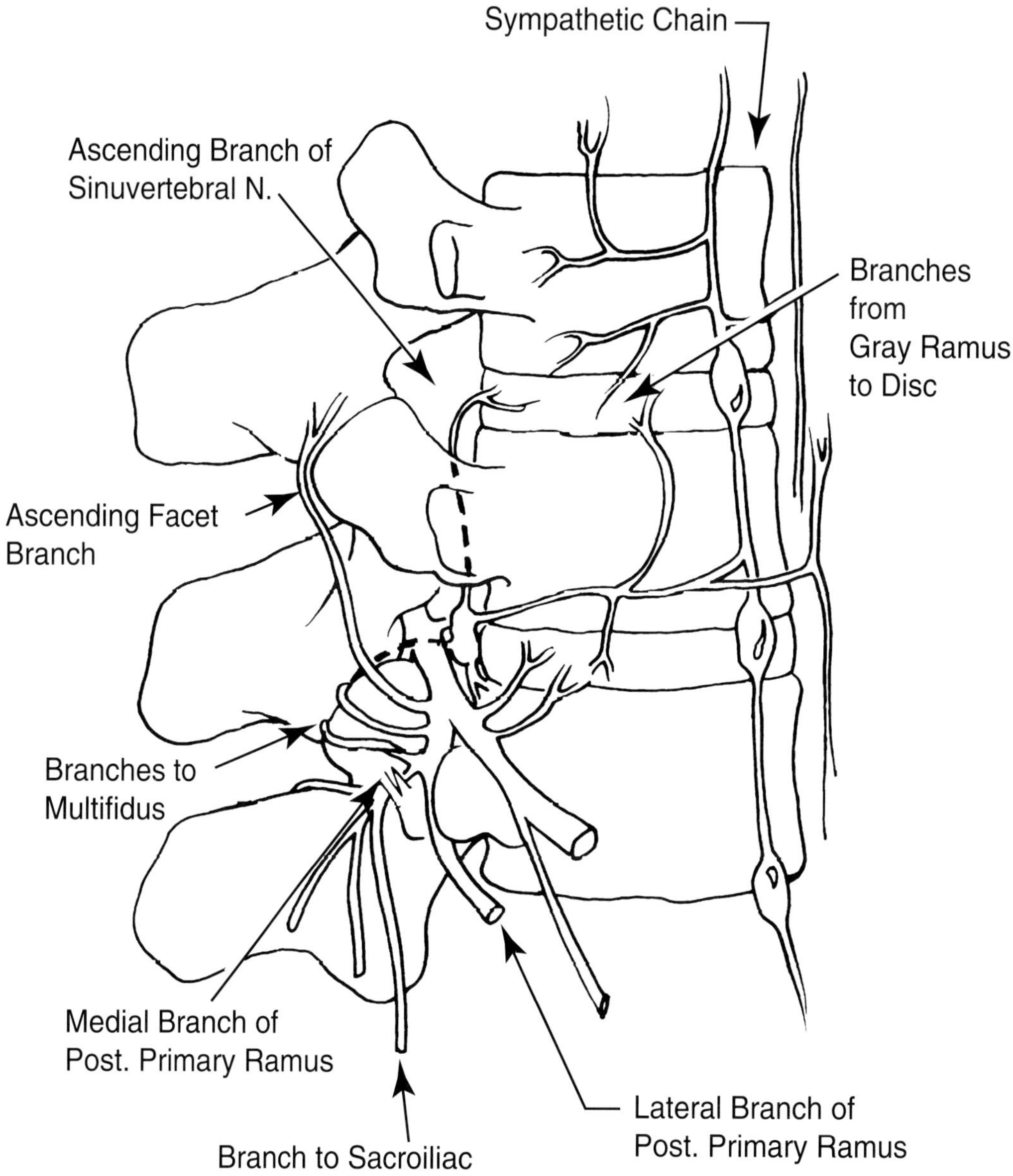

Figure 9. The paravertebral neural network.

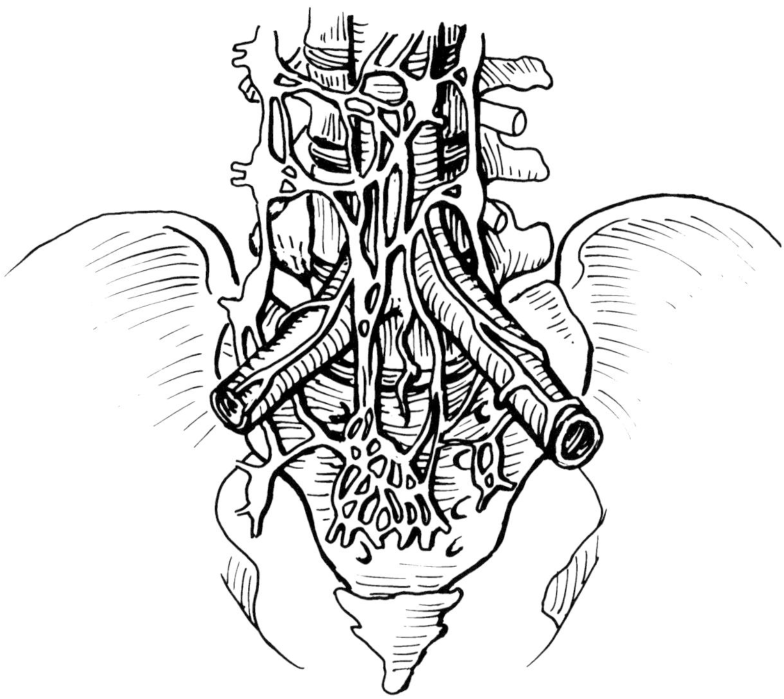

Figure 10. The low lumbar and presacral arterial and neural networks.

As one progresses caudally, the ilium obstructs the lateral approach to the L5-S1 intervertebral space. The major neurovascular structures course laterally, diverging from the hypogastric plexus (sympathetic innervation to the urogenital system). The smaller middle sacral artery and vein often course within the hypogastric plexus (Figure 10).

Chapter 4

Ventral Exposures of the Upper Cervical Spine

Arnold H. Menezes, MD, FACS, FAAP

Early and traditional surgical treatment of pathology of the craniocervical region was performed via a dorsal route. Subsequently, operative procedures based on the understanding of the complex anatomy, craniocervical dynamics, and the site of encroachment of the neural elements were developed. Advances in neurodiagnostic imaging and microsurgical instrumentation have opened new vistas, placing the entire circumference of the foramen magnum within the neurosurgeon's reach. The varied and extensive pathology includes congenital, acquired, and developmental lesions.[10]

The craniocervical junction encompasses the foramen magnum, the C1 and C2 vertebrae, and the structures contained within the confines of these bony landmarks, including the cervicomedullary junction, the cerebellum, the lower cranial nerves, vascular structures, and cerebrospinal fluid (CSF) spaces. The factors influencing specific treatment are:[11] 1) the etiology of the lesion (e.g., basilar invagination, rheumatoid cranial settling, intra- and extradural tumors, etc.); 2) vascular abnormalities, such as syrinx and Chiari malformation; 3) the mechanics of compression and the orientation of the encroachment; 4) the presence of ossification centers and epiphyseal growth plates in certain congenital abnormalities; and 5) reducibility. The latter is the most important factor. It determines the efficacy of nonoperative reduction of compressive lesions affecting the cervicomedullary junction via the restoration of normal anatomical relationships between neural and offending structures. Surgical decompression is performed on patients with an irreducible pathological process.

Surgical decompression should be achieved via the same orientation as the relationship between the offending lesion and the affected neural elements. Thus, if a ventral neural element encroachment is present, a ventral or ventrolateral surgical route is chosen. With dorsal neural element encroachment, a dorsal or dorsolateral approach is mandated.

If decompression is achieved via closed reduction techniques, surgical decompression is not usually warranted. However, for reducible craniocervical junction lesions, surgical stabilization is the treatment of choice.[11]

Diagnostic Imaging

The diagnostic procedures performed for the evaluation of craniocervical junction lesions are governed by the factors that influence treatment. Magnetic resonance imaging (MRI) is, perhaps, the most common diagnostic tool utilized for craniovertebral junction assessment. MRI fails, however, to completely visualize the osseous pathology and is unable to delineate the true extent of congenital and developmental abnormalities in this region. Therefore, MRI alone is not an adequate diagnostic tool. The diagnostic procedures utilized must complement each other in order to achieve a full understanding of the pathophysiology, as well as the extent of the lesion. Thus, the imaging of the craniocervical junction should include computed tomography (CT) of the craniocervical region, followed by MRI in the flexed and extended positions. The effect of traction is also ascertained. In selected patients, vertebral angiography is necessary, and the effects of rotation, flexion, and extension of the head should be documented. Thin-section CT may be essential for the identification and localization of abnormalities, and may be supplemented by intrathecal contrast enhancement with iohexol.

Decision-Making and the Extent of Exposure

The transoral-transpalatopharyngeal approach to the craniocervical junction provides an effective, safe, and rapid exposure of the ventromedial 3.5 cm of the spine, from the midclivus to the C2-3 interspace.[2,10] A more rostral access via median glossotomy may be combined with a labiomandibular split.[5,7] A transpalatal approach, with limited resection of the caudal hard palate, provides further rostral exposure, from the sphenoid and paranasal sinuses to the upper border of the C3 vertebra. One option is the lateral rhinotomy, combined with the transoral-transpharyngeal approach.[7,10,11]

The lateral extrapharyngeal route is a safe and effective access to the upper cervical spine.[3,8,9] Entry into the preclival and the high retropharyngeal space is limited by the parotid gland with the facial nerve rostrally, the angle and ramus of the mandible ventrally, the hyoid bone and the hypoglossal nerve caudally, and the structures of the carotid sheath dorsally. Dissection of the caudal branches of the facial nerve and their elevation, together with displacement of the mandible, allows for a limited exposure.[10] This procedure, however, can achieve satisfactory visualization of the clivus.

The dorsolateral approach to the upper cervical spine has been recognized for many years.[4,6,10,13] Recently, skull base surgeons have altered the nomenclature, thus adding to the confusion. This approach combines a standard dorsal midline with the lateral cerebellar approach, and includes the partial resection of the mastoid process and the occipital condyle to achieve exposure from the jugular bulb laterally to the midline. It also accesses the vertebral artery in the foramen magnum and in the posterior fossa, as well as in the vertebral canal (at the foramen transversarium) in the upper cervical spine. The major advantage of this approach is the ability to attain an occipitocervical or atlantoaxial fusion, should that be necessary. This exposure begins at the level of the lateral atlantal masses laterally and proceeds medially past the midline. The approach into the posterior fossa is both in the midline and dorsolaterally along the cerebellopontine angle, and can be extended to the petrous bone rostrally. The caudal margin is extended as needed.

Thus, the entire circumference of the foramen magnum can be exposed with the three aforementioned standard approaches. The extension of these approaches includes the direct lateral transcondylar approach,[12] the mandible-splitting midline approach,[5,7] and the ventral transnasal maxillotomy.[1] The subtemporal, infratemporal fossa, pre-auricular, and postauricular exposures offer the facility of an intracranial operative procedure while providing the ability to dissect caudally as extensively as necessary.[10]

A distillation of the surgical approaches to the craniovertebral junction is presented below.

The Transoral-Transpharyngeal Approach

Indications

The primary indication for the transoral approach is the presence of an extradural lesion that is located between the midclivus and the C3 vertebral body, and up to 2 cm laterally from the midline. Usually, intra-arachnoid pathology is best approached from a dorsal or dorsolateral orientation. Osseous abnormalities must be documented to be irreducible prior to the consideration of a ventral or ventrolateral surgical approach.

Preoperative Assessment

Nutritional assessment is an important aspect of preoperative and perioperative management. Oral intake is not permitted during the first week after operation. In circumstances such as rheumatoid arthritis affecting the temporomandibular joint, the ability to open the mouth may be limited. It is important to be able to achieve an operative working distance of 2.5 to 3 cm between the upper and lower incisor teeth. If this is not possible, an alternative route must be sought. If this is not achievable, a mandible-splitting approach with a midline glossotomy is an essential adjunct to a transoral operation. Oropharyngeal cultures are obtained 3 days before surgery, and no antibiotics are administered unless pathological flora are present. It is imperative that a preoperative assessment of swallowing and respiratory function be made. If significant lower cranial nerve dysfunction is present, a tracheotomy should be performed at the time of the transoral operation.

Operative Technique

Fiberoptic oral endotracheal intubation is performed in the awake patient. The patient is examined following intubation in order to ensure that no neurological changes have occurred during positioning. The supine position, with the head in mild extension on a padded horseshoe headrest, is used. Traction is maintained via a pulley bar with mild extension of the neck. Once it has been established that no neurological deficit has occurred, general endotracheal and intravenous anesthesia ensues. A tracheotomy is performed only when the operation involves the craniocervical junction and more rostral structures in a patient with brain stem compression.

A modified Dingman self-retaining mouth retractor secures the endotracheal tube and allows exposure of the oral cavity and pharynx. Operative procedures involving the clivus and foramen magnum make it essential to split the soft palate to provide the necessary exposure.

After the oral cavity is cleansed with 10% povidone-iodine and hydrogen peroxide, the mouth is rinsed with saline. A midline incision in the soft palate extends from the hard palate to the base of the uvula and then to the right or the left side, preserving the base (Figure 1A). Stay sutures hold the leaves of the soft palate apart in order to expose the high nasopharynx, which is anesthetized with topical cocaine while the median raphe is infiltrated with a solution containing 0.5% lidocaine and 1:200,000 epinephrine. The dorsal pharyngeal midline is incised and the pharyngeal flaps swept away to either side in order to expose the clivus and the upper three cervical vertebrae. Again, stay sutures provide for the self-retaining exposure (Figure 1B). In the prevertebral space, the longus colli and the longus capitis muscles are dissected free of the osseous and ligamentous attachments, thus exposing the clivus and the atlas and axis vertebrae.

The lateral exposure must be limited to 1.5 cm to the right and left of the midline in the region of the foramen magnum in order to prevent injury to the hypoglossal nerve and to 2 cm to either side of the midline below the foramen magnum. The latter preserves the integrity of the eustachian tubes and the vertebral arteries.

The anterior aspect of the arch of the atlas, as well as the caudal clivus, is removed with a high-speed burr (Figure 1C). The soft tissues ventral to the odontoid

A

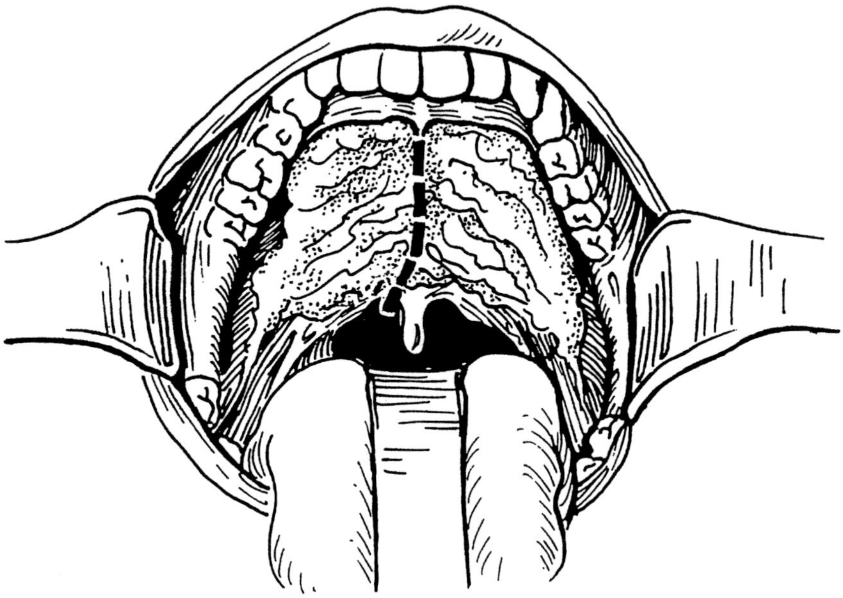

Figure 1A. The transoral-transpalatopharyngeal approach. A self-retaining mouth retractor is in place and the tongue depressed. The *dotted line* denotes the incision in the soft palate extending onto the hard palate.

B

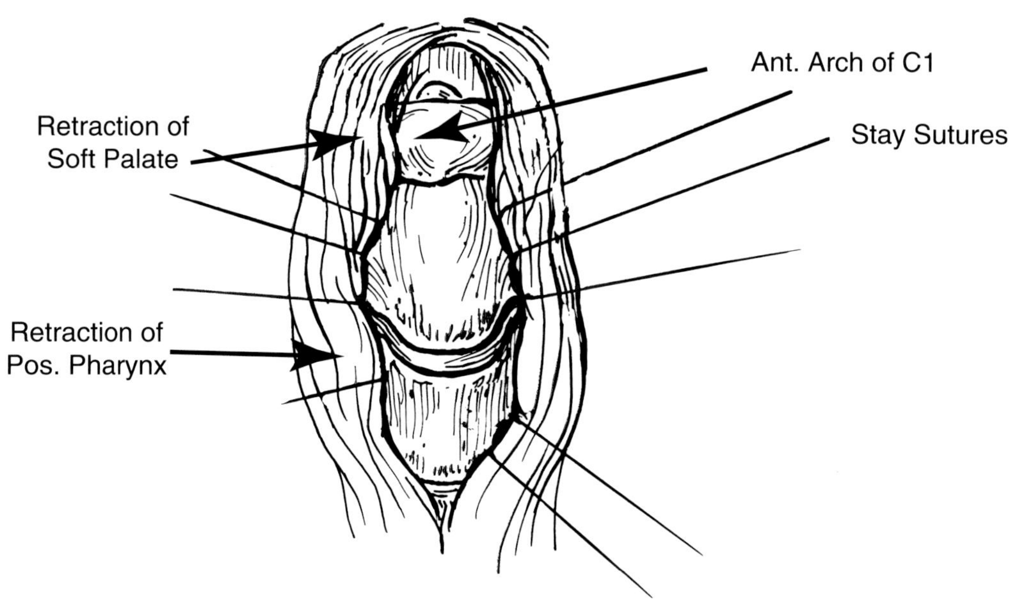

Figure 1B. The soft palate is retracted with stay sutures, as are the dorsal pharyngeal wall and the longus colli muscles, which have been separated from the medial attachment.

C

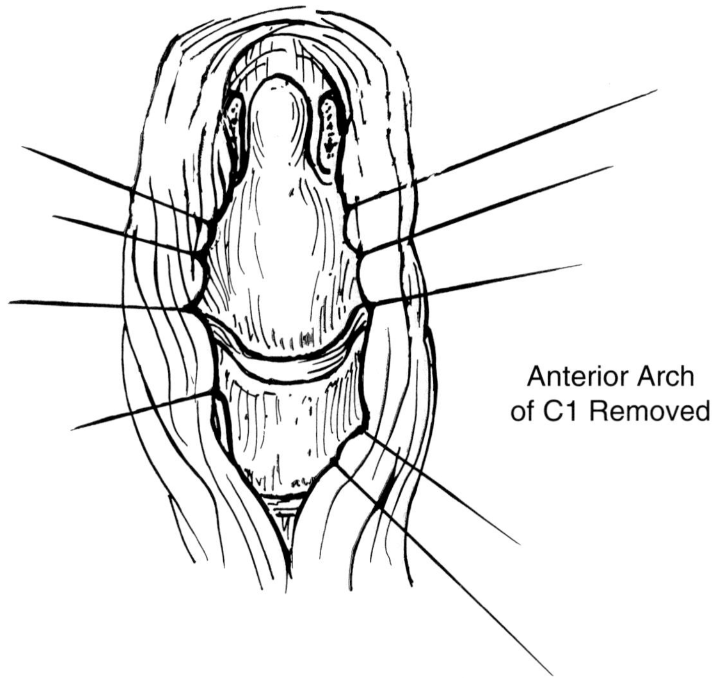

Figure 1C. The caudal clivus, the anterior arch of the atlas, and the base of the dens are exposed. The lateral presentation shows removal of the anterior arch of the atlas.

D

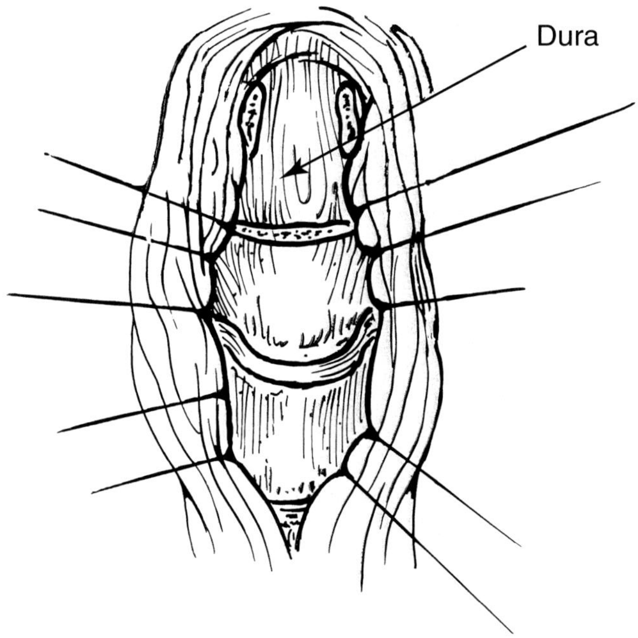

Figure 1D. Resection of the clivus and the odontoid process has occurred. The ventral indentation of the cervicomedullary junction by the tough tectorial membrane and pannus requires resection.

process are removed with rongeurs. Odontoid process removal is then begun, using a high-speed cutting burr, followed by a diamond burr, with periodic pannus removal, if appropriate (Figure 1D). The division of the odontoid process at its base by caudal retraction must be avoided. This is especially fraught with danger if the pannus is attached tenaciously to surrounding structures or if the odontoid process has migrated into the subarachnoid space and anchored itself to the brain stem or juxtaposed vascular structures. The tectorial membrane is then incised to obtain adequate decompression. Dural pulsations herald the completion of the decompression.

If the subarachnoid space has been entered, it is imperative that the dura mater be closed. In this situation, fascia may be laid against the closed dural defect, which is reinforced with a fat pad prior to closure of the wound. Spinal drainage is essential for the first 10 days after operation.

In many cases, the bony pathology is greater than that of an odontoid process that has migrated rostrally or laterally. The extent of bone resection is governed by the preoperative diagnostic studies. Extradural tumors, such as chordoma or plasmacytoma, often require careful correlation of the diagnostic studies in order to locate the position of intra-arachnoid vessels.

Next, the longus capitis and longus colli muscles and the dorsal pharyngeal musculature are approximated in the midline using 3-0 polyglycolic sutures in an interrupted fashion. The dorsal pharyngeal mucosa is brought together with interrupted sutures of a similar strength. The muscularis and the oral mucosa of the soft palate are approximated with interrupted vertical mattress sutures.

The rostral extent of this operative procedure may be extended by resection of the hard palate. This permits high nasopharyngeal exposure without splitting the mandible or incising the tongue. Postoperative caloric intake is provided by placement of a soft nasogastric feeding tube under direct vision into the esophagus and stomach during the operative procedure and prior to closure of the soft palate.

Postoperative Care

No oral intake is permitted in the immediate postoperative period. The head of the bed must be elevated. The endotracheal tube is left in place for the first 48 to 72 hours, until lingual swelling has receded. A soft cervical collar is used. When appropriate, oral intake of a clear liquid diet is permitted usually after 1 week, followed by a gradual increase in feedings until a regular diet is achieved by the end of the third postoperative week. Postoperative intravenous antibiotic administration is maintained only for the first 24 hours. If the subarachnoid space has been violated, an intravenous antibiotic regimen (including methicillin, metronidazole, and cefotaxime) and spinal drainage are maintained for 10 days after the operation.

Postoperative stability is evaluated with pleuridirectional lateral tomography at 5 to 7 days after the procedure. This is performed with the patient in the flexed and extended positions in order to ascertain the extent of stability. An offset at the lateral occipitoatlantal articulation or vertebral displacement is indicative of instability, in which case dorsal occipitocervical fixation is necessary. All patients with rheumatoid cranial settling require dorsal fixation. Of the remaining patients, 90% require operative dorsal fixation.

Complications

The most dreaded complication of the transoral operative procedure is CSF leakage. To handle this complication, a lumbar drain is placed preoperatively if intradural pathology is recognized; otherwise, postoperative drainage is necessary. An attempt to approximate the dural leaves should be made using a cover of fascia, a fat pad, and possibly tissue gel. Careful closure of the wound must then ensue.

Severe tongue swelling may occur, especially in rheumatoid arthritis patients. An intermittent release of the retractor during the operation may assist in relieving the venous and lymphatic compression. Decadron (dexamethasone) administration has been useful. Postprocedure massaging of the tongue encourages the reconstitution of normal venous and lymphatic flow following long and complicated cases.

Bleeding during the transoral exposure accumulates in the surgical field, and can only be controlled by clipping both leaves of the venous circular sinuses. Careful packing with Avitene and Oxycel may also be performed. Bleeding from the vertebral artery branches is secured by use of microbipolar forceps under saline irrigation. On rare occasions, occlusion of the vertebral artery with a clip may be required; this, however, is obviously a treatment of last resort.

Palatal dehiscence requires immediate reclosure. The occurrence of meningitis implies CSF leakage, which must be attended to after intravenous antibiotics have been instituted.

Pharyngeal wound dehiscence that occurs after the first postoperative week signifies improper closure and the need for the closure to be redone. Pharyngeal wound dehiscence after 2 weeks indicates a retropharyngeal abscess. The most unrecognized complication is postoperative craniovertebral instability.

Neurological worsening after a transoral operation signifies loss of alignment, possible meningitis, retained bone, or an abscess formation. In rare instances, the vertebrobasilar system may have an occlusion.

Lateral Transcervical Extrapharyngeal Approach to the Craniocervical Junction

Indications

The ventral retropharyngeal approach does not enter into the oral cavity. Furthermore, it allows for the utilization of a ventral fusion procedure, if necessary.

The author has used a modification of this procedure for exposure from the clivus to the lower cervical spine. The patient is intubated awake via the nasal endotracheal route. The oral cavity is kept free of any tubes because the upper and lower dentition are kept in their occluded state. The same precautions are taken as with the transoral route regarding intubation and anesthesia.

Operative Technique

The patient is positioned supine, with the head maintained in traction resting on a padded doughnut. During surgery, the head is turned slightly to the patient's left by a right-handed surgeon. The cervical incision begins behind the ear, over the mastoid process, and extends about 1.5 to 2 cm below the angle of the mandible. It is then brought to the midline at the level of the hyoid bone and extended slightly upward (Figure 2A). A caudal extension of the rostral limb converts the transverse incision to a "T." This incision is brought down to the level of the omohyoid muscle along the sternocleidomastoid muscle. The incision traverses the subcutaneous tissue and platysma muscle. Dissection is made with mobilization in a subplatysmal plane over the superficial fascia. The caudal division of the facial nerve is identified and dissected forward to allow for elevation of the parotid gland and the facial nerve. The superficial draining veins are dissected free and ligated before entry to the common facial vein.

By elevating the fascia around the parotid gland and the facial nerve, the dissection proceeds more deeply. The deep fascia at the ventral border of the sternocleidomastoid muscle is incised, allowing for visualization of the carotid sheath. The jugular digastric nodes in the carotid triangle are then resected, and the dissection is taken ventral to the carotid sheath (Figure 2B). The submandibular salivary gland is elevated and retracted ventrally, and may be resected without consequence if the duct is sutured to prevent a salivary fistula. The dorsal belly of the digastric muscle is traced to its tendon at the hyoid bone and then transected. This will be reapproximated at the time of closure. The stylohyoid muscle is divided, allowing for medial retraction

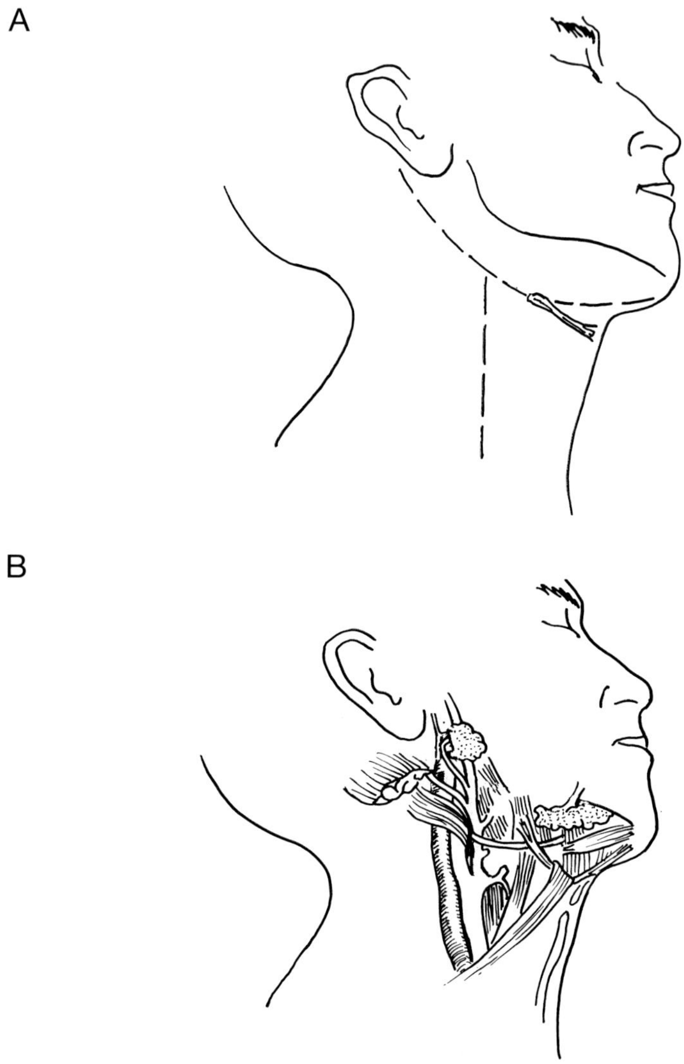

Figure 2A-B. The lateral extrapharyngeal approach to the clivus and the upper cervical spine. **A)** The *dotted line* denotes the incision, which starts at the mastoid tip and extends about 2.5 cm below the angle of the mandible. It proceeds to just above the greater cornu of the hyoid bone toward the midline and symphysis mentis. An extension of the rostral limb caudally converts the incision into a T. **B)** The skin flaps have been developed in a subplatysmal plane and the deep fascia opened. The hypoglossal nerve is seen entering between the internal and external carotid arteries. The rostral belly of the digastric muscle has been sectioned. The facial nerve is identified in the tail of the parotid gland and dissected rostrally to allow for further retraction. The submandibular salivary gland may be elevated rostrally.

of the nasopharynx and laryngopharynx. The hypoglossal nerve swings between the internal and external carotid arteries at the greater cornu of the hyoid bone. The hypoglossal nerve is mobilized rostrally, taking care to preserve the descendens hypoglossi. The retropharyngeal space is then exposed using blunt dissection. Any veins crossing the operative field into the jugular vein need to be sectioned (Figure 2C).

As with the transoral operation, the prevertebral fascia must be incised in a

C

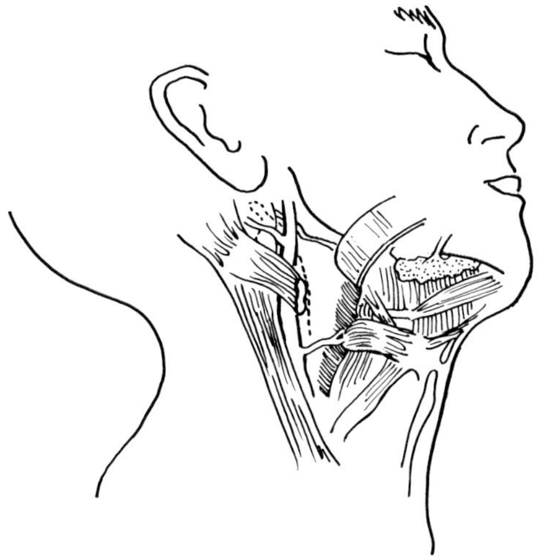

Figure 2C. Retraction and exposure are achieved medial to the carotid sheath and lateral to the pharynx with elevation of the hypoglossal nerve. Further exposure is accomplished by sectioning the stylohyoid muscle.

vertical fashion, and the longus colli and the longus capitis muscles are dissected free of their medial origin, thus exposing the anterior arch of the atlas. Blunt Cloward or Caspar retractors may be used to maintain the exposure. It is important to orient oneself to the midline at all times. Ventral decompression is accomplished as with the transoral operation. Once decompression has been achieved, fusion may be carried out using a tricortical iliac crest graft or a fibular strut interposed between the caudal clivus and the caudal aspect of the axis vertebra.

The closure of the cervical wound is first accomplished by approximating the longus colli muscles in the midline with 3-0 polyglycolic sutures. The digastric tendon is approximated with 3-0 or 4-0 nonabsorbable sutures, such as silk or woven nylon. The deep fascia of the ventral border of the sternocleidomastoid muscle is likewise approximated with 4-0 polyglycolic sutures. The platysma muscle and subcutaneous tissue are approximated in layers with the subsequent approximation of the skin in a standard fashion. No drains are used.

Complications

This procedure is not tolerated as well as a transoral operation due to pharyngeal dysfunction. There is a high risk of injury to the hypoglossal and the glossopharyngeal nerves. It is difficult to visualize deep midline structures at the true craniovertebral junction. However, this procedure is ideal for extradural lesions below the axis level.

This approach requires dissection along the carotid sheath and its dorsal displacement. It is important that the carotid artery be imaged prior to embarking on such a procedure, since intraoperative stroke with embolization is a well-recognized, and potentially avoidable, complication.

Dorsolateral (Far Lateral) Transcondylar Approach

The terms "extreme lateral transcondylar approach," "lateral suboccipital approach," "transjugular approach," "extreme lateral approach," "dorsal lateral suboccipital condylar approach" have all been used to describe the dorsolateral approach. Although the technique utilized in each of these approaches varies slightly, they all represent an attempt to expose the lower clivus, foramen magnum, craniovertebral junction, and upper cervical spine without retracting the cerebellum or spinal cord. This exposure is accomplished by performing an extensive dorsal and lateral bony resection, including the lateral rim of the foramen magnum and the dorsal occipital condyle. It is necessary at times to remove the posterior arch of the atlas vertebra, together with the dorsal aspect of the foramen transversarium and the lateral atlantal mass. If one is approaching lesions that are solely within the upper cervical canal, resection of the occipital condyle is unnecessary.

The far lateral approach allows for control of the extracranial vertebral artery from the foramen transversarium into the posterior fossa. The benefit of this approach is that the depth of field is relatively short, considering that the dorsal cervical musculature is retracted to an extreme lateral position.

Indications

The indications for the dorsolateral approach are intradural neoplasms located entirely ventral to the brain stem and cervical spinal cord, and aneurysms of the vertebral artery and proximal basilar trunk. Extradural lesions of the clivus and upper cervical canal also may be approached by this exposure. This route, combined with the dorsal retrosigmoid and presigmoid approach, allows for control of both intradural and extradural tumors that involve the jugular foramen and the upper clival region.

Operative Technique

This procedure has been performed with the patient in the sitting, lateral, and modified decubitus or park bench positions. With the prone position, the head is turned slightly to the side of the exposure and fixed in a multipin headrest. The patient is secured on an adjustable operating table so as to allow for a 45° rotation of the table intraoperatively. The sitting position places the patient at risk for air embolism, but provides excellent access. The technique, however, is fraught with danger and requires the skills of a competent neuroanesthesiologist and placement of a right atrial and pulmonary artery catheter, as well as Doppler ultrasound monitoring of the heart and end-tidal CO_2 monitoring. The lateral position allows for the cerebellum to fall away from the site of the operative field and for the head to be tilted upward in order to provide for venous drainage without the concern of air embolism. The placement of a central venous catheter, however, is still recommended. The author prefers the straight dorsal approach with the head rotated 20° toward the side of the lesion and slightly elevated. The shoulders are taped downward and the patient is firmly secured to the operating table.

The incision has many variations, including a straight dorsal cerebellar craniectomy incision. The author prefers an inverted U-shaped skin incision or an inverted hockey stick incision that starts at the mastoid prominence and proceeds beneath the rostral nuchal line and extends caudally to the midline (Figure 3A). The advantage of this incision is that a cuff of nuchal fascia and muscle caudal to the incision can be left for closure, thus preventing CSF leakage. The paraspinal muscles are split along the spinous process and dissection is then carried laterally to the side of the lesion. A cuff of muscle attached to the rostral nuchal line is maintained for subsequent approximation and closure of the muscle flap. The paraspinal musculature is then retracted laterally with fish hooks and weights. A self-retaining retractor should never be used because the bulk of the cervical musculature obliterates the avenue of exposure. Special care should be taken when dissecting in the vicinity of the lateral portion of the C1 lamina and the lateral mass of C1. This area of loose connective tissue is caudal to the caudal border of the inferior oblique muscle. The ventral ramus of the C2 nerve root runs transversely and crosses the vertebral artery between the C1 and C2 vertebrae. At times the vertebral artery may be redundant, especially in the elderly, and the venous plexuses may produce troublesome bleeding. Once the vertebral artery is fully exposed between C1 and C2, the oblique muscle is detached from the transverse process of C1 and C2. The vertebral artery is followed from C1 to its entry into the dura mater. In 35% to 50% of individuals, the artery is completely surrounded by bone at the posterior arch of C1. The vertebral artery gives off radical and muscular branches in this region, which may supply an intradural or extradural tumor and should be obliterated.

The subperiosteal plane of dissection minimizes bleeding from the vertebral venous plexus. Bleeding is controlled with bipolar cauterization under saline irrigation.

The ipsilateral occipital bone is then removed. This resection includes the condylar fossa, the dorsal rim of the occipital condyle, and the dorsal lateral rim of the foramen magnum (Figure 3B and C). The posterior arch of the atlas, including the transverse process and the ipsilateral lamina of C2, may be exposed as necessary. If the dissection is carried into the posterior fossa, it is important that the resection of bone expose the sigmoid and transverse sinuses to the jugular bulb. In circumstances where the lesion is in the cerebellopontine angle or where clival exposure is necessary, a mastoidectomy must be performed to expand the exposure. The vertebral artery is elevated from the sulcus arteriosis and dissected free from the transverse foramen of the atlas to the zone where it penetrates the atlanto-occipital membrane in the dura mater. Small branches to the surrounding musculature and the posterior meningeal artery are interrupted after bipolar cauterization.

During exposure of the vertebral artery, the flexure of the vertebral artery as it leaves the groove of the atlas to join the dura mater requires special attention. Control of the vertebral arteries is an important step in the lateral extension of the dorsal approach.

Further lateral exposure into the posterior fossa as well as the upper cervical canal is obtained by vertebral artery transposition, which requires exposure and section of the second cranial nerve and extension of the subperiosteal dissection inside the foramen transversarium. The C1 foramen transversarium is removed from its dorsal aspect and the vertebral artery unroofed and dissected caudally to C2. The vertebral artery can then be mobilized from C2 to its intracranial portion and gently displaced (Figure 3D). Surgical maneuvers can then be carried out laterally. When dealing with lesions within the cerebellopontine angle and the cervical canal, the craniectomy extends from the junction of the transverse and sigmoid sinuses rostrally to just beyond the midline, including the foramen magnum. The opening is wider caudally and laterally. The lateral extent of the exposure proceeds into the mastoid air cells and is completed caudally by resection of the medial aspect of the occipital condyle. A C1 laminectomy is then performed ipsilateral to the lesion. The extreme lateral resection of bone into the condylar fossa and, at times, into the medial aspect of the occipital condyle is the key to the approach to the ventral aspect of the brain stem and cervical spinal cord without retraction. The resection of the lateral edge of bone must be accomplished with a drill. The author prefers using the Midas Rex M8 diamond drill or a Bien drill with a 4-mm drill bit. At times, a small emissary branch of the vertebral artery is encountered, which perforates the bone behind the condyle in the condylar fossa. Further lateral exposure can be realized with division of the sigmoid sinus, if the exposure is essential. The vertical and horizontal portions of the sigmoid sinus are exposed through a dorsal mastoidectomy and the sigmoid sinus is occluded at the junction between the horizontal and vertical segments; however, this is rarely necessary. Further ventral exposure is limited by the ninth and 10th cranial nerves at the jugular foramen.

Once the craniectomy is completed, the capsule of the atlanto-occipital joint is cauterized and the dorsal medial aspect of the occipital condyle and the lateral mass of the atlas is drilled away as the vertebral artery is protected with a small spatula. Bone removal should be performed to create a 1-cm gap between the resected occipital condyle and the dural entry of the vertebral artery, which

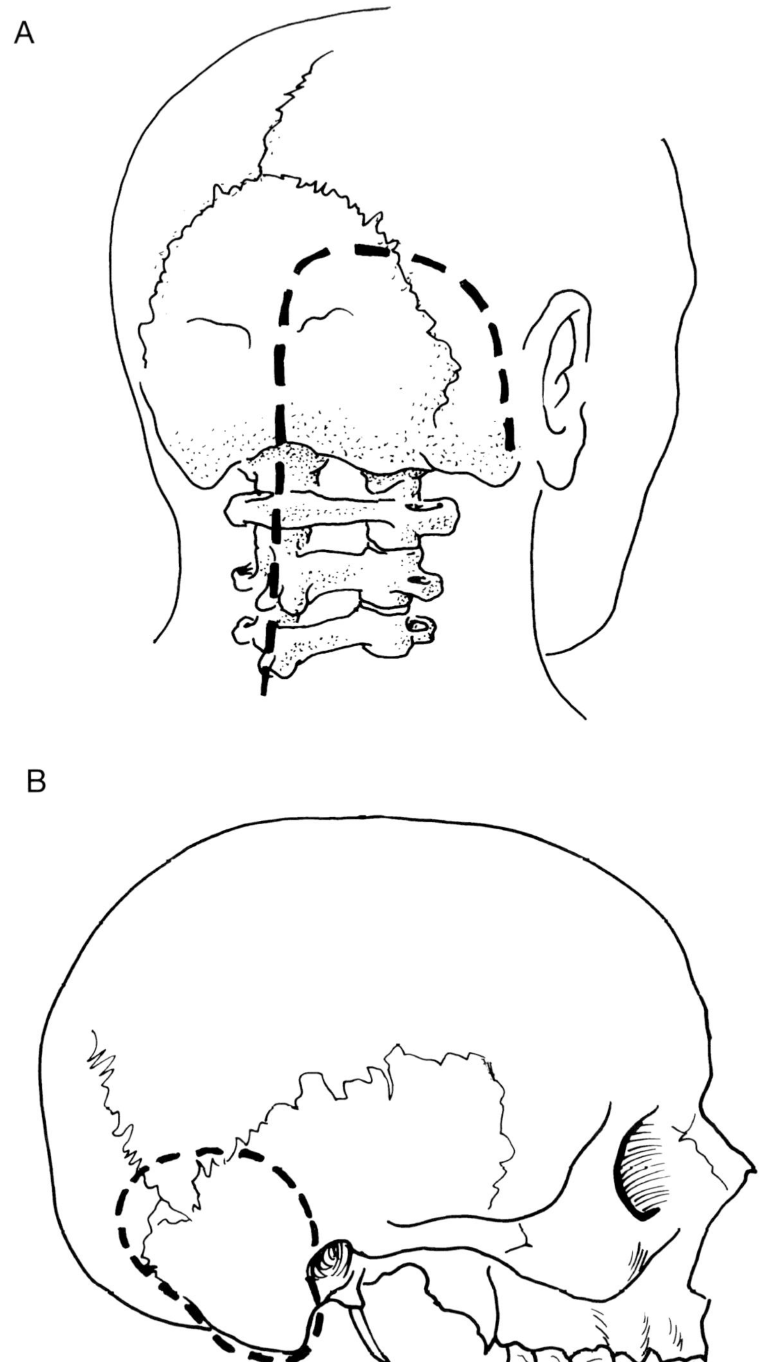

Figure 3A-B. The dorsolateral (far lateral) transcondylar approach to the ventral foramen magnum. **A)** The skin incision *(dotted line)* is made from the external occipital protuberance to the spinous process of C4 and then extended rostrally and laterally to the mastoid process, creating an inverted hockey stick incision. **B)** The extent of bone removal needed to gain access to the caudal clivus and upper cervical spine necessitates a partial mastoidectomy and removal of the medial aspect of the occipital condyle.

C

D

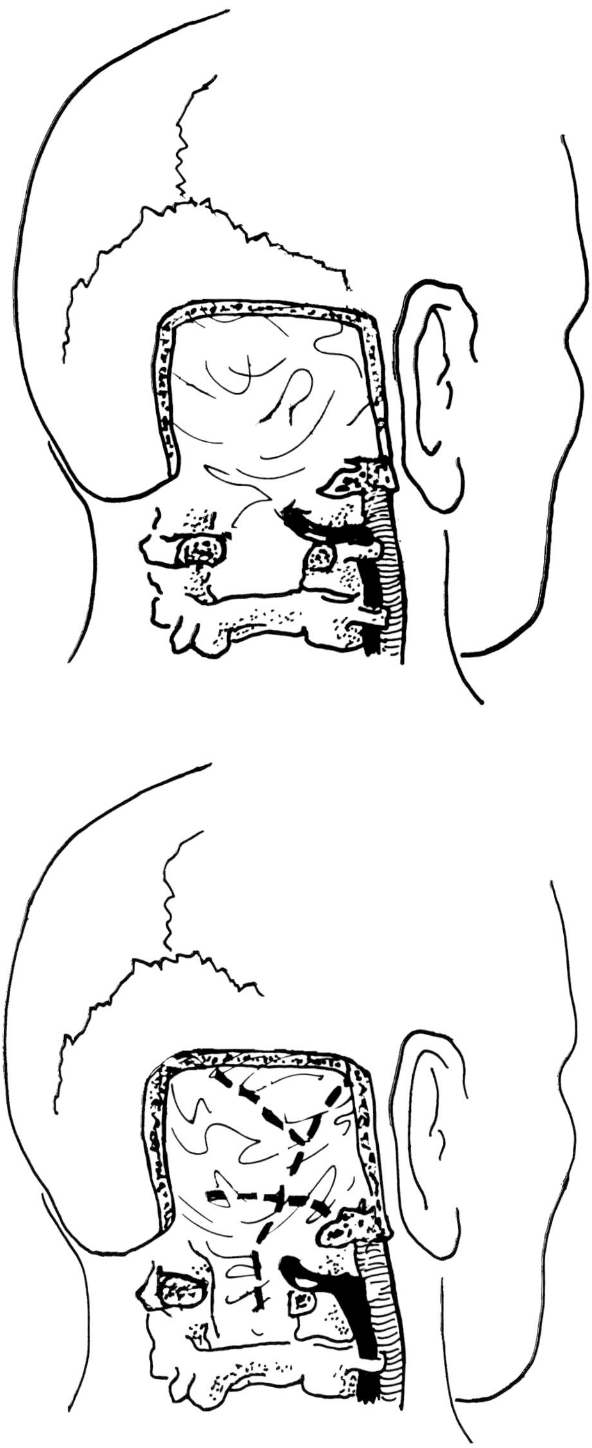

Figure 3C-D. C) A posterior fossa craniectomy exposes the transverse and sigmoid sinus as well as the jugular foramen. The entrance of the extradural vertebral artery into the dura mater is identified. **D)** A laminectomy of the atlas is accomplished on the affected side. The vertebral artery is unroofed by removal of the dorsal aspect of the transverse atlas process and dissection at the foramen transversarium, thus allowing for elevation of the vertebral artery. Dural incisions are represented by the *dotted lines*.

E

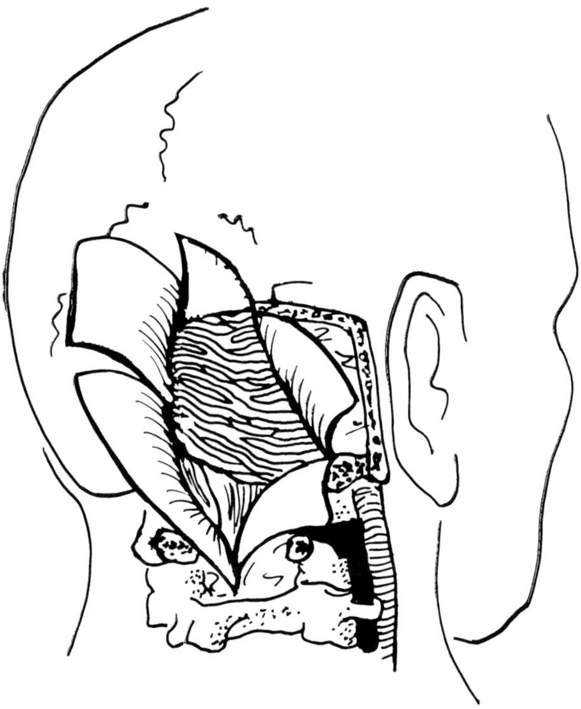

Figure 3E. The dura mater is exposed and the leaves held apart with stay sutures to visualize the cerebellum, the brain stem, and the upper cervical spinal cord. The intra-arachnoid vertebral artery and its branches are exposed, as well as the cerebellopontine angle.

usually involves removing only the dorsal two-thirds of the condyle. Dissection ventral to this leads one to the hypoglossal canal, where significant venous hemorrhage may occur from the vertebral plexus accompanying the condylar emissary veins in the hypoglossal plexus.

When a dumbbell neurilemmoma is encountered, the neural foramen of the involved level is exposed by drilling away the adjacent superior and inferior articular facets. The intradural extent of the neurilemmoma determines the level at which the dorsal facetectomies are performed.

A curvilinear dural incision extends from the sigmoid sinus to the lateral cervical exposure (Figure 3E). This incision runs medial to the vertebral artery. Several secondary incisions are made perpendicular to the primary incision to allow for retraction and intracranial and intraspinal exposure.

Once the dura mater is opened, the operating microscope is essential for magnification and for the attainment of a concentrated light source. The intradural vertebral artery is immediately encountered. The dentate ligament is sectioned and the cervicomedullary junction rotated rostrally and away from a ventrally placed lesion. In rare circumstances, the dorsal rootlets of C1 and C2 may be sacrificed. In the case of clivus meningiomas, the involved clival dura may be resected close to the entrance of the lower cranial nerves into the parietal dura.

The specific pathology encountered is now addressed. Hemostasis must be exact. The mastoid air cells are carefully closed with wax and a fat pad, if necessary. A meticulous dural closure is essential, and may be supplemented by a fascial graft. Paraspinal musculature is approximated anatomically in layers. If there is a concern about CSF leakage, a lumbar subarachnoid catheter may be needed for drainage of CSF in the early postoperative period.

In circumstances when only the medial aspect of one occipital condyle has been resected, instability does not occur. However, if a significant portion of the lateral mass of C1 is resected and a facetectomy is performed at C2, postoperative instability will result. Stability can be achieved by contralateral fusion or an ipsilateral fusion that spans the operative defect, extending to one vertebral level caudal to the disrupted stability. Instrumentation may consist of a contoured threaded Steinmann pin loop or a bent-angled plate secured to the occiput as well as the upper cervical spine wherever possible and at times may be supplemented with the use of lateral mass-transarticular C1-2 screw fixation. It is imperative that instrumentation be supplemented with fresh autologous bone for the achievement of a solid osseous fusion at a later stage.

Complications

The far lateral transcondylar approach has been fraught with complications, including vertebral artery complications in the case of involved neoplasm, as well as CSF leakage. In the series by George et al,[4] three of 14 patients died. In one case, death was due to a massive air embolism with the patient in a sitting position.

Lower cranial nerve palsies have been described after excision of tumors in the foramen magnum. However, this complication is due to the dissection of the tumor from the cranial nerve itself and not to the operative exposure.

References

1. Archer DJ, Young S, Uttley D: Basilar aneurysms: a new transclival approach via maxillotomy. **J Neuro-surg 67:**54-58, 1987

2. Crockard HA, Pozo JL, Ransford AO, et al: Transoral decompression and posterior fusion for rheumatoid atlanto-axial subluxation. **J Bone Joint Surg (Br) 68:**350-356, 1986

3. De Andrade JR, MacNab I: Anterior occipito-cervical fusion using an extrapharyngeal exposure. **J Bone Joint Surg (Am) 51:**381-392, 1969

4. George B, Dematons C, Cophignon J: Lateral approach to the anterior portion of the foramen magnum. Application to surgical removal of 14 benign tumors: technical note. **Surg Neurol 29:** 484-490, 1988

5. Hall JE, Denis F, Murray J: Exposure of the upper cervical spine for spinal decompression by a mandible and tongue-splitting approach. **J Bone Joint Surg (Am) 59:**121-123, 1977

6. Heros RC: Lateral suboccipital approach for vertebral and vertebrobasilar artery lesions. **J Neurosurg 64:**559-562, 1986

7. Krespi YP, Sisson GA: Transmandibular exposure of the skull base. **Am J Surg 148:**534-538, 1984

8. Lesoin F, Jomin M, Pellerin P, et al: Transclival transcervical approach to the upper cervical spine and clivus. **Acta Neurochir 80:**100-104, 1986

9. McAfee PC, Bohlman HH, Riley LH Jr, et al: The anterior retropharyngeal approach to the upper part of the cervical spine. **J Bone Joint Surg (Am) 69:**1371-1373, 1987

10. Menezes AH: Surgical approaches to the craniocervical junction, in Frymoyer JW (ed): **The Adult Spine: Principles and Practice.** New York: Raven Press, 1991, pp 967-985

11. Menezes AH, VanGilder JC: Platybasia, basilar invagination and cranial settling, in Apuzzo MLJ (ed): **Brain Surgery: Complication Avoidance and Manage-ment.** New York: Churchill Livingstone, 1992, pp 2029-2053

12. Sen CN, Sekhar LN: An extreme lateral approach to intradural lesions of the cervical spine and foramen magnum. **Neurosurgery 27:** 197-206, 1990

13. Spetzler RF, Grahm TW: The far-lateral approach to the inferior clivus and the upper cervical region: technical note. **BNI Q 6(4):**35-38, 1990

Chapter 5

Ventral Exposures of the Subaxial Cervical Spine

Richard L. Saunders, MD

There are three principal exposures of the ventral subaxial spine that should be familiar to spine surgeons.[1,5,10] By far the most important of these is the medial approach, popularized by Cloward[4] and Robinson.[11] Facility with this operation is fundamental to the less often required cervicothoracic extension[9] and the so-called "lateral approach" to the vertebral artery and nerve root foramen.[6,14] A table-fixed retraction system allows the surgeon to realize the full potential of the surgical approach employed.[12] Without this adjunct, the need for a fixed exposure necessitates the impaling of soft tissues by self-retaining retractors, or the uncertain security of hand-held retractors in the midst of the potentially treacherous anatomy of the carotid sheath, esophagus, cranial nerves, nerve roots, sympathetic chain, thoracic duct, great vessels, and a lung apex. The disadvantage of not using table-fixed retraction is compounded by the differential tissue resistance between the relatively unyielding midline structures and the easily retracted more lateral anatomy. These newer retractors do not impale and have the immediacy of one that is hand-held, without the consequence of fatigue or inattention.

The emphasis of this chapter is on the mainstay of subaxial exposures for visualizing vertebral bodies from C2 through T1, i.e., the medial approach. A description of more lateral strategies to access the nerve root foramen and more caudal exposure to T3 are built upon the foundation of this mainstay.

Surgical Indications

Simply stated, any pathology located ventral to the cervical spinal cord from the body of C3 to that of T2 is usually best approached ventrally. In the case of cervical spondylosis, there are some provisos, such as the importance of a lordotic curve, that must be considered during the decision-making process.[3] In this regard, the presence of a cervical kyphosis is a specific indication for the ventral approach. With tumor surgery, it is usually a mistake to approach intraspinal lesions ventrally. Conversely, this is the approach of choice for tumors of the vertebral body. Nerve root lesions can be dealt with ventrally or dorsally. With trauma, the ventral approach is definitive for corpectomy of a comminuted vertebral body fracture with spinal canal compromise; however, decisions regarding simultaneous stabilization procedures are required. Simple corpectomy and strut graft alone is not a stable construct for the majority of posttrauma situations. As such, it represents an incomplete strategy.

In considering surgery for critical cervical stenosis, whether acute traumatic or chronic spondylotic, the clinical picture is the deciding factor. In the patient with a complete motor and sensory myelopathy, the significance of stabilization is all-important, whereas that of spinal canal decompression is arguable. In patients with an incomplete myelopathy, there is some controversy relating primarily to the timing of surgery, not its indications.

Spondylotic spinal canal stenosis, unassociated with symptoms or signs, is not unusual, and increasingly common, with advancing age. The literature on the natural history of spondylotic spinal cord compression is simply not supportive of expectant management when compared with modern outcomes. For example, the minimally impaired group reported by Nurick[8] was not properly interpreted. It was suggested that this group be primarily managed by nonsurgical methods. By modern statistical analysis, however, his data support surgery, not "conservatism."[2] Today, the primary debate is over the proper surgical strategy and selection criteria. For ventral surgery, especially corpectomy, the critical factor is the presence of a straightened or kyphotic spine.

Lateral approaches to the ventral cervical spine are principally for nerve root decompression[7,14] and the rare symptomatic spondylotic vertebral artery compression. Manabe et al[7] have described using this strategy for a transforaminal ventral spinal canal decompression to treat myelopathy. The advantage of such a method lies in the avoidance of weakening or destabilizing the spine, while achieving spinal cord decompression. In the case of congenital spinal canal stenosis, however, such an avenue would probably not be prudent. Since the lamina are not disturbed and the intervertebral disc as a unit is not removed, no subsequent fusion is necessary.

Indications for extending the ventral cervical approach into the thoracic inlet are not unlike those of the subaxial cervical spine.[9] The normally kyphotic thoracic spine angles away from the surgeon at the T1 and T2 levels. Accordingly, the need for access to the ventral spinal canal for vertebral body tumor or spondylotic spinal cord compression, ossification of the posterior longitudinal ligament, and bony spinal canal intrusion necessitates a more caudal exposure that complements the ventral cervical exposure. By such an inlet extension, surgery to the T3 vertebral body is feasible, although somewhat confining. The alternative is thoracotomy, or a variant thereof. One should bear in mind that with the neck extended, the removal of T1 and fusion to T2 is feasible through the standard ventral cervical approach.

Regional Anatomy

The sternocleidomastoid muscle is the surface landmark that should be followed with either a transverse or a longitudinal incision (Figure 1). Although some accesses are lateral to the sternocleidomastoid muscle, an access medial to the muscle is preferred. Critical to a full exposure of the spine is the sectioning of the fascial attachments to the ventral sternocleidomastoid muscle throughout its surgical exposure. This landmark allows the identification of the carotid sheath, which lies along the medial border and is protected with the fingers of the surgeon's nondominant hand. At the rostral and caudal extremes of soft tissue dissection are the 12th cranial nerve and the recurrent laryngeal nerve, respectively. Virtually all of the anatomy between these two extremes is tolerant of sacrifice, including the ansa hypoglossi, common facial vein, and the vascular pedicle to the thyroid. The tubercle on the caudal ventral edge of C2 is a categoric landmark for the midline, unique to C2. A ligamentous extension rostral to this tubercle creates a sharp keel, further identifying the C2 body.

The thoracic duct is on the left side, usually more lateral than most spine dissections, at least with exposures medial and

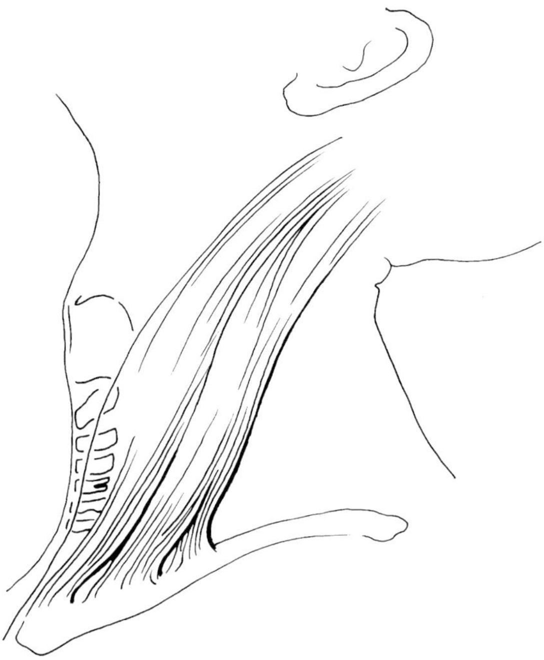

Figure 1. The surface landmark for ventral cervical incisions is the sternocleidomastoid muscle.

ventral to the sternocleidomastoid muscle. The brachiocephalic vein lies behind the rostral edge of the manubrium and is a potential source of major blood loss, if it is not identified during the dissection into the thoracic inlet. The longus colli muscles run on either side of the vertebral bodies from the rostral extreme of the cervical spine to T3. These muscles approach the midline at C2 and are variably spaced more caudally. The sympathetic chain lies between the carotid sheath and the middle one-third of the longus colli muscles in their midcervical position. The muscle overlies the uncinate and transverse processes.

Adjuncts to Surgery

The importance of retraction decisions has already been addressed. Positioning for subaxial cervical spine surgery is ordinarily with the patient's head and neck in a neutral position, secured by tape. Neck extension facilitates access to the upper thoracic spine. If the thoracic inlet is entered, turning the head away from the surgeon is facilitating. Anesthetic technique is best accomplished without paralytic agents to enable the monitoring of surgically induced motor responses due to undue or unappreciated surgical irritation of the spinal cord or nerve roots. The preoperative placement of Gardner-Wells tongs, without traction, allows a "handle" for spine distraction at the time of strut grafting. The unstable spine may be treated with a varying degree of traction during the procedure, as indicated. The preoperative placement of a lumbar drain is a consideration in those cases in which ossification of the posterior longitudinal ligament or trauma cause an increased likelihood of cerebrospinal fluid (CSF) leakage.

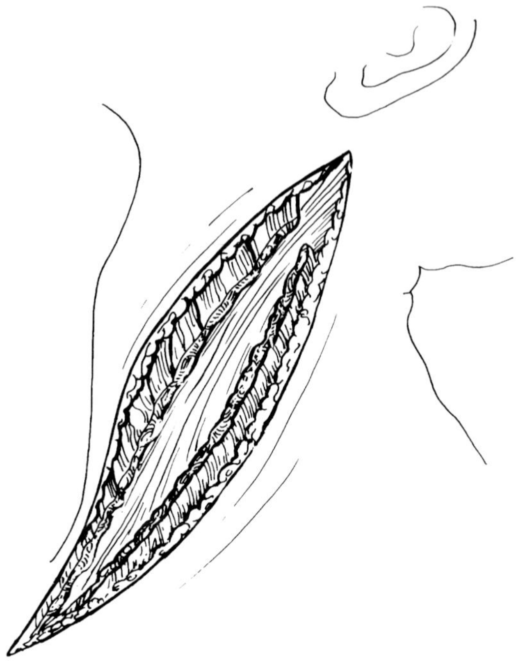

Figure 2. The platysma muscle is cut to reveal the ventral edge of the sternocleidomastoid muscle.

The Ventromedial Approach for Corpectomy

The Approach

Surgery is performed with the patient's head and neck in a neutral position. Nonparalytic anesthesia, as previously mentioned, is employed. The side of the surgical approach is dictated by the laterality of symptoms, signs, and/or radiographic asymmetry. It is best to approach the patient from the side opposite that with the greatest spinal canal encroachment, whether right or left. Being right-handed, it is the author's preference to approach the symmetrical problem from the right side. A transverse incision is used for the thick short neck and a sternocleidomastoid incision for the long thin one. A sharp incision through the dermis is made, and the wound deepened through the platysma muscle, with cutting monopolar current. The fascia along the ventral border of the sternocleidomastoid muscle is then sharply incised to as great a length as possible (8-9 cm) (Figures 2 and 3). This usually exposes the omohyoid muscle, which when transected permits blunt dissection access to the prevertebral space. Holding the carotid artery lateral with the nondominant hand, the prevertebral space is widened with blunt and sharp dissection (Figure 4). Hemostasis is obtained. The tubercle that is readily palpable on the caudal ventral aspect of the mid-C2 vertebral body and its associated sharp midline keel dictate the direction of exposure, pending x-ray confirmation (Figure 5). At least 8 to 9 cm of prevertebral exposure between two fingers perpendicular to the spine should be created for long exposures. Definition of the hypoglossal nerve, section of the ansa cervicalis, and section of the common facial vein may be needed for exposure of the C2 vertebra.

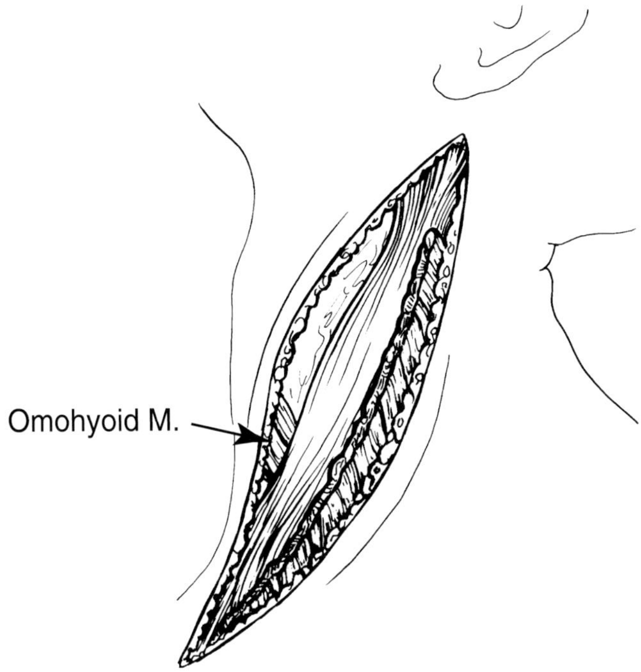

Figure 3. The omohyoid muscle is exposed for sectioning of the deep fascial attachments on the ventral border of the sternocleidomastoid muscle. The omohyoid muscle is then transected to access the prevertebral space.

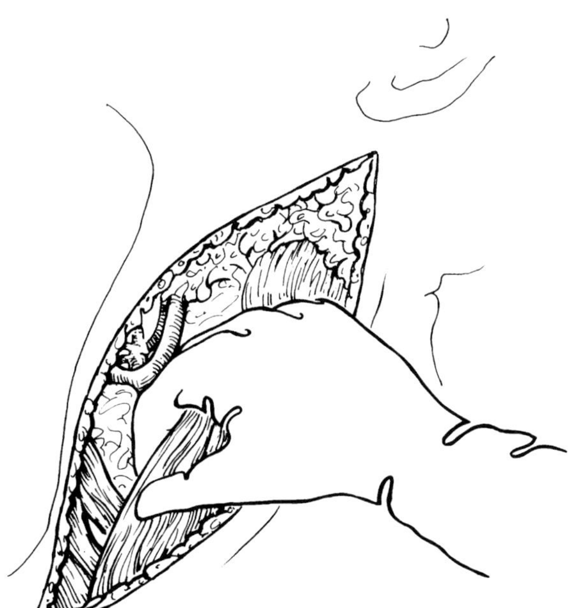

Figure 4. The prevertebral space is entered medial to the carotid sheath, which is protected and retracted by the surgeon's nondominant hand.

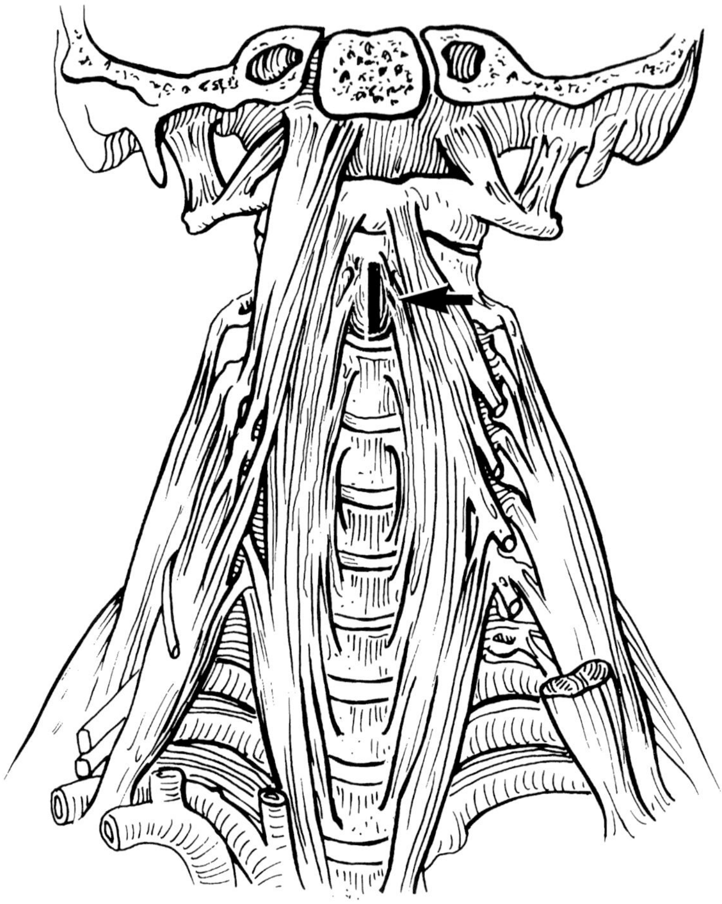

Figure 5. The soft tissues of the ventral surface of the cervical spine. A key landmark in this prevertebral space is the midline keel on the ventral surface of the C2 vertebral body *(arrow)*.

Retraction

A table-fixed retractor system is positioned, placing the midline blade first, then the low lateral retractors, followed, as necessary, by the rostral and caudal blades (Figure 6). The critical retraction points are: maintaining vertical retraction of the trachea and esophagus, directing the lateral retraction loosely toward the table, and lifting rostral tissues away from the spine, so as to create a short narrow tunnel toward C2. The resulting exposure should appear wide and shallow, not trenchlike. Soft tissues should not be tensely stretched. The midline retractors are relaxed hourly.

The spinal level and extent of exposure is dependent upon the purpose of the operation. For the purpose of this discussion, a multi-level corpectomy is considered. A complete discectomy of the rostral and caudal disc spaces relative to the planned decompression is performed. The uncinate processes are carefully defined, because they represent reliable markers of the lateral extremes of the spinal canal. The width of the decompression should be no greater than the greatest diameter of the graft.

The Corpectomy

Having defined the uncinate processes bilaterally, rostrally, and caudally, the central corpectomy trough is created expediently with rongeur and Midas Rex AM8 burrs (Midas Rex, Fort Worth, Texas) (Figure 7). Diamond burrs are not necessary. Adjoining vertebrae are taken simultaneously in long

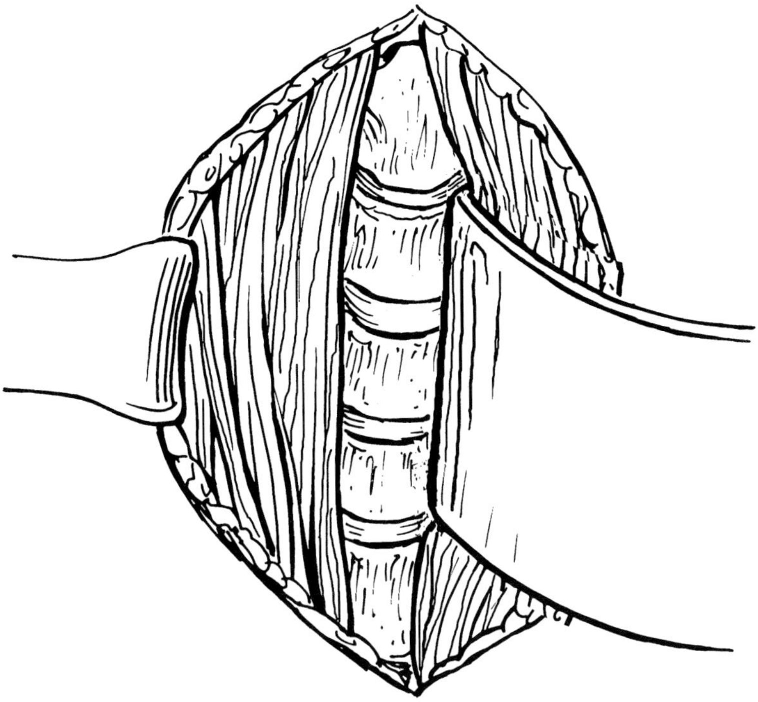

Figure 6. Exposure of the ventral spinal surface for midline decompression. Note that the wide medial retractor protects the viscera.

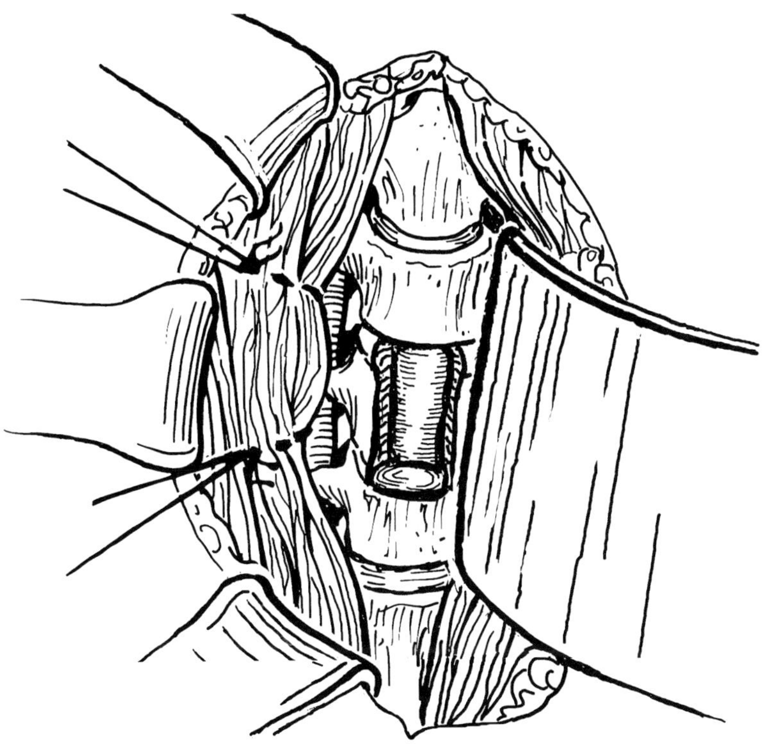

Figure 7. After mobilizing the longus colli muscle, bilateral stay sutures are placed for local retraction. Single-level central corpectomy prior to mortising is illustrated.

wiping sweeps of the drill, first with loupe magnification, then under the operating microscope as the trough is deepened. Premeasured sections of wood applicator sticks (8, 10, and 15 mm) are used frequently to calibrate the exact desired width of the resection and dimensions of mortises.

Substantial bleeding occurs from bone surfaces. Bone wax and Gelfoam can be used in this situation. However, it is usually best to simply move along rapidly, quickly accessing the posterior longitudinal ligament, where definitive bipolar coagulation of venous bleeders is usually effective. The sides of the bone trough can at this point be "waxed" with Gelfoam. The decompression trough is up to 15 to 16 mm in width.

Since the surgeon's side of exposure is often obliquely angled toward the opposite side (consequent to the angle of view), the surgeon's assistant (from the opposite side of the table) can correct this trough obliquity to achieve the final decompression width. This makes the surgeon's side of the decompression more vertical and ensures adequacy of the decompression itself. Efforts directed at foraminotomies beyond the width of the corpectomy trough are not made.

The posterior longitudinal ligament is opened and excised if imaging suggests disc sequestration or ossification of the posterior longitudinal ligament. In the lateral gutters, this ligament is usually thin and harbors troublesome varices. It is, accordingly, not removed. Sharp incision of the ligament away from the annulus fibrosus will almost always allow a definition of the epidural space, even in the face of ligament-dural adhesions. There is often a trace of moisture as the glistening dura is visualized. If the posterior longitudinal ligament is ossified, it can be readily drilled away with a Midas Rex AM8 burr to a point where the plaque "floats" loosely. The dura mater is often invaded by the ligament in this circumstance. The field may become filled with CSF. If this is anticipated preoperatively, a lumbar drain is placed after induction of anesthesia. If not and CSF is then observed with or without ossification of the posterior longitudinal ligament, a drain is placed postoperatively, if possible.

With completion of the decompression, mortises are fashioned in the opposing endplates of the rostral and caudal vertebra, using a high-speed burr and an angled curette to measure approximately 8 to 9 mm in the ventrodorsal dimension, 3 mm deep, and 11 mm wide in the rostral vertebra. The caudal mortise is made only 1 to 2 mm deep. In creating the mortises, the dorsal lips are made 2 mm longer than the ventral counterpart (Figure 8). If the graft fractures or is displaced dorsally, the longer dorsal mortise lips ensure that any graft movement is directed away from the spinal cord into the prevertebral space. The thickness of the mortise lips is 1 to 2 mm.

The length of the graft is determined with a caliper or a broken applicator stick with and without manual cranial traction. Usually 1 mm of distraction can be achieved. More distraction is not necessary and indeed may place excessive load on the graft and hyperextend the neck.

The Bone Graft

When anticipating the use of an iliac crest graft, the surgeon should note that the width of the iliac crest narrows dorsally toward the edge of the crest. Accordingly, with a short decompression, a tricortical strut graft harvested close to the anterior superior iliac spine is optimal. Similarly, the natural curve of the iliac crest may be utilized to an advantage, allowing the graft to conform to the curvature of the cervical spine.

The harvesting technique is critical from two perspectives, especially in the osteoporotic patient. 1) Use of a saw or burr, rather than an osteotome, avoids microcracks in the cortical surfaces, which may lead to graft fracture. The clinical significance of this, however, has not been shown. 2) Care should be taken during harvest to avoid undercutting the anterior superior

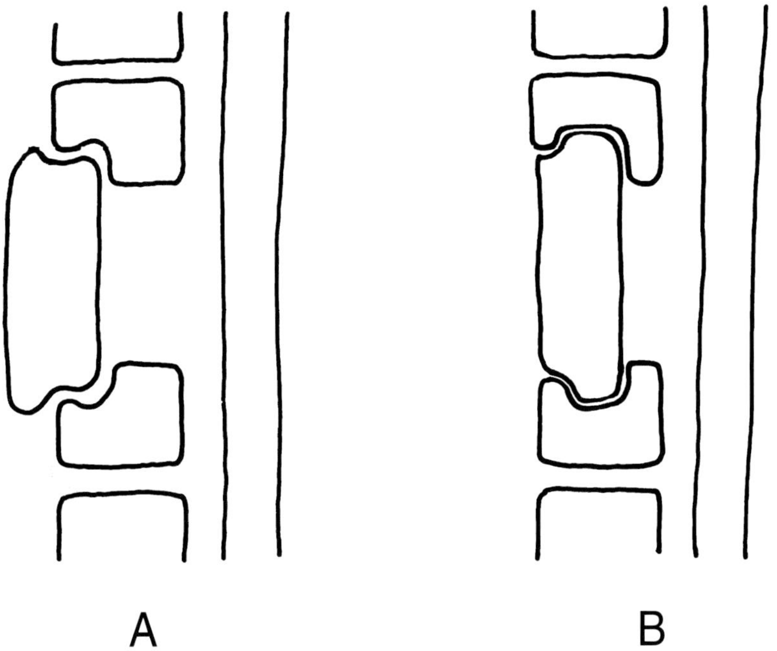

Figure 8. A schematic of mortise design from a lateral perspective. **A)** Dovetail method. **B)** Keystone method.

iliac spine. Postoperative fracture of the anterior superior iliac spine adds to the pain of an already painful donor site.

Fibula harvest is from the middle one-third of the shaft, through the lateral muscle septum. The periosteum is preserved. After fibula harvest, a short period of compressive leg wrapping, depending upon venous and vascular history, will minimize swelling and discomfort. Leg elevation during the first postoperative week is also beneficial.

When using an iliac crest graft, a tricortical construct is ideal. If necessary, a bicortical graft with the two cortical surfaces in continuity is sufficient. The cortical bone of either end of the graft is carefully preserved, which prevents weakening of the most stressed portion of the graft. In its final position, the ideal graft measures approximately 12 to 14 mm in the ventrodorsal dimension, lies in line with the neutral axis of the spine, and is tightly opposed to the sides of the decompression trough.

The Fusion

The graft, either iliac crest or fibula, is inserted into the cephalad mortise and then tapped gently into its final caudal position, while manual traction achieves 1 to 2 mm of distraction. There is usually substantial epidural venous bleeding during the traction for graft placement. This, however, stops when traction is released, requiring no specific address. Rarely is Gelfoam, Surgicel, or collagen left in the decompression trough. A suction drain may be left in the prevertebral space for 24 hours. Neck wound closure involves loose apposition of the platysma muscle with absorbable suture and subcuticular pull-out suture or skin tapes. A rigid collar is placed prior to reversal of anesthesia if the neck is otherwise thought to be stable.

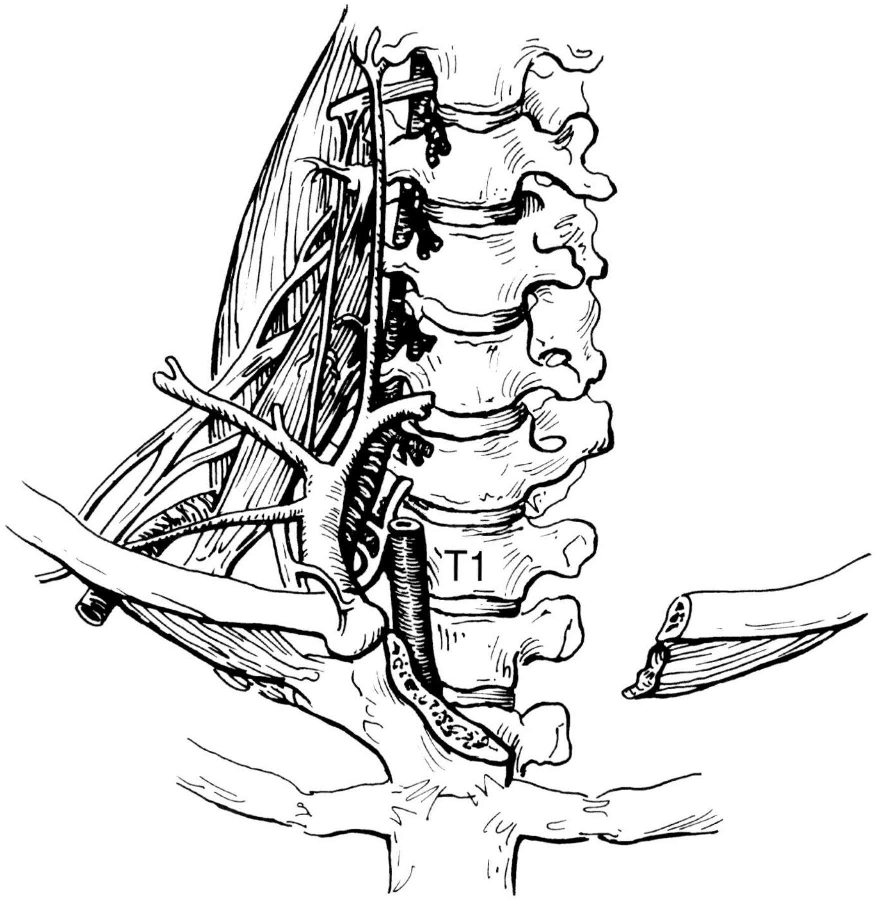

Figure 9. Access to the cervicothoracic junction to the T3 level requires resection of the medial clavicle and manubrium.

The Cervicothoracic Approach

The cervicothoracic approach is an extension of the ventromedial exposure of the subaxial spine.[9] Depending upon the patient's habitus and the nature of the shoulder girdle, exposure of the T1 and T2 vertebrae is usually feasible through the thoracic inlet, without violation of the sternoclavicular joint. If this is not the case, the opening of the sternoclavicular joint at the manubrium allows access to T3. The sternocleidomastoid skin incision is simply extended in the midline across the jugular notch and down the sternum.

Two practical considerations impact the complexity of the effort of entering the thoracic inlet: the recurrent laryngeal nerve and the degree of thoracic kyphosis. In general, the thoracic duct is lateral enough to be ignored. Usually, the recurrent nerve is lower on the left side, making a left-sided approach to the inlet preferable, with the neck turned toward the opposite side by 10° or more.

The clavicles and sternum can be traversed by either transsection or resection. The angle of view of the T1, T2, and T3 vertebrae is made less oblique by removing the upper portion of the manubrium and the head of the left clavicle, using a Leksell rongeur (Figure 9). Alternatively, the sternoclavicular joint and manubrium may be split, using an oscillating saw, and then spread with a ratcheting-type rib retractor. The key point with either of these strategies is the recognition that the brachiocephalic vein lies immediately behind the jugular notch. Rather than risk the tearing of this vein, it is best to doubly ligate and incise it.

Because the left recurrent nerve is at a lower level, the approach from the left side is preferable (unless there are compelling reasons to the contrary). The angle of view into the thoracic inlet approaches that of the upper thoracic spinal axis. It is by opening the sternoclavicular junction that this angle is made more perpendicular to the thoracic kyphosis. The sternal notch of the manubrium lies in the same horizontal plane as the T2-3 interspace. It may be unwise to attempt exposure of the spine caudal to T3 via the thoracic inlet route, as this might place the great vessels at an excessive risk of injury. Retraction of the innominate artery, trachea, and esophagus toward the right, in a fashion similar to the ventromedial exposure of the cervical spine, is quite simple.

After the upper thoracic spine and the cervicothoracic junction of the spine have been exposed, the angle of view may still be such that the angle of the intervertebral disc is away from the surgeon. If this is the case and the surgical indication is a thoracic disc, the resection of one or two vertebral bodies in the fashion of a corpectomy is simpler than attempting a discectomy through this awkward angle. The subsequent strut graft can be placed in the caudal mortise first and then tilted into the rostral mortise while hyperextending the neck.

Where the spinal pathology crosses the cervicothoracic spinal junction, the author has been hesitant to attempt a long decompression of the cervical component. Although five- and six-level corpectomies have been described (by definition implying strut grafts from C2 across the inlet), the author expects the long graft lever arm to be dangerously stressed, thereby risking graft displacement. Attempting to tailor such a long graft to the configuration of the cervicothoracic curve reversal might be challenging as well.

It is said that the thoracic duct may be an anatomical stumbling block with left-sided low approaches. However, the duct is usually lateral enough to not be problematical during medial surgery. A fatty meal ingested by the patient the night prior to surgery has been suggested as helpful in identifying the duct, if need be. If a chyle leakage point is encountered, it is simply best clamped and tied. Another problem at the thoracic inlet is that of a tear of the apical pleura. Such a tear can be sutured and tested by the Valsalva maneuver; failing this or if a lung parenchymal tear occurs, a tube thoracostomy may be required.

The Lateral Approach

The lateral approach to the cervical spine has not been a common surgical strategy in North America. It is essentially a medial approach, without midline exposure.[7,14] The choice of a skin incision is similar to that of midline exposures and is based on neck configuration and the extent of surgery. The key landmark after palpating the intervertebral disc medial to the carotid sheath is the anterior tubercle of the transverse process, which lies just lateral to the foramen transversarium of the vertebral artery.

After the anterior tubercle has been palpated at the level of the desired uncinate process, the level is confirmed radiographically. The most prominent tubercle is at the C6 level (the so-called "Chassaignac's tubercle"). Access to the longus colli muscle and the final lateral position is affected by opening the prevertebral fascia, as in the usual medial approach. The lateral surface of the uncinate process lies immediately medial to the vertebral artery and approximately 1 cm medial to the anterior tubercle. With a retractor positioned just lateral and in the same plane as the tubercle, a second retractor is positioned just medial to the uncinate process, exposing the full width of the longus colli complex. The sympathetic chain lying on

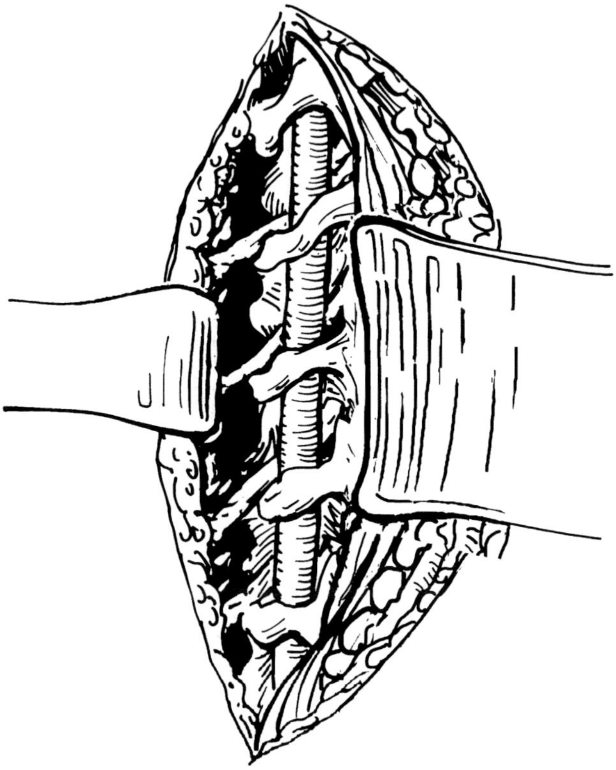

Figure 10. Mobilizing the longus colli muscle medially exposes the lateral uncinate processes and facilitates access to a single lateral nerve root foramen.

the longus colli muscle is mobilized with the muscle from lateral to medial, sectioning the insertions of the muscle to the anterior tubercles and transverse process. The muscle is then stripped subperiosteally across the costotransverse lamellae to the uncinate process (Figure 10). The tubercle and lamellae associated with the uncinate of interest are removed with angled Kerrison rongeurs to expose the vertebral artery. There is always substantial venous oozing from both the venous plexus surrounding the vertebral artery and the emissary veins from the base of the uncinate process on the lateral vertebral body. Bipolar coagulation and Gelfoam and bone wax packing are usually effective in controlling the bleeding. The region encompassed by the uncinate process to the lateral spinal canal can now be visualized, facilitated by an operating microscope. The extent of visualization is dependent upon the degree of uncinate process hypertrophic changes. Following 1 to 2 mm of lateral retraction of the vertebral artery with a Penfield elevator, uncinate resection and a dorsolateral discectomy is feasible, using a diamond burr and/or a small angled Kerrison rongeur.

Manabe et al[7] have recommended following the margins of the disc space and osteophytes across the ventral spinal canal through the expanded foramen. A key concept is the avoidance of more than 1 or 2 mm of vertebral artery retraction, which minimizes bleeding. The nerve root is visible as it passes behind the vertebral artery and along the lateral uncinate process.

Wound closure is over a suction drain, with a layer of sutures in the platysma muscle and a subcuticular running pull-out suture for skin. No orthosis is necessary.

A variation on the lateral approach is to approach the spine lateral (dorsal) to the sternocleidomastoid muscle, retracting the carotid sheath and muscle medially (ventrally). This is fairly restrictive, but has the advantage of avoiding traction on the recurrent laryngeal nerve when lower cervical uncinate processes are approached. If performed from the left side, the thoracic duct may be jeopardized.

Complications and Avoidance of Pitfalls

Medial Approach for Corpectomy

There are three elements of perioperative morbidity: complications relating to soft tissue manipulation and bone grafting, and postoperative radiculitis. Soft tissue problems stem from inadequate soft tissue dissection and exposure. If the tissues on either side of the retractor feel solid, they are under undue tension. Stridor, hoarseness, and dysphagia are possible consequences. Dissection should be such that the exposure is always more than needed. Nevertheless, retractors apply significant force on the midline structures and should, therefore, be relaxed regularly on the clock (e.g., 30 seconds every hour, on the hour).

Bone grafting requires care in harvesting and obsessive tailoring. Dougherty has shown that osteotomes cause cortical microcracks in iliac crest grafts (Cervical Spine Research Society Meeting, December, 1992). The use of an oscillating saw and/or the Midas Rex AM8 burr for harvest and graft shaping avoids this weakening effect. As previously discussed, no clinical evidence is available to support this, however.

Delayed postoperative C5 radiculitis is common after corpectomy, although not generally acknowledged. Restricting decompression to a 15- to 16-mm width has eliminated this problem.[13] The presumption is that decompression greater than this allows an excessive degree of spinal cord displacement, such that traction is placed upon the relatively fixed cervical nerve roots. Exactly why the C5 root is predisposed to this effect is not known.

Lateral Approach

Theoretically, because this approach is similar to that of the medial access to the prevertebral space, but with less midline retraction, there should be less retractor morbidity. The sympathetic chain is manipulated substantially, along with the longus colli muscle, creating the distinct possibility of a complicating Horner's syndrome. The best way to avoid this is lengthy mobilization of the sympathetic chain and longus colli muscle prior to retraction medially. The risk of major vascular injury is greater with this approach, in light of the more substantial retraction of the carotid sheath and the opening of the foramen transversarium. Retraction of the vertebral artery away from the uncinate process should be no more than 1 or 2 mm during the uncinate process and lateral disc resection. The nerve root is usually injured lateral to the uncinate process, not at the level of the uncinate process itself. Restricting lateral dissection to a plane no deeper than the anterior tubercle may avoid such injury.

Suction drains, employed for 24 hours postoperatively, may significantly diminish wound hematomas. Pseudomeningoceles and spinal fluid fistulas are best managed prophylactically by postoperative lumbar drains whenever CSF leakage is anticipated or visualized in the operative field. If the dura mater is deliberately opened, suture closure is usually feasible, and a lumbar drain is not necessary. If the dura mater is atretic, as in ossification of the posterior longitudinal ligament, elaborate efforts at grafting are not necessary, provided a lumbar drain is used. Gelfoam and a thin layer of muscle held in place by the bone graft is all that is necessary. If a pseudomeningocele develops, expectant management will usually result in its resolution.

References

1. Bailey RW, Badgley CE: Stabilization of the cervical spine by anterior fusion. **J Bone Joint Surg (Am) 42:**565-575, 1960

2. Ball PA, Saunders RL: Subjective myelopathy, in Saunders RL, Bernini PM (eds): **Cervical Spondylotic Myelopathy.** Boston: Blackwell Scientific, 1992, pp 48-55

3. Batzdorf U, Batzdorff A: Analysis of cervical spine curvature in patients with cervical spondylosis. **Neurosurgery 22:**827-836, 1988

4. Cloward RB: New method of diagnosis and treatment of cervical disc disease. **Clin Neurosurg 8:** 93-103, 1962

5. Hodgson AR: An approach to the cervical spine (C-3 to C-7). **Clin Orthop 39:**129-134, 1965

6. Louis E, Ruge D: Lateral approach to the cervical spine, in Wiltse LL, Ruge D (eds): **Spinal Disorders.** London: Henry Kimpton, 1977, pp 132-136

7. Manabe S, Tateishi A, Ohno T: Anterolateral uncoforaminotomy for cervical spondylotic myeloradiculopathy. **Acta Orthop Scand 59:**669-674, 1988

8. Nurick S: The natural history and the results of surgical treatment of the spinal cord disorder associated with cervical spondylosis. **Brain 95:** 101-108, 1972

9. Perry J: Surgical approaches to the spine, in Pierce D, Nichol V (eds): **The Total Care of Spinal Cord Injuries.** Boston: Little, Brown & Co, 1977, pp 53-79

10. Riley LH Jr: Surgical approaches to the anterior structures of the cervical spine. **Clin Orthop 91:**16-20, 1973

11. Robinson RA: Approaches to the cervical spine C1-T1, in Schmidek HH, Sweet WH (eds): **Current Techniques in Operative Neurosurgery.** New York: Grove & Stratten, 1978, pp 205-302

12. Saunders RL: Anterior reconstructive procedures in cervical spondylotic myelopathy. **Clin Neurosurg 37:**682-721, 1991

13. Saunders RL: On the pathogenesis of the radiculopathy complicating multilevel corpectomy. **Neurosurgery 37:**408-413, 1995

14. Verbiest H: Anterolateral operations for fractures and dislocations in the middle and lower parts of the cervical spine. Report of a series of forty-seven cases. **J Bone Joint Surg (Am) 51:**1489-1530, 1969

Chapter 6

Lateral Exposures of the Cervical Spine and Vertebral Artery

John A. Anson, MD

Although the standard ventral approach to the cervical spine is frequently performed by most spine surgeons, many are less comfortable with lateral approaches. These surgical approaches provide improved exposure of the lateral elements of the cervical spine, including the vertebral artery, uncinate processes, and neural foramina, as well as lateral pathology, such as lateral herniated discs, foraminal tumors, and vertebral artery lesions.

The lateral approaches have been developed over a number of years and modified by many surgeons. There remains, however, a somewhat confusing nomenclature regarding the description of the various approaches, some of which differ only minimally from others. In the interest of simplifying the descriptions of these surgical approaches, it is easiest to consider three different lateral approaches to the middle and lower cervical spine, and three to the upper cervical spine. At both levels, there is a ventral approach, a ventrolateral approach, and a more truly lateral approach to the lateral cervical spine. This chapter describes these surgical approaches and illustrates their use.

Some of the surgical procedures described in this chapter have been outlined in previous chapters. Redundancy allows for a more complete coverage of the anatomical and surgical principles. It is in this vein that this chapter provides a comprehensive overview of the surgical approaches to the lateral aspect of the cervical spine.

Surgical Anatomy

The obliquely oriented sternocleidomastoid muscle divides the neck into its anterior and lateral triangles. The prominent difference between the three lateral approaches is the dissection relative to this muscle and the carotid sheath. With the ventral approach to the lateral spine, the dissection is ventral to both the sternocleidomastoid muscle and the carotid sheath. The ventrolateral approach is directed dorsal to the carotid sheath, but remains ventral to the muscle. More lateral approaches either pass dorsal to the sternocleidomastoid muscle or divide it (Figure 1).

The superficial anatomy of the ventrolateral neck is described in Chapter 1. An understanding of the lateral anatomy of the cervical vertebral column and the vertebral artery, however, is of crucial importance in safely approaching lesions in this area.

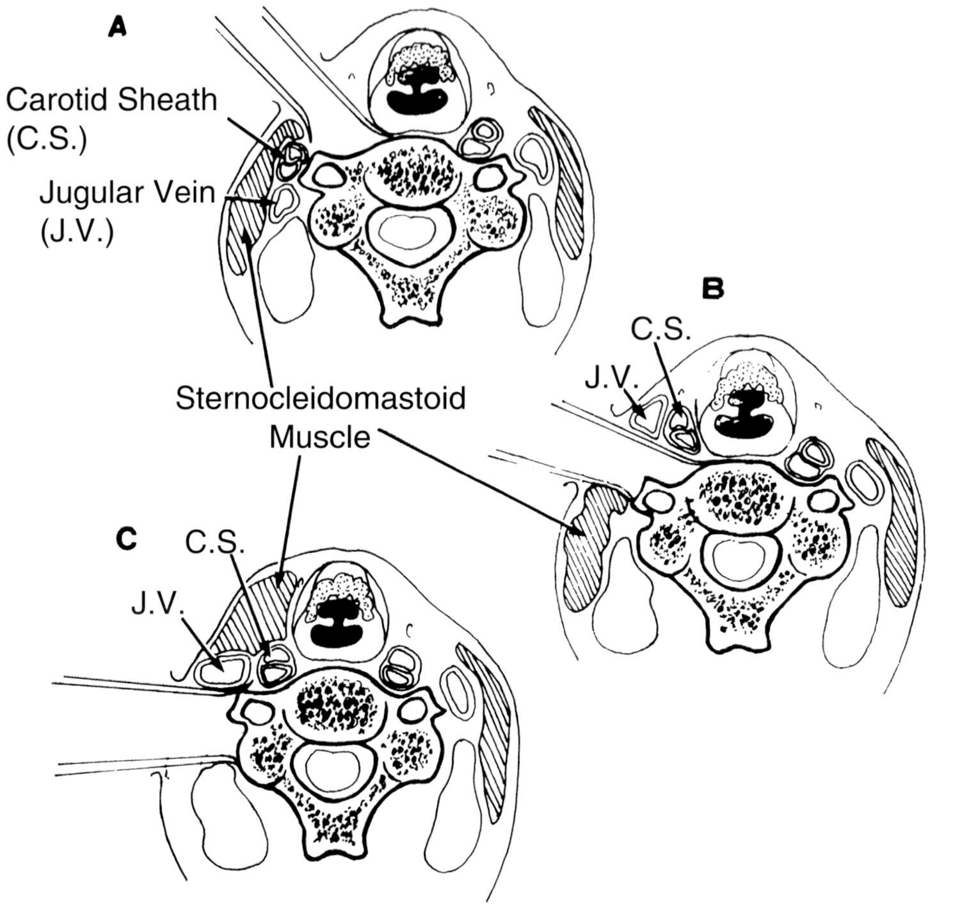

Figure 1. Cross-sectional anatomy of the midcervical spine demonstrating the three anatomical approach planes to the lateral cervical spine: **A)** ventral to the sternocleidomastoid muscle and great vessels; **B)** ventral to the sternocleidomastoid muscle, dorsal to the vessels; and **C)** dorsal to the sternocleidomastoid muscle and the vessels, with a direct orientation to the neuroforamen.

The transverse processes become increasingly prominent from C3 through C7. The transverse foramen lies just lateral to the vertebral body. Its dorsal margin is formed by the pedicle (Figure 2). The anterior and posterior tubercles of the transverse process are separated by the costotransverse bar. The anterior tubercle at C6 is known as Chassaignac's tubercle and can be identified by palpation as the most caudal anterior tubercle, lying in line with its more rostral counterparts. The C7 tubercle is situated more dorsally because of the normal cervical lordosis.

The longus colli and longus capitus muscles lie along the anterior tubercles of the transverse processes and must be sectioned prior to surgical dissection of the transverse process. The cervical sympathetic trunk extends along the deep side of the longus colli muscles in the ventral recess of the transverse processes. It is very important to protect the sympathetic chain in this region, since injury can result in a Horner's syndrome. Enlargements of the superior cervical ganglion are located ventral to the C2 and C3 vertebrae. Similarly, for the middle cervical ganglion, an enlargement is located ventral to C6 and for the inferior cervical ganglion, an enlargement is located ventral to C7. The inferior ganglion often is fused with the first thoracic ganglion and forms the stellate ganglion.

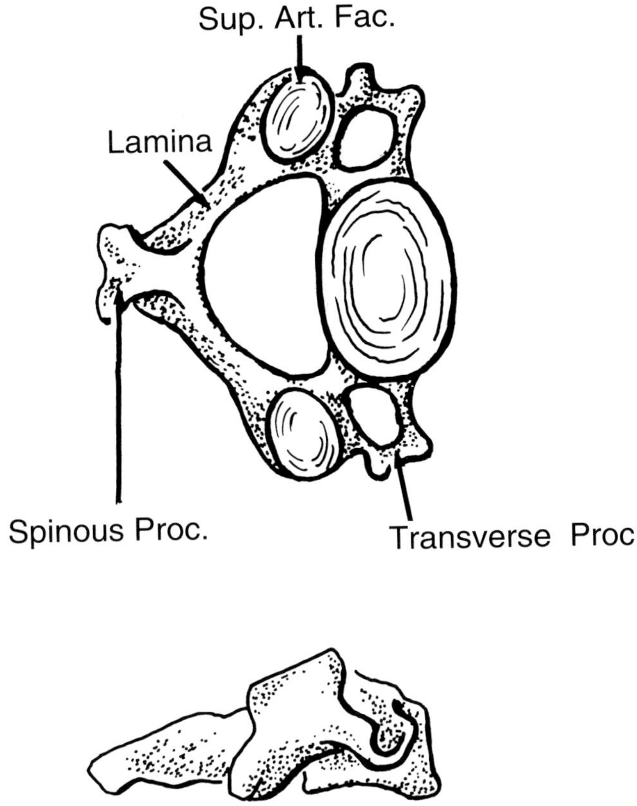

Figure 2. Bony anatomy of a midcervical vertebral body demonstrating the relationship of the transverse process and foramen to the body and canal.

A vertebral nerve originates from the cervical portion of the stellate ganglion and enters the C6 transverse foramen. From there, the nerve accompanies the vertebral artery into the cranial cavity.[10] It typically runs behind the vertebral artery and contains fibers that connect the sympathetic trunk to the cervical nerves. Stimulation of the vertebral nerve can cause pupillary changes, headache, and dizziness,[15] and injury can potentially cause a Horner's syndrome.

At each intervertebral foramen, the cervical nerve root passes immediately behind the vertebral artery between the adjacent transverse processes. These nerve roots continue laterally to form the anterior rami of the brachial plexus. Care must be taken to avoid injuring the nerve roots immediately behind the vertebral artery; they are most frequently damaged during blind attempts to control bleeding from surgical injury to the vertebral artery. It has also been observed that many of the fibers of the anterior scalene muscle originate from the nerve sheaths of the anterior rami.[13,21] Careful separation of the scalene muscles should be performed if exposure of the anterior rami is needed.

The vertebral arteries are, of course, the most important vascular structure in the lateral cervical spine. After originating as the first branches of the subclavian arteries, they course rostrally and dorsally between

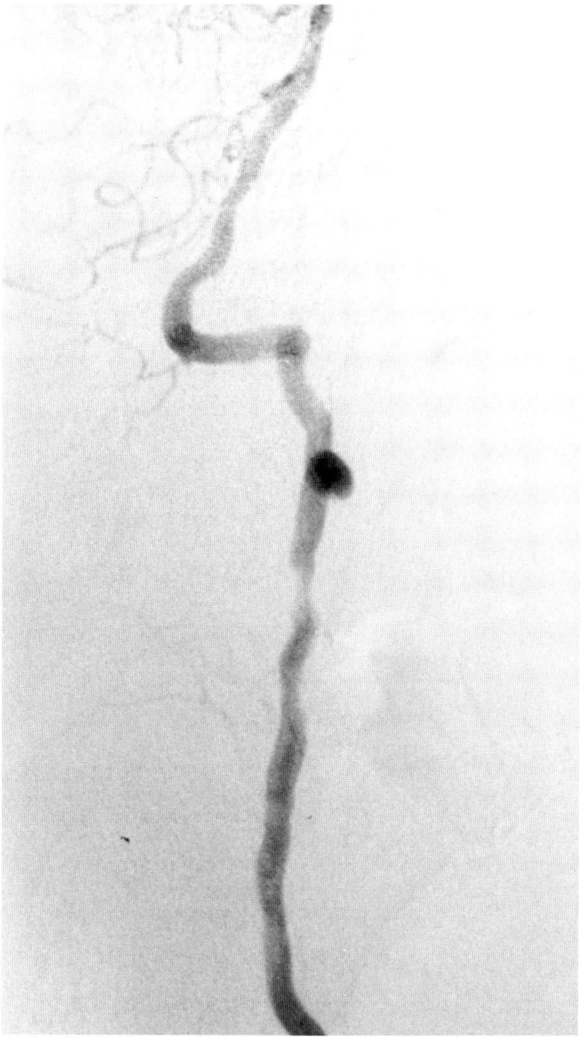

Figure 3A. Preoperative vertebral angiogram in a 58-year-old man who suffered vertebrobasilar transient ischemic attacks with head turning. A large uncinate process spur caused compression of the artery at the C4-5 level. The opposite vertebral artery was occluded.

the longus colli and anterior scalene muscles before ascending rostrally within the transverse foramen. The proximal vertebral artery enters the transverse foramen at C6 in 90% of cases, at C5 in 7%, and at C7 in 3%.[3]

The midportion of the vertebral artery within the transverse foramen is immediately adjacent to the facet joints from C6 to C3. These articulations are dorsomedial to the artery and subluxation or osteoarthritic changes can cause compression of the vessel.[2] The uncovertebral joints are just medial to the vertebral artery in the transverse foramen and are often affected in cervical spondylosis. The degenerative changes can produce bony prominences that displace the vertebral artery laterally, sometimes causing severe distortion.[16] These changes can cause dorsal circulation symptoms related to neck motion, since the vertebral artery can be compressed medially by the uncovertebral bony spurs while being held relatively fixed both rostrally and caudally in the transverse foramen[12,16] (Figure 3).

There are numerous small branches of the extracranial vertebral artery that are seldom

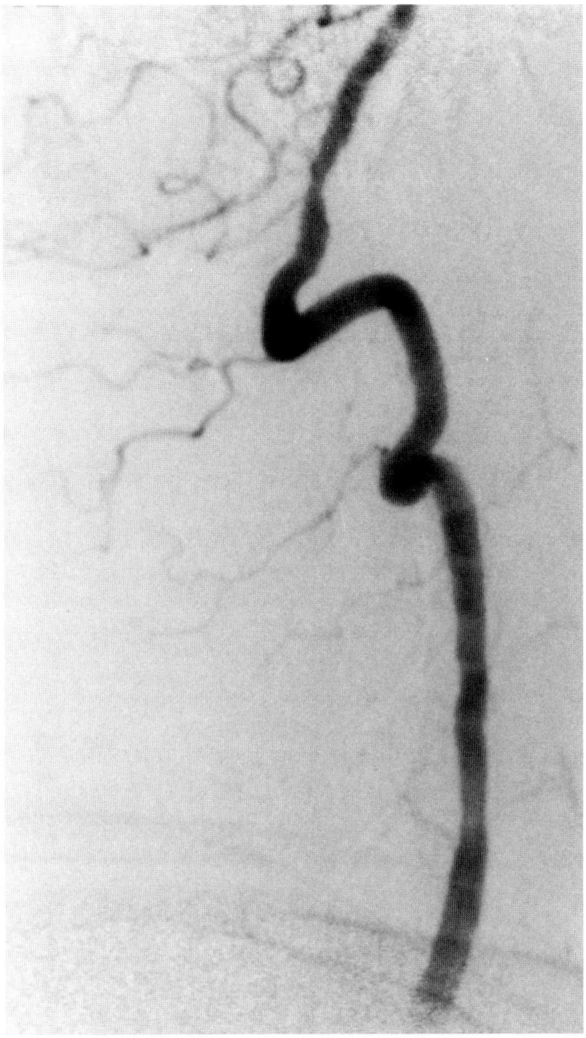

Figure 3B. Postoperative angiography after unroofing the C4 and C5 transverse foramina and drilling off the uncinate process spur.

of surgical significance. Spinal branches enter the vertebral canal through the intervertebral foramen to anastomose with other spinal cord arteries. Branches from the distal vertebral artery also anastomose with the occipital artery and the ascending and deep cervical arteries to supply the deep neck muscles as the artery curves dorsally. Lastly, one or two small meningeal branches exit the vertebral artery, just as it penetrates the dura mater below the foramen magnum. Any of these branches can be safely divided to allow mobilization of the artery.

The vertebral artery is also surrounded by a plexus of venous channels that forms the vertebral vein at the lower neck. This venous plexus can be troublesome during surgery, but can be controlled by stripping it back along the artery and packing with Surgicel. It is this immediate proximity of the vertebral artery to the surrounding venous plexus that predisposes it to the formation of vertebral arteriovenous fistulas. Historically, several of the early descriptions of lateral approaches to the cervical spine were for treating vertebral artery fistulas.[6,20,21]

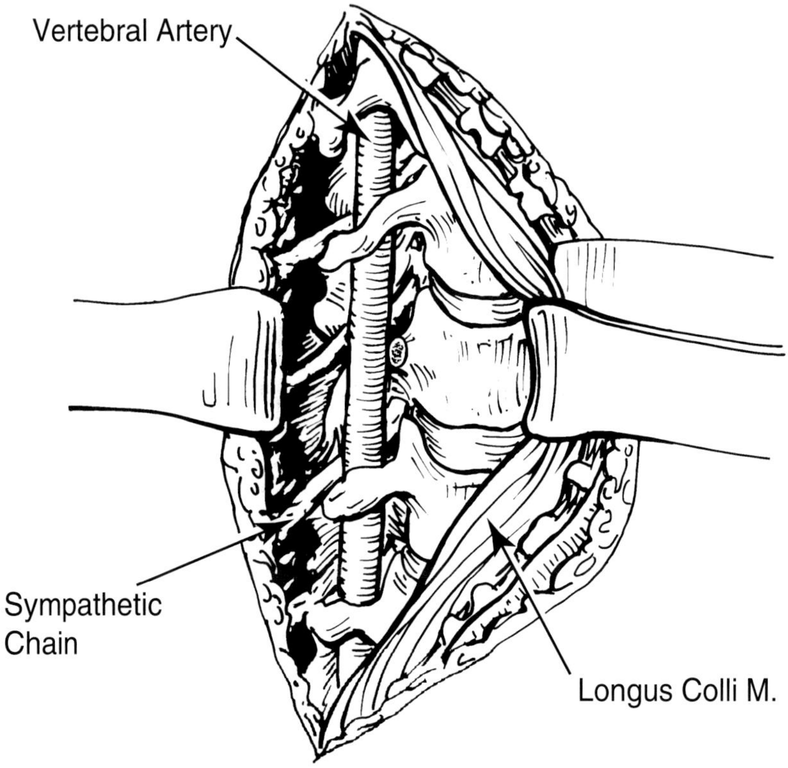

Figure 4. Diagram of the operative view of the lateral aspect of the cervical spine with the C3 transverse foramen opened.

Surgical Exposures of the Middle and Lower Cervical Spine

Ventral Approach to the Lateral Cervical Spine

The ventral approach to the lateral cervical spine uses the typical medial soft tissue dissection, but with a final lateral exposure of the cervical spine (Figure 1A). Verbiest[19-21] extensively described this approach for treatment of vertebral artery and lateral spinal pathology. He developed it as a modification of Henry's classic technique.[8] An angled skin incision is made along the ventral border of the sternocleidomastoid muscle. Caution should be taken during the turning of the patient's head away from the side of surgery if spondylotic compression of the vertebral artery is present, as this can exacerbate the compression or occlude the artery.

The sternocleidomastoid muscle and carotid sheath are retracted laterally, and the trachea and esophagus medially. Upon exposure of the prevertebral fascia, the anterior tubercles of the transverse processes can be palpated and the appropriate level confirmed radiographically.

The longus colli muscle is then dissected medially from the anterior tubercles in the subperiosteal plane along the transverse processes, taking care to avoid injuring the sympathetic chain running along the underside of the muscle. The sympathetic chain should be mobilized and left juxtaposed to the dorsal surface of the longus colli muscle. The dissection is continued until medial to the uncinate processes (Figure 4). Alternatively,

Verbiest[20] has suggested initial exposure of the anterior rami of the brachial plexus before dissecting the longus colli muscle. Visualization of the nerve roots helps protect them from inadvertent injury. Furthermore, they provide a landmark for the identification of the intervertebral foramina.

The transverse foramina are then unroofed by removing the anterior tubercle and the costotransverse bar (Figure 4). This can be accomplished with angled rongeurs or with a drill, using a diamond burr to thin the bone and curettes or a small Kerrison rongeur to remove the final dorsal remnants. Bleeding always occurs from the perivertebral venous plexus during this portion of the dissection. It is best managed by stripping back the plexus rostrally and caudally, and packing with Surgicel or Gelfoam. After the foramina are unroofed above and below the level of interest, the vertebral artery can be gently dissected free of its confines and retracted laterally a few millimeters, thus allowing visualization of the lateral aspect of the vertebral bodies and completely exposing the uncinate processes and uncovertebral joints. The ventral nerve roots are also visible immediately behind the vertebral artery and can be followed back into the intervertebral foramina. Uncovertebral osteophytes compressing the vertebral artery can now be removed using a high-speed drill with a small diamond burr. Likewise, a dorsolateral discectomy can be performed, if indicated, using the drill or small angled rongeurs.

Besides osteophytes, fibrous adhesions within or between the transverse processes also may constrict the vertebral artery and should be removed. Similarly, the periosteum along the transverse foramina should be removed because it can cause persistent constriction of the artery, even after bony decompression.[5] Gentle mobilization of the artery allows inspection of the dorsal aspect of the foramina. Additional osteophytes from degenerative disease of the apophyseal joints may be present in this area and should be removed. After completing the decompression and releasing all fibrous bands, the vertebral artery should be observed to expand to its full size and not be compressed or compromised by turning the head. In selected patients with focal areas of atherosclerotic stenosis, the vertebral artery can be endarterectomized through this exposure.[4,5]

This exposure also allows treatment of medial pathology at the same time. Many patients with spondylotic disease compressing the vertebral artery may have symptomatic foraminal narrowing or disc disease as well. This procedure is easily combined with a standard cervical discectomy or corpectomy without additional exposure.

Wound closure is straightforward, using absorbable sutures to reapproximate the platysma muscle, followed by skin closure. A drain can be left, if indicated. No cervical collar or other orthosis is necessary.

Ventrolateral Approach to the Lateral Cervical Spine

The ventrolateral, or oblique, approach is also performed through a skin incision along the ventral border of the sternocleidomastoid muscle, but then proceeds through the anatomical plane between the sternocleidomastoid muscle and the internal jugular vein (Figure 1B). The great vessels are retracted medially, along with the trachea and esophagus. Once the dissection reaches the prevertebral tissues, dissection of the lateral cervical spine is similar to the ventral approach.

The lateral aspect of the vertebral bodies can be removed to achieve exposure of the ventral aspect of the spinal canal with good control and protection of the vertebral artery. This is done by drilling from the ipsilateral ventrolateral corner and proceeding toward the opposite dorsolateral corner. George et al[7] have described this approach in 15 patients, with good results and no instability. Because only a wedge of bone is removed, there is no resultant destabilization and bone grafting is unnecessary.[7]

Lateral Approach to the Lateral Cervical Spine

A more lateral approach is seldom required, and the lesser familiarity of most surgeons with the lateral anatomy and orientation makes it more difficult and potentially dangerous. The true lateral approach divides, or dissects dorsally to, the sternocleidomastoid muscle. Hodgson[10] described a variation of the lateral approach that takes advantage of the loose tissue planes in the prevertebral space, where the visceral compartment of the neck, including the esophagus, thyroid gland, and trachea, is very loosely attached to the prevertebral fascia. This facilitates rostrocaudal movement during swallowing, which, in turn, creates a natural cleavage plane that allows access from a lateral route to the ventral aspect of the spine.

One approach uses a transverse incision over the posterior triangle of the neck.[10] After dividing the subcutaneous tissue and platysma muscle, dissection is continued dorsally to the sternocleidomastoid muscle through the fat pad of the posterior triangle. If necessary, the dorsal one-third of the muscle can be divided. It is usually necessary to divide the external jugular vein near the dorsal terminus of the incision. The dissection is continued dorsal to the carotid sheath and leads directly into the loose cleavage plane ventral to the prevertebral fascia, which is opened in the usual manner. Muscular branches of the vertebral artery may be encountered during dissection through the posterior triangle and can be divided without risk. The sympathetic trunk is also present as dissection deepens. It should be carefully preserved in order to avoid a Horner's syndrome.

Elkin and Harris,[6] in their landmark description of surgical treatment of vertebral artery fistulas, used a vertical incision directly over the space between the sternal and clavicular heads of the sternocleidomastoid muscle to gain access to the first portion of the vertebral artery. It could also be used to gain access to the lateral aspect of C6 and C7. The heads of the muscle are separated and retracted and the dissection continued through the triangular space between the longus colli and anterior scalene muscles. The inferior thyroid artery crosses ventral to the first portion of the vertebral artery on the right side, whereas the thoracic duct crosses ventral to it on the left.

Surgical Exposures of the Upper Cervical Spine

Lateral Approach

The approaches to the lateral aspect of the upper cervical spine and vertebral artery described above provide adequate exposure from C3 to C7. To gain lateral exposure of C1 and C2, however, a modification of these approaches or a separate approach is necessary. The ventrolateral approaches to the upper cervical spine are essentially extensions of the ventrolateral midcervical approaches. These approaches are usually indicated for pathology that includes C1 and C2, along with lower cervical levels. When only ventral pathology at C1 and C2 is present, a transoral approach is often adequate. Conversely, exposure of the vertebral arteries at this level can be achieved with a dorsal or far lateral (transcondylar) approach.

The lateral approach to the upper cervical spine was first described by Henry,[8] and elaborated by Whitesides and Kelly.[22] In this procedure, the usual skin incision along the ventral border of the sternocleidomastoid muscle is made, but then extended dorsally across the base of the temporal bone and mastoid process. After dividing the platysma muscle and deep fascia, the sternocleidomastoid muscle is divided at its mastoid origin (Figure 5). The splenius capitis muscle is partially divided in the same area as well. The sternocleidomastoid muscle should be reapproximated after the operation. This can be done with a U-shaped stitch through the muscle to keep from pulling through the longitudinal fibers. The muscles are then mobilized and retracted caudally and dorsally until the spinal accessory nerve is identified entering the deep side of the muscle, approximately 4 cm below the mastoid tip. Arterial branches to the muscles can be divided and the carotid sheath retracted ventrally.

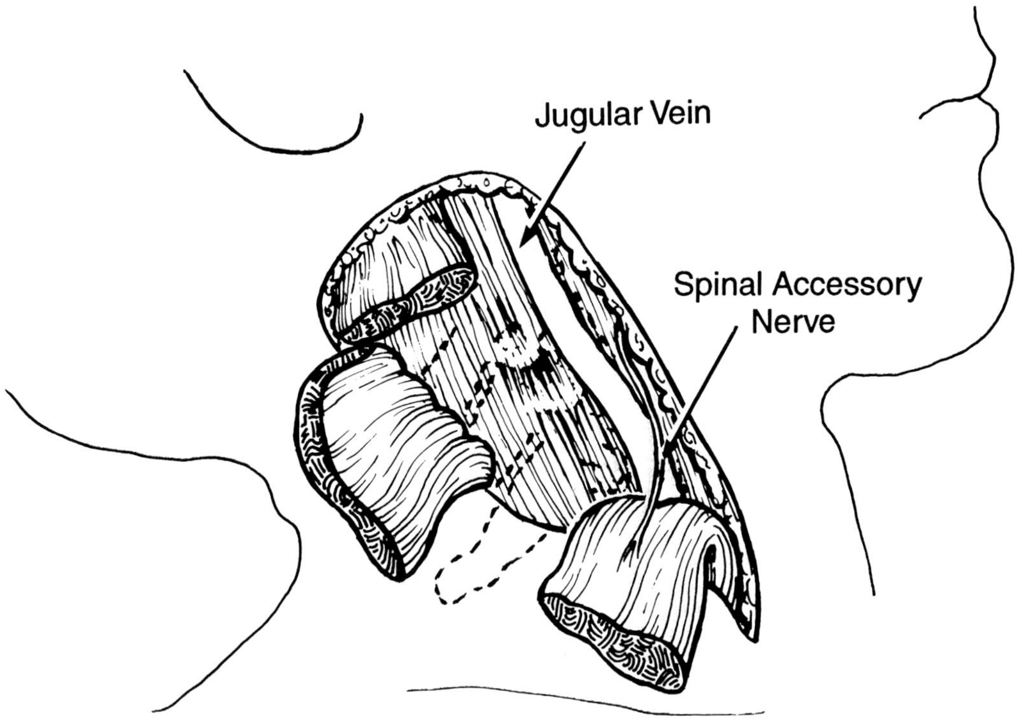

Figure 5. Diagram of the operative view of the lateral approach to the upper cervical spine. The incision along the sternocleidomastoid muscle curves dorsally, at its rostral end, to the mastoid process. The sternocleidomastoid muscle is divided below its mastoid attachment, taking care to preserve the spinal accessory nerve along its deep surface. The splenius capitis muscle is divided. The lateral tubercles of C1 and C2 are palpable through the overlying fascia.

The tip of the transverse process of C1 can usually be palpated at this point, approximately 1 cm caudal and 1 cm ventral to the mastoid tip. The shorter tip of the C2 transverse process is less easily felt. The deep fascial layer over the transverse processes is opened in a vertical fashion. The attachments of the levator scapulae and splenius cervicis muscles to the C1 transverse process are identified and carefully divided. The vertebral artery runs immediately behind these muscles and is exposed after the muscles are separated. Additional muscle attachments to the C2 transverse process are also divided and small curettes used to reflect the muscles off the lateral aspects of C1 and C2, including the lamina to nearly the midline. Again, care should be taken to stay in the subperiosteal plane in order to protect the vertebral artery. By extending the incision and dissection caudally, the lateral aspect of the entire cervical spine can be exposed caudally to T1.[22]

The lateral aspects of the vertebra and lamina are then removed using a high-speed drill with a diamond burr and fine rongeurs. The foramen transversarium of C2 can be opened, if necessary, to further mobilize the vertebral artery. In this fashion, the lateral aspect of the dura mater can be exposed from the foramen magnum to C3. The dura mater can be opened with a lateral longitudinal incision for intradural lesions. Tumors located lateral to the spinal cord or ventral to the spinal cord with dorsal displacement of the spinal cord are readily accessible for removal.[18]

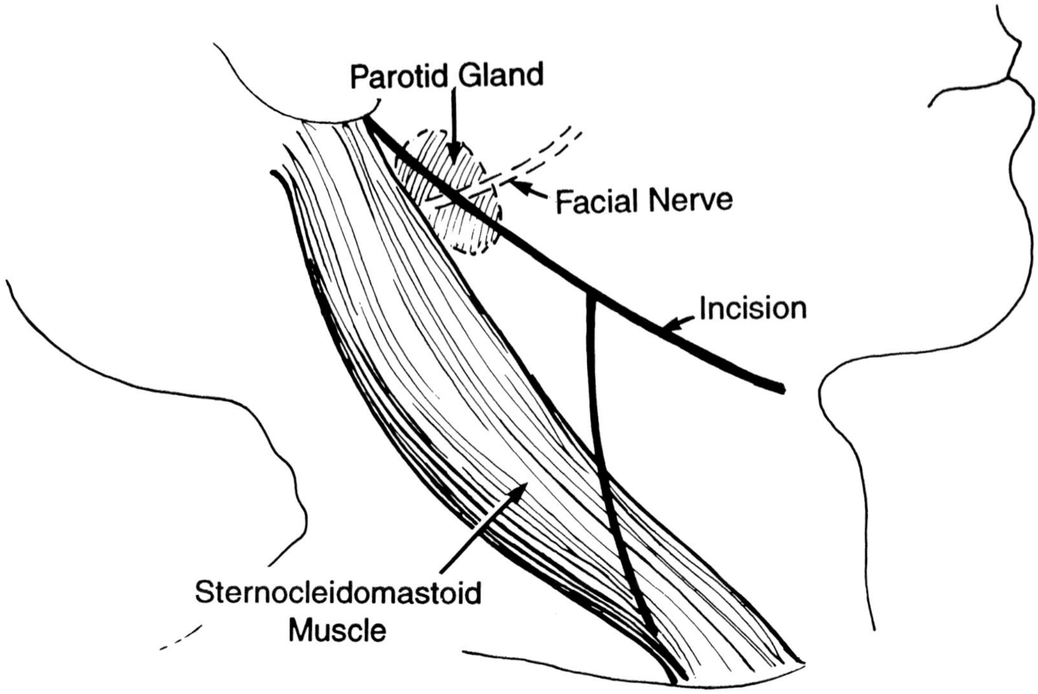

Figure 6. Diagram of the skin incision for the lateral extrapharyngeal approach of Menezes[14] to the upper cervical spine.

One very helpful modification of this approach is to position the patient in the true lateral position with the head turned 10° toward the floor.[18] This provides a direct line of vision to the lateral aspect of the thecal sac after exposure, an important factor for optimizing the use of the operating microscope in intradural procedures.

Fusion should not be necessary if the joints are preserved. When indicated because of underlying pathology, onlay bone grafts have been used along the denuded ventral surface of C1 and C2, with good results.[22] The most common complications associated with this approach are injury to the vertebral artery and the spinal accessory nerve. The vertebral artery can usually be identified early in relation to prominent landmarks, and should be carefully protected. The spinal accessory nerve is easily visualized early in the dissection. It is unlikely, therefore, to be cut; however, it can easily suffer stretch injury by excessive retraction of the sternocleidomastoid muscle.

Lateral Extrapharyngeal Approach

The lateral extrapharyngeal approach of Menezes[14] provides a more ventrolateral exposure of the craniocervical junction than the classic lateral approach and allows exposure of the lower clivus as well, without violating the oral cavity. The patient is positioned supine, with the head in traction and turned slightly away from the surgeon. Nasotracheal intubation is used so that the teeth can remain occluded in order to maximize retraction of the mandible. An angled transverse incision is made below the angle of the mandible from the mastoid process to the midline. A T-shaped incision is extended caudally along the border of the sternocleidomastoid muscle (Figure 6). After dividing the platysma muscle, dissection is continued in the subplatysmal plane until the caudal division of the facial nerve is freed, allowing elevation of the parotid gland and facial nerve.

Deeper dissection is continued along the ventral aspect of the sternocleidomastoid muscle and then ventral to the carotid sheath. Veins crossing the operative field into the internal jugular vein are divided. The dorsal belly of the digastric muscle is divided at its tendinous attachment to the hyoid bone. It is reapproximated during closure, using non-absorbable suture. The stylohyoid muscle is also divided, allowing greater medial retraction of the laryngopharynx. The carotid artery is dissected along its ventral border, and the hypoglossal nerve freed where it courses over the carotid bifurcation. The hypoglossal nerve can be mobilized rostrally and dorsally, taking care to preserve the descendens hypoglossi. In order to further retract the carotid artery laterally, all of the anterior branches of the external carotid artery are ligated and divided.

The prevertebral fascia is widely exposed and opened vertically. The longus colli and longus capitis muscles are divided at their medial origin and reflected laterally. The ventral aspects of C1 and C2 are exposed and can be removed with a drill and fine curettes. Exposure can potentially be extended caudally as far as necessary down the entire length of the cervical spine. If needed, a bone graft can be placed between the lower clivus and C2.

The extensive dissection required for this approach is not without risk. There is a greater risk of pharyngeal dysfunction than with a transoral operation. Injury to the hypoglossal nerve is possible, as well as to the glossopharyngeal nerve medially. Significant mobilization and displacement of the carotid artery predisposes to embolic stroke in the presence of atherosclerotic disease. Preoperative imaging of the carotid artery is helpful to identify patients at increased risk.

Dorsolateral Approach

The various lateral approaches described above provide access to nearly the entire course of the vertebral artery, as well as the lateral aspect of the vertebral column. Because of its dorsal swing around C1, however, the most distal aspect of the rostral extracranial vertebral artery is best exposed from a dorsolateral orientation. The far lateral approach is best suited for this exposure and for lesions of the intracranial vertebral artery as well as certain other lesions of the upper cervical spine and foramen magnum.[1,9,17]

The far lateral approach is performed with the patient in a modified park-bench position. The head is rotated downward, flexed, and tilted away from the ipsilateral shoulder. The inverted J-shaped incision curves medially from the mastoid tip and extends caudally in the midline to the C6 level (Figure 7A). After dividing the nuchal fascia, the paraspinal muscles are elevated laterally from the spinous processes and lamina. The muscle flap is dissected suboccipitally to the mastoid and the entire flap retracted laterally. The dorsal arch of C1 is removed with a high-speed drill, making the ipsilateral cut at the extreme lateral aspect of the C1 ring. The rostral cervical vertebral artery can be dissected free, if necessary, in its course around the lateral aspect and over the top of C1. The extensive venous plexus surrounding the artery bleeds profusely; however, the bleeding can be controlled by packing with Surgicel.

For exposure of the intradural vertebral artery, a suboccipital craniotomy is performed that extends as far to the ipsilateral side as possible. Additional bone is then removed, including the rim of the foramen magnum to the occipital condyle. The dorsal one-third of the occipital condyle and the rostral lateral mass and facet of C1 are removed using the drill (Figure 7B). The safest technique involves drilling out the center of the condyle, leaving a thin shell of cortical bone to protect surrounding structures, particularly the vertebral artery. This remaining shell of bone is then carefully removed with small curettes and rongeurs while protecting the vertebral artery with a small dissector. The hypoglossal canal is located in the ventromedial one-third of the

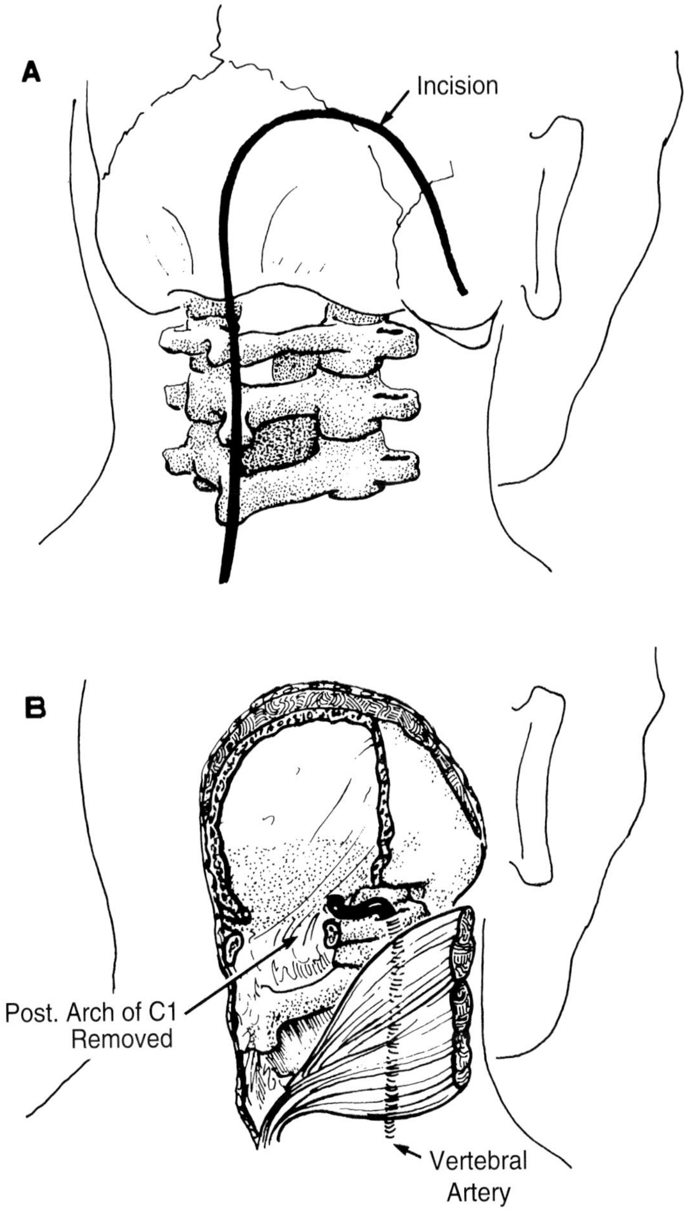

Figure 7. A) Skin incision for the far lateral approach curves rostrally from the mastoid tip and caudally to the midline, at approximately the C6 level. **B)** Bone removal for exposure of the distal vertebral artery includes the ipsilateral portion of the dorsal arch of C1, and a lateral suboccipital craniotomy with additional lateral bone removal through the dorsolateral one-third of the occipital condyle.

occipital condyle and is not threatened by removal of the dorsal portion.

The dura mater opening is made along the midline and curved to the ipsilateral side at the caudal end. Rostrally, the dural incision is curved to the rostral and lateral aspect of the craniotomy. The dura mater is reflected laterally, thus exposing the caudal intradural vertebral artery. Minimal retraction of the cerebellum improves exposure of the distal vertebral artery. This approach is excellent for vertebral artery aneurysms and tumors of the foramen magnum and lower clivus, and has been used for intradural vertebral artery endarterectomy.[1,9,17]

Conclusion

Although the need to approach the lateral aspect of the cervical spine arises infrequently, pathology in this region, such as lateral disc or osteophytic disease, vertebral artery lesions, or neural foramen dumbbell tumors, are best exposed by an appropriate lateral approach. Because most spine surgeons are very comfortable with a standard ventral approach, performing one of the ventrolateral approaches to the lateral spine is usually the most familiar initially, and can be followed by progressively dorsal and lateral dissections, as experience increases. Knowledge of the anatomy of the transverse process and vertebral artery aids the surgeon regarding safe dissection around these structures. In this fashion, an approach that provides the most direct surgical route and widest exposure of the lateral cervical spine can be used for nearly any laterally situated pathological process.

References

1. Anson JA, Spetzler RF: Endarterectomy of the intradural vertebral artery via the far lateral approach. **Neurosurgery 33:**804-811, 1993

2. Brain L: Some unsolved problems of cervical spondylosis. **Br Med J 1:**771-777, 1963

3. Brink B: Approach to the second segment of the vertebral arteries, in Berguer R, Bauer RB (eds): **Vertebrobasilar Arterial Occlusive Disease. Medical and Surgical Management.** New York: Raven Press, 1984, pp 257-264

4. de los Reyes RA, Ausman JI, Diaz FG, et al: The surgical management of vertebrobasilar insufficiency. **Acta Neurochir 68:**203-216, 1983

5. Diaz FG, Ausman JI, Shrontz C, et al: Surgical correction of lesions affecting the second portion of the vertebral artery. **Neurosurgery 19:**93-100, 1986

6. Elkin DC, Harris MH: Arteriovenous aneurysm of the vertebral vessels. Report of ten cases. **Ann Surg 124:**934-951, 1946

7. George B, Zerah M, Lot G, et al: Oblique transcorporeal approach to anteriorly located lesions in the cervical spinal canal. Technical note. **Acta Neurochir 121:**187-190, 1993

8. Henry AK: **Extensile Exposure, ed 3.** Baltimore: Williams & Wilkins, 1966, pp 53-89

9. Heros RC: Lateral suboccipital approach for vertebral and vertebrobasilar artery lesions. **J Neurosurg 64:** 559-562, 1986

10. Hodgson AR: An approach to the cervical spine (C-3 to C-7). **Clin Orthop 39:**129-134, 1965

11. Hoffman HH, Kuntz A: Vertebral nerve and plexus. Components, anatomical relationships, and surgical implications. **Arch Surg 74:**430-437, 1957

12. Hutchinson EC, Yates PO: The cervical portion of the vertebral artery. A clinico-pathological study. **Brain 79:**319-331, 1956

13. Kirgis HD, Reed AF: Anatomical relations of possible significance in the production of the scalenus anticus syndrome. **Anat Rec 97:**348, 1947 (Abstract)

14. Menezes AH: Surgical approaches to the craniocervical junction, in Frymoyer JW (ed): **The Adult Spine: Principles and Practice.** New York: Raven Press, 1991, pp 967-985

15. Nagashima C, Iwama K: Electrical stimulation of the stellate ganglion and the vertebral nerve. **J Neurosurg 36:**756-762, 1972

16. Pallis C, Jones AM, Spillane JD: Cervical spondylosis. Incidence and implications. **Brain 77:** 274-289, 1954

17. Sen CN, Sekhar LN: An extreme lateral approach to intradural lesions of the cervical spine and foramen magnum. **Neurosurgery 27:** 197-204, 1990

18. Shucart WA, Kléríga E: Lateral approach to the upper cervical spine. **Neurosurgery 6:**278-281, 1980

19. Verbiest H: Anterolateral operations for fractures and dislocations in the middle and lower parts of the cervical spine. Report of a series of forty-seven cases. **J Bone Joint Surg (Am) 51:** 1489-1530, 1969

20. Verbiest H: The lateral approach to the cervical spine. **Clin Neurosurg 20:**295-305, 1973

21. Verbiest H: A lateral approach to the cervical spine: technique and indications. **J Neurosurg 28:** 191-203, 1968

22. Whitesides TE Jr, Kelly RP: Lateral approach to the upper cervical spine for anterior fusion. **South Med J 59:**879-883, 1966

Chapter 7

Ventral Exposures of the Thoracic Spine

Stephen M. Papadopoulos, MD

Ventral surgical approaches to the thoracic spine provide excellent visualization and access to the ventral spinal elements, with minimal manipulation of the neural structures, and the opportunity for direct reconstruction of the ventral spinal column in instances of trauma, tumor, and infection, or for the treatment of scoliosis. Hodgson and Stock[10] reported the first extensive description of the ventral exposure of the thoracic spine via thoracotomy for the debridement of tuberculous abscesses. The reported mortality and morbidity rate was 2.9%, providing the impetus for other surgeons to use this approach for a variety of pathological conditions (Table 1).

Approaches to the ventral thoracic spine may be grouped into four general categories (Table 2).

1. The lower cervical and upper three thoracic vertebrae (C7-T3) may be exposed via a direct ventral cervical approach, extended caudally, with an accompanying median sternotomy or upper sternal resection. This approach is particularly useful in the setting of ventrally situated pathology without significant paraspinal or lateral involvement. For the management of thoracic disc disease, the most caudal disc space that may be routinely approached is T2-3 because of the sweeping kyphosis of the upper thoracic spine and the inclination of the disc space. For the management of vertebral body disease (i.e., tumor or infection), adequate exposure for a T3 corpectomy with subsequent reconstruction may be accomplished via this approach.
2. The T2 through T5 segments can be approached via a right dorsolateral thoracotomy. The left side of the upper thoracic spine is relatively less accessible because of the location of the aortic arch and great vessels. The right side, however, may provide some additional hemostatic difficulties due to the fragility of venous structures.
3. Exposure of the T6 vertebra through the T10 segment may be approached from either a left or a right thoracotomy. Many authors believe that the left side is preferred because mobilization of the aorta is technically easier and safer than mobilization of the vena cava or azygos venous system. However, one should be guided by the optimal approach for neural decompression, if that is the primary goal

Table 1. **Historical Aspects of Ventral Spinal Surgery**

Authors	Year	Approach
Hodgson & Stock[5]	1956	Transthoracic approach
Cauchoix & Binet[1]	1957	Median sternotomy for C7 to T4
Nanson[9]	1957	Neck approach for T1 to T3
Hodgson et al[6]	1960	Transthoracic approach
Dwyer et al[2]	1969	Transthoracic approach (scoliosis)
Perot & Munro[10]	1969	Transthoracic approach (disc)
Harrington[3]	1981	Transthoracic approach (cancer)
Sundaresan et al[11]	1984	Clavicular resection for T1 to T3
Lesoin et al[7]	1986	Transsternal approach for T1 to T4
Heitmiller[4]	1988	Thoracolumbar approach
Leventhal[8]	1992	Thoracolumbar approach

of the operative procedure. When dealing with scoliosis or other deformities, the choice of laterality favors the side of the apex or convexity of the curve. In cases where severe aortic atherosclerosis or an aortic aneurysm are coexistent with the spinal pathology, the left side should be avoided.

4. Exposure of the thoracolumbar junction (T10-L2) can be achieved through a left thoracotomy combined with a dorsal detachment of the diaphragm and entrance into the retroperitoneal abdominal space. The left side is preferred because of the favorable vascular anatomy and to avoid liver retraction.

Cervicothoracic Junction (C7-T3)

Ventral lesions from C7 through T3 may be approached by a standard ventral cervical exposure, paralleling the medial border of the sternocleidomastoid muscle. This approach is combined with an upper sternal osteotomy to approximately T2 or a median sternotomy to T4, allowing the optimum exposure of this level without significant risk of injuring surrounding structures. The left side is preferred because of the lower "recurrence" of the left recurrent laryngeal nerve (aorta on the left vs. innominate on the right, Figure 1). This approach provides for a direct ventral approach to the spine, but may be limited if there is significant lateral or paravertebral involvement.

Table 2. **Ventral Approaches to the Thoracic Spine**

Levels	Approach
C7-T3	Ventral cervical/median sternotomy
T2-5	Right thoracotomy
T6-T10	Left (or right) thoracotomy
T10-L2	Left (or right) thoraco-abdominal/retroperitoneal

Surgical Anatomy

The thoracic inlet is oval-shaped, with a ventrodorsal diameter of approximately 5 cm and a transverse diameter of approximately 10 cm in adults. The sternocleidomastoid muscle attaches to the sternum and clavicle by two heads. The oblique sternohyoid muscle arises from the dorsal surface of the medial portion of the clavicle and sternoclavicular junction. Key vascular structures in the superior mediastinum include the innominate vein and artery, common carotid and left subclavian arteries, internal jugular vein, and the arch of the aorta. The innominate artery and vein and the aortic arch limit the caudal extent of exposure. The recurrent laryngeal nerve arises from the vagus nerve

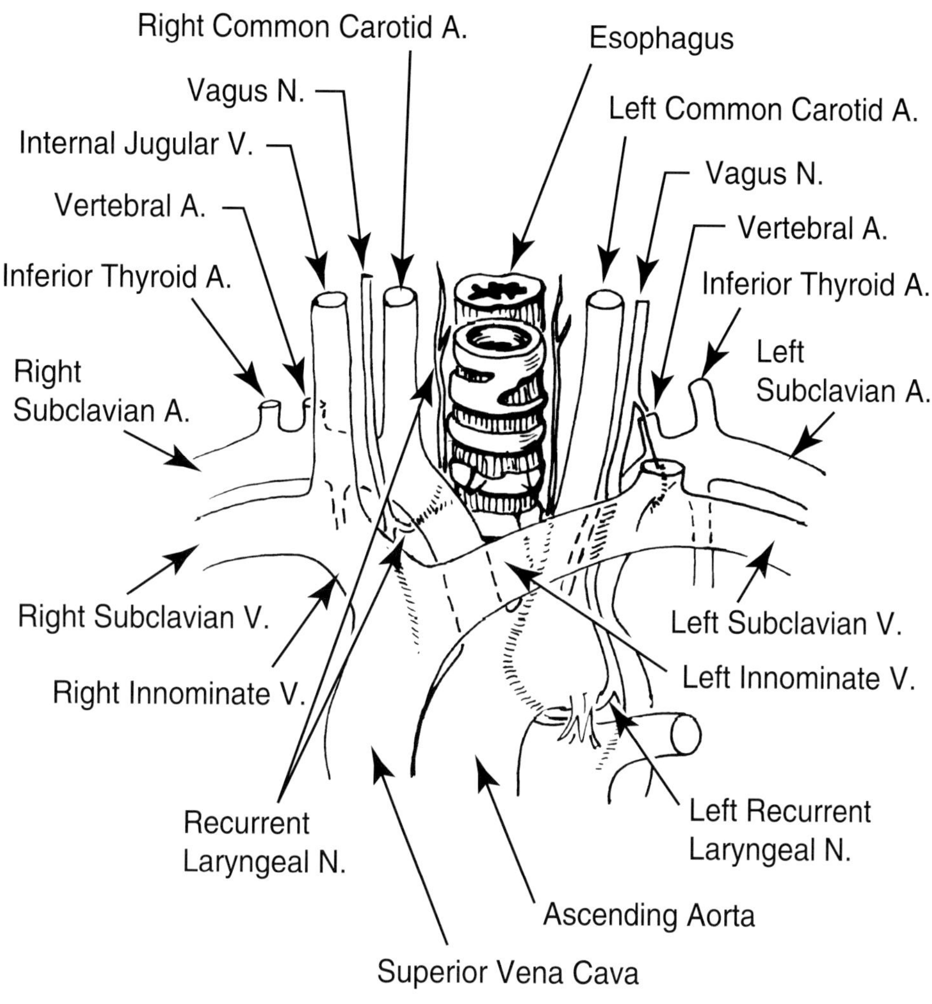

Figure 1. Vascular relationships of the upper mediastinum.

and courses under the innominate artery on the right and under the aortic arch on the left. The recurrent laryngeal nerve typically courses obliquely and ascends in the tracheo-esophageal groove. A 1% incidence of nonrecurrence of the right laryngeal nerve should be carefully considered. For these reasons, a left-sided approach is preferred for this exposure. The only significant disadvantage of the left-sided exposure is the position of the thoracic duct.

The blood supply of the spinal cord in the cervicothoracic region is derived from radicular arteries that take origin from the vertebral, thyrocervical, and costocervical branches of the subclavian artery. A ventral midline approach should not encounter these vessels.

Operative Technique

The patient is positioned in the supine position, with the neck slightly extended and the chin up. The skin incision is made parallel to the ventral border of the sternocleidomastoid muscle, and carried caudally along the midline over the sternum to approximately

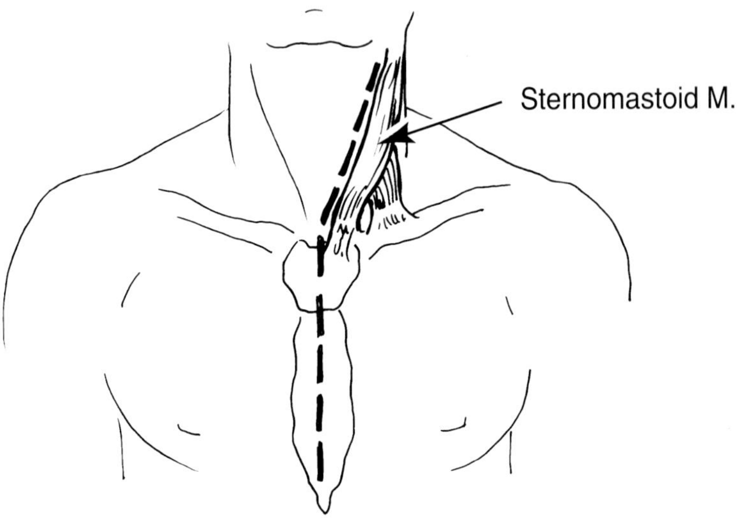

Figure 2. Skin incision used for the ventral exposure of the cervicothoracic junction via the transsternal route.

the level of the angle of Lewis (Figure 2). The platysma muscle is divided along its fibers in the direction of the incision. A plane is developed along the ventral border of the sternocleidomastoid muscle, retracting the carotid sheath laterally and the trachea and esophagus medially (Figure 3). The sternohyoid muscle is identified and then detached from the medial clavicle and sternum. A plane is then developed by finger dissection underneath the sternum into the upper mediastinum. Thymus tissue may be encountered, but can be swept away. The superior thyroid artery should be identified and ligated. A median sternotomy to the angle of Lewis is then performed using an oscillating saw. The mediastinum is opened with a crank retractor, and the pleura is carefully dissected on both sides and retracted. It is essential to stay within the confines of the mediastinal space. The left innominate vein may be divided with ligatures in order to obtain adequate caudal exposure. A plane is developed beneath the esophagus and above the prevertebral fascia. Self-retaining mediolateral retractors are placed under the elevated longus colli muscles. However, in the upper thoracic spine, the longus colli muscles are atretic and the attainment of good footing for the retractor blades may be difficult. A table-mounted retractor may be helpful in achieving and maintaining proper exposure. One should take great care not to place undue stretch on the recurrent laryngeal nerve at this level. The prevertebral fascia is then cleared of all surrounding connective tissue (Figure 4). The proper level can generally be identified by counting rib heads that are palpable lateral to the ventral spine; however, definitive confirmation with an intraoperative radiograph is suggested. The appropriate resection and/or reconstruction is then performed.

Upper Thoracic Spine (T2-5)

Lesions of the upper thoracic spine are best approached via a right dorsolateral thoracotomy through the interspace above the rib localized to the appropriate level of the spinal pathology. For example, exposure of the T3-4 disc space would be approached through a

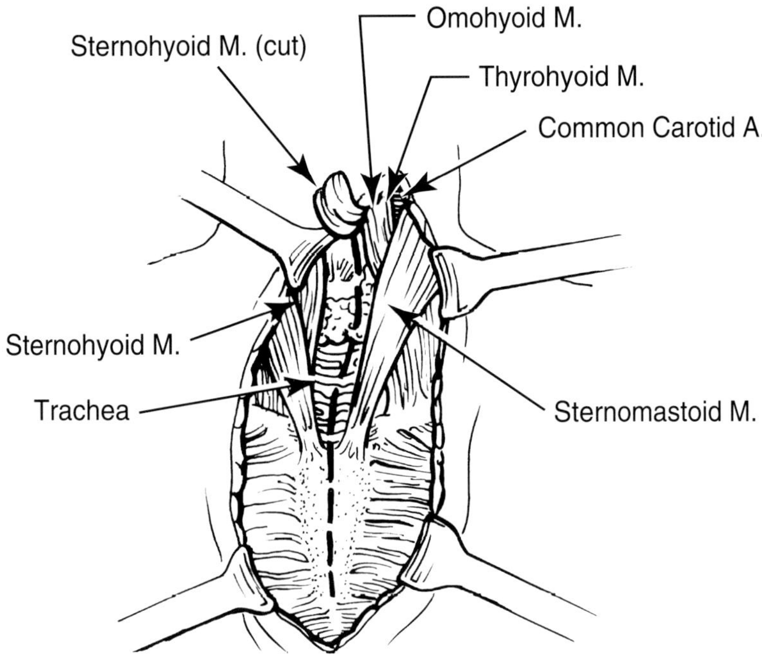

Figure 3. A view of the anatomy exposed during descent into the upper mediastinum for exposure of the upper thoracic spine.

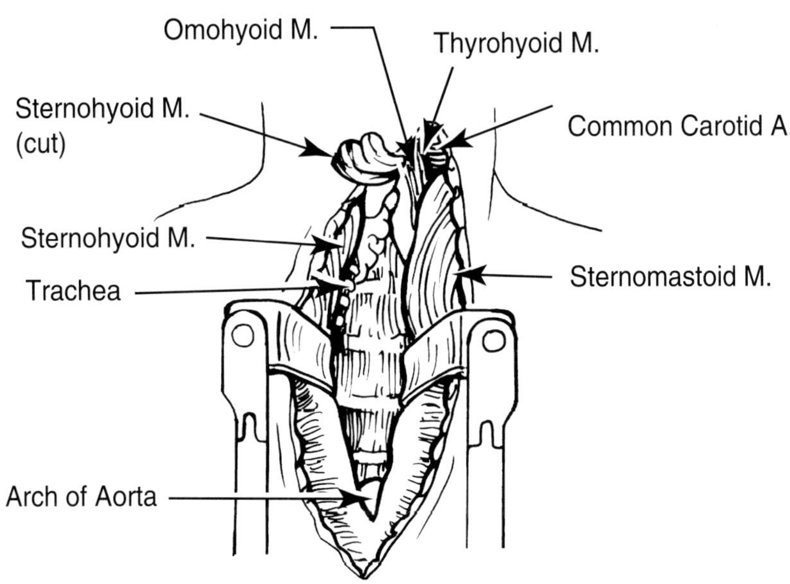

Figure 4. The upper thoracic spine, as viewed from a transsternal operative exposure.

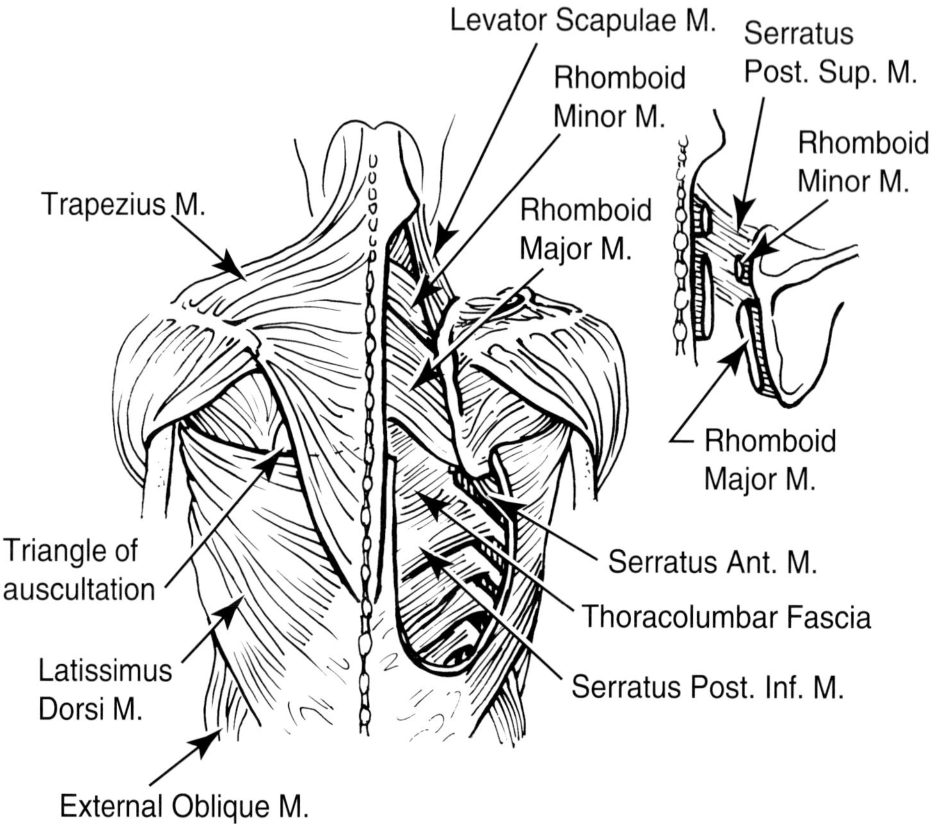

Figure 5. The dorsal paravertebral muscles of the thoracic and upper lumbar spine.

right T3-4 intercostal space exposure. In general, the intercostal space entered should represent the rostral margin of the spinal pathology. Left-sided exposure of this upper portion of the thoracic spine is limited by the position of the aortic arch and great vessels.

Surgical Anatomy

The right upper dorsolateral thoracotomy requires the identification and division of several important structures. The trapezius muscle extends from the spinous processes and attaches to the spine of the scapula throughout the length of the cervical and thoracic spine. Its fibers run obliquely and laterally to the scapular spine. Deep to the trapezius muscle is the rhomboid muscle group, which arises from the spinous processes of C6 to T5. Midline attachment of the latissimus dorsi muscle is also deep to the trapezius muscle from approximately T6 through T12. The serratus posterior inferior muscle arises as muscular bundles from the lower four ribs, whereas the serratus posterior superior muscle arises from the upper three ribs medially (Figure 5).

In addition to the muscular anatomy, a series of ligaments join the ribs, transverse processes, and vertebral bodies. The costotransverse ligaments run from the transverse process of a vertebra to the rib attached to the same vertebra. They are divided into superior, posterior, and inferior costotransverse ligaments. In addition, the capsular ligaments secure the neck of the rib to the front of the transverse process (Figure 6).

Understanding the complex three-dimensional anatomy of the head of the rib, the

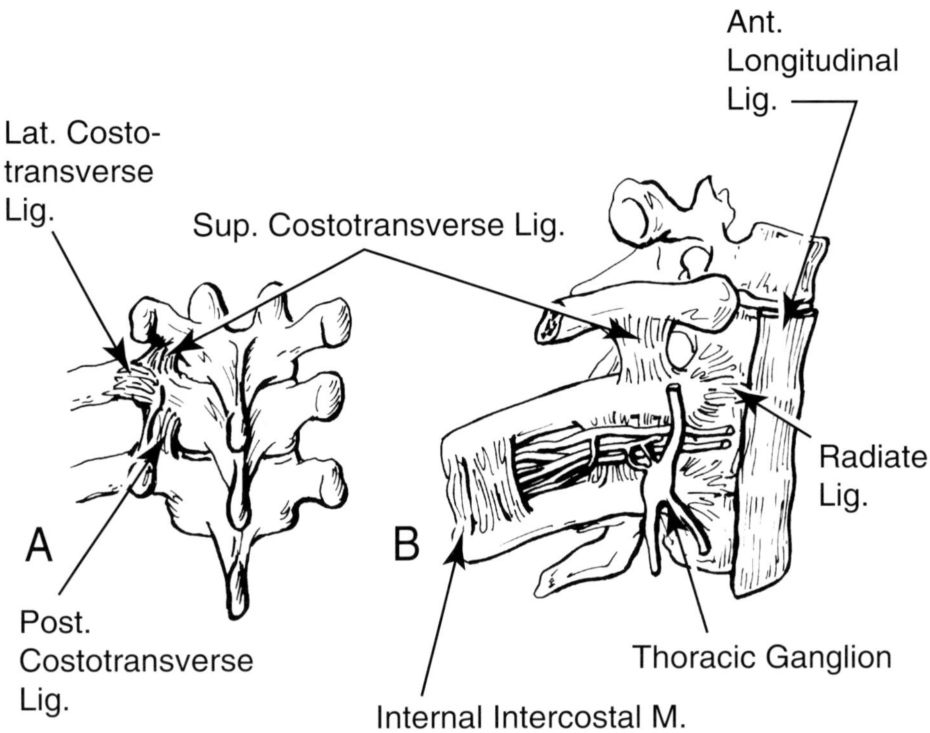

Figure 6. Dorsal **(A)** and lateral **(B)** views of the ligamentous attachments of the rib to the vertebral body and transverse process, as well as other structurally significant ligamentous attachments.

transverse process, the pedicle, the neuroforamen, the rib articulation with the vertebral body and disc, and the intercostal neurovascular bundle is essential to proper and safe exposure of this region. The head of the rib articulates with the corresponding vertebral body, as well as the disc space adjacent to the body above. At the T11 and T12 levels, the rib head articulates with the corresponding vertebral body, but the level of rib articulation migrates to a position that overlaps the rostral adjacent disc space in the middle and upper thoracic spine. The pedicle lies directly ventral to the base of the transverse process and directly medial to the head of the rib. The neuroforamen is bounded by the rostral margin of the pedicle below, the caudal margin of the pedicle above, the dorsal margin of the vertebral body and disc, and the ventral portion of the corresponding facet joint (Figure 7). The corresponding intercostal vein and artery arise from the aorta and the azygos vein on the right. This vascular bundle lies in the middle portion of the vertebral body. The disc space may be identified as the intervening space between the intercostal vessels and directly beneath the rib head. The intercostal vessels join the intercostal nerves exiting the neuroforamen and form the subcostal neurovascular bundle below the corresponding rib. The sympathetic trunk runs parallel to the thoracic spine, splaying over the region of the rib heads.

Operative Technique

The patient is placed in a lateral decubitus position and tilted forward approximately 15°. An axillary roll is placed beneath the

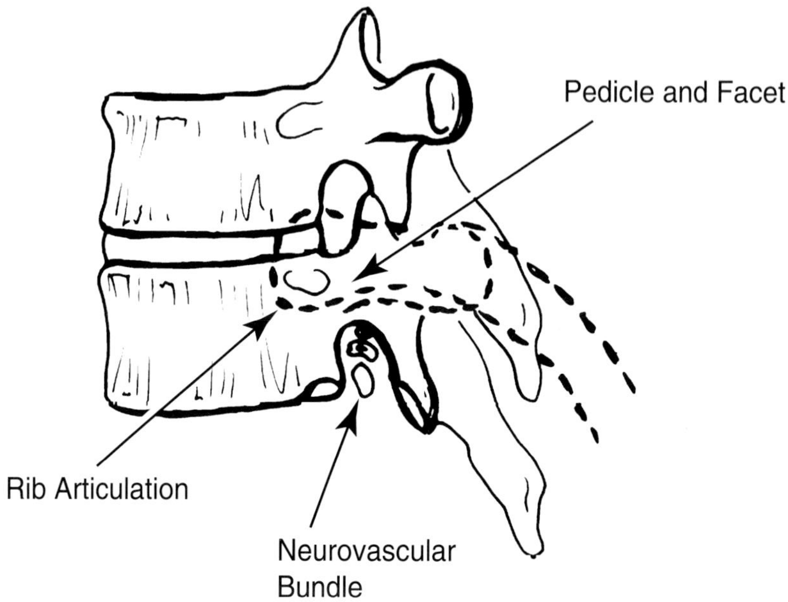

Figure 7. The anatomy of the thoracic neuroforamen, as observed from a lateral view.

axilla and a pillow is placed between the legs. The lower leg is kept extended and the upper leg flexed slightly. A vacuum bean bag may be used to mold around the body. Tape is placed over the hip and secured to the table on both sides (Figure 8).

A double-lumen endotracheal tube may be used so that selective lung deflation can be achieved, if necessary. The skin preparation is carried over the top of the shoulder so that the shoulder and scapula can easily be mobilized within the sterile field. The skin incision is carried medial to and below the angle of the scapula (Figure 8). Careful sequential identification of the muscle layers is necessary so that a proper closure can be performed. The trapezius muscle is divided lateral to its midline attachment. The rostral portions of the latissimus dorsi, the rhomboid major, and serratus posterior muscles also are divided. As the muscle layers are divided, the scapula is further retracted rostrally in order to identify medial muscular tissue on stretching. This tissue requires division for proper scapula retraction and exposure of the upper ribs. A plane is then developed deep to the scapula, and the first rib is located with a gloved hand. Identification and palpation of the first rib is essential. The first rib can be recognized by its downward and inward slope. The ribs are then sequentially counted until the appropriate space is identified. The interspace should be confirmed with a radiopaque marker and an intraoperative radiograph. The periosteum of the appropriate rib is stripped circumferentially with the Doyan periosteal elevator and carried as medial as possible. The rib is then cut at approximately 3 to 4 cm from the rib head, and the interspace is opened above the cut rib. For example, to expose the T3-4 interspace, the T4 rib is cut and the chest is entered at the T3-4 intercostal space.

The parietal pleura may be opened at this juncture or, if limited exposure is needed, the operation may be performed extrapleurally. If the pleura is opened, the lung is deflated and the ventrolateral portion of the thoracic spine is identified. The azygos vein is readily identified along the ventrolateral border of the spine on the right (Figure 9).

To expose the pertinent paravertebral structures, a pleural flap is made adjacent to the spine. The pleura is raised with a medial

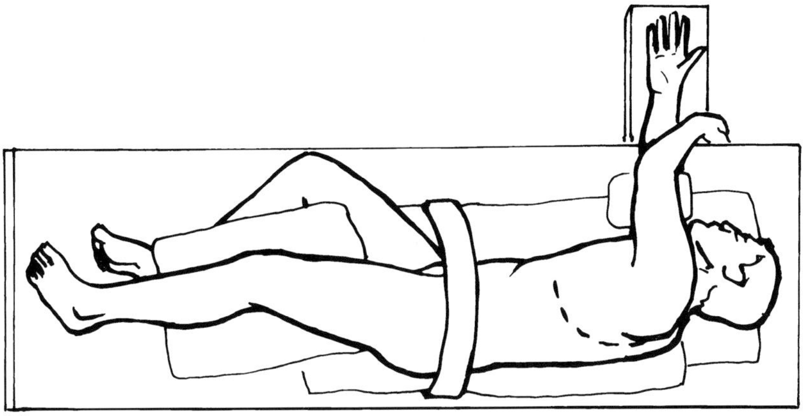

Figure 8. The positioning of the patient and the skin incision used for approaching the upper thoracic spine via the transthoracic route.

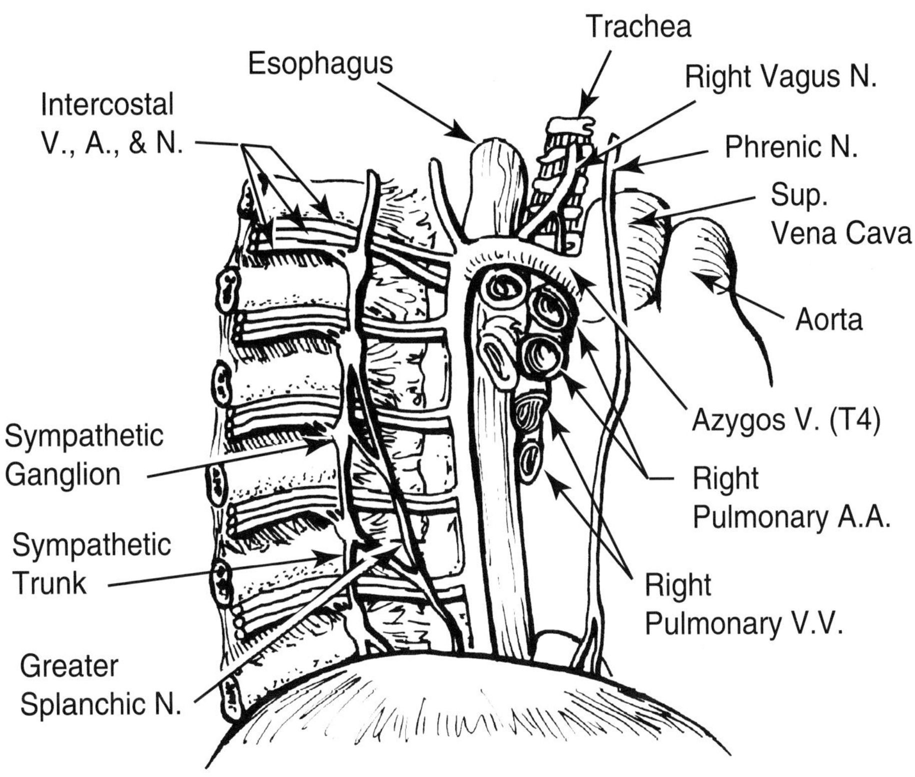

Figure 9. The view gained by a right upper transthoracic approach. Note that the venous structures partially obstruct the view of the spine.

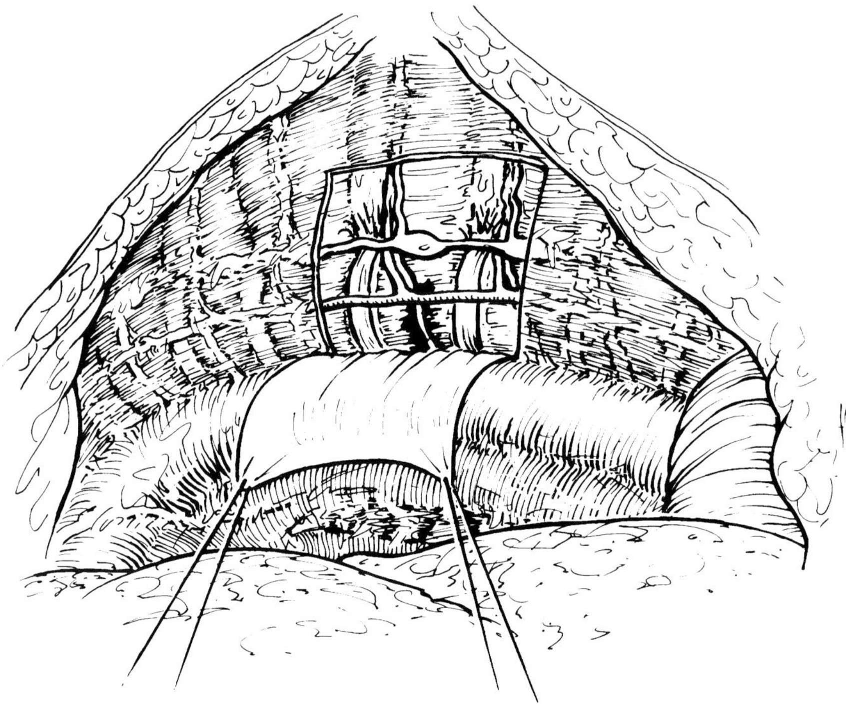

Figure 10. In order to gain access to the spine through the transthoracic approach, a parietal pleural flap is made.

base (Figure 10), and the intended ribs and vertebral bodies to be exposed are identified subpleurally. It is important to have a clean subpleural exposure so that the intercostal vessels, sympathetic trunk, rib head, and neuroforamen may be identified. The appropriate intercostal vessels are then ligated close to the origin of the azygos vein and aorta, which provides appropriate collateral flow to the radicular and subcostal vascular bundles. The corresponding rib heads are removed to identify the disc space, pedicle, and transverse processes. After the appropriate disc space is identified, a discectomy is performed as the initial step. Appropriate decompression and reconstruction may then be performed. Sequential ligation of intercostal vessels should be limited to the minimum needed for the appropriate exposure (Figure 11).

After the operation is completed, the pleural flap is replaced and tacked with sutures. A tube thoracostomy is performed, the chest is closed, and the wound is closed in the usual fashion.

Midthoracic Spine (T6-10)

Surgical Anatomy

The pertinent surgical anatomy on the left side, as compared with the right side, is related to the aorta and great vessels. On the left, the aortic arch reaches the level of the T4 vertebra and is closely applied to the ventrolateral aspect of the vertebral bodies to the left of midline. Rostral to the level of the aortic arch, the esophagus, thoracic duct, and subclavian artery are in close proximity to the vertebral body. In the lower thorax, the aorta

A

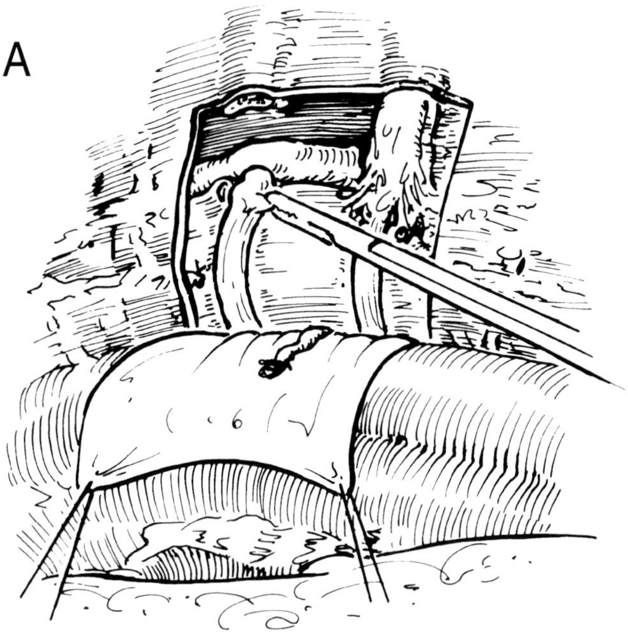

B

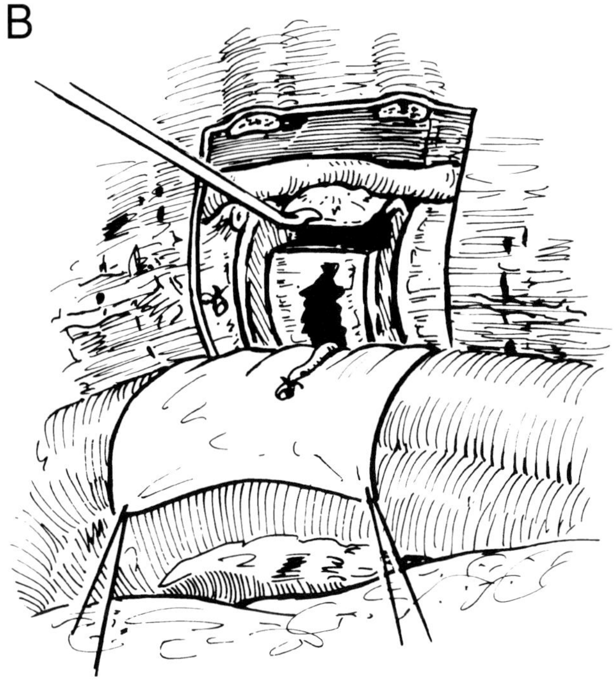

Figure 11. Thoracic discectomy **(A)** and dural sac decompression **(B)** via the transthoracic approach.

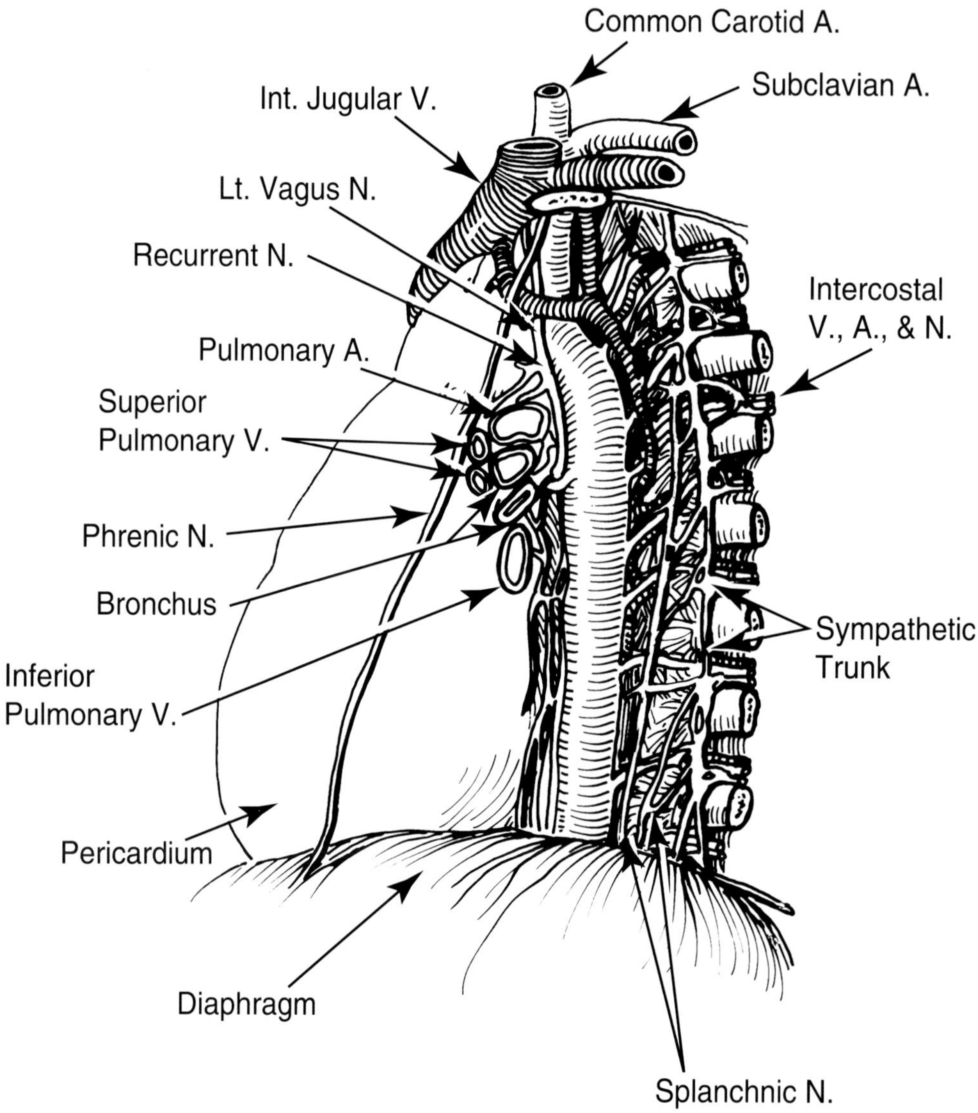

Figure 12. The view gained by a left transthoracic approach.

lies to the left of midline with short radicular vessels coursing across the middle body and anastamosing with the intercostal vessels at the level of the neuroforamen (Figure 12). Thoracic spine exposure uses a similar technique of ligation of the radicular vessels close to the aorta and vena cava. The aorta is then elevated from the ventrolateral aspect of the vertebral body.

Operative Technique

The position is similar to the right-sided approach. The patient is placed in a lateral decubitus position and tilted forward approximately 15°. The bed may be flexed, but must be returned to the neutral position before spine reconstruction. An axillary roll is placed beneath the lower axilla and a pillow beneath the legs. Generally, the lower

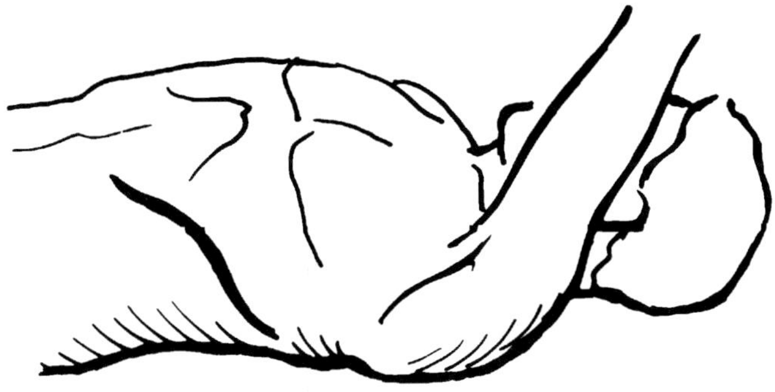

Figure 13. The skin incision used for the ventrolateral approach to the thoracolumbar junction.

leg is kept extended at the knee and the upper leg is flexed. The patient is again secured to the operating table with wide adhesive tape across the hip. If lung retraction is anticipated, a double-lumen endotracheal tube may be used for anesthesia. The skin incision should be overlying the level of the intended rib resection (Figure 13). Both the latissimus dorsi muscle and the anterior serratus muscle are mobilized by blunt finger dissection underneath the muscles and transected with electrocautery along the line of the incision. Dorsally, the division of the trapezius and rhomboid muscles may be necessary for higher exposures. Retracting the scapula, a plane is developed by blunt dissection beneath the scapula and above the chest wall. The first rib is generally inside the second rib; therefore, when palpating from the dorsal chest, it may be difficult to identify. It is essential to confirm the level with an intraoperative radiograph. The rib below the interspace to be entered is then cut approximately 3 to 4 cm from the rib head. Either an extrapleural or interpleural operation may be performed. If an extrapleural operation is preferred, the pleura is dissected from the medial portion of the rib and vertebral body to be exposed, thus providing direct exposure to the radicular vessel, sympathetic chain, rib head, and vertebral body. If the chest is entered and the spine is observed from the pleural side, then a pleural flap is gently elevated to expose the underlying structures. The parietal pleura is typically quite delicate and should be carefully reflected. After the pleura is reflected, the intercostal vessels, as they course over the vertebral body, should be identified and ligated as previously described. Disc spaces are then identified and the appropriate resection is carried out. Following the procedure, the pleural flap is laid back and tacked in place. The wound is then closed in the usual fashion.

Thoracolumbar Junction (T10-L2)

Surgical Anatomy

A variety of transthoracic/extrapleural/retroperitoneal approaches may be used for surgical access to the thoracolumbar junction. For thoracolumbar exposure, the dorsolateral costal attachment of the diaphragm may be divided to allow entrance into the retroperitoneal space and exposure of the ventral spine. The typical approach involves a thoracotomy with the resection of the 10th or 11th rib. The dorsolateral portion of the diaphragm is detached from the lower costal

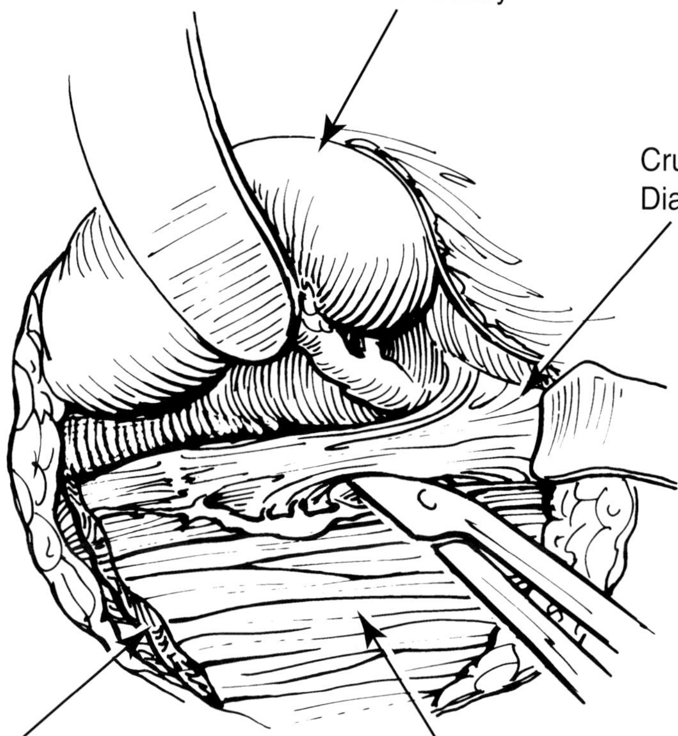

Figure 14. The exposure of the immediate paravertebral thoracolumbar region via the ventrolateral approach.

attachment and a plane is developed in continuity with the retroperitoneal space.

The diaphragm is a dome-shaped muscle that is muscular at its periphery and tendinous centrally. Ventrally and laterally, it attaches to the lower six ribs and xiphoid cartilage. Dorsally, it originates from the upper lumbar vertebra through the crura and the arcuate ligaments of the 12th ribs. The medial arcuate ligament arises from the crura and crosses over the psoas muscle and into the transverse process of the L1 vertebra. The lateral arcuate ligament arises from the transverse process of the L1 vertebra and extends over the quadratus lumborum muscle to the tips of the 12th ribs. The right crus extends down the right side of the L1, L2, and L3 vertebral bodies, and the left crus attaches to the left side of the L1 and L2 vertebral bodies. The esophagus, vena cava, azygos vein, and thoracic aorta ascend through the diaphragm near the ventrolateral portion of the spine. The esophageal hiatus is at the level of the T10 vertebra (Figure 14).

Operative Technique

After positioning and preparation as described for a left thoracotomy, the skin incision is made in the region of the 10th or 11th rib. The incision is carried more ventrally, depending on the length of caudal exposure required (Figure 13). Subperiosteal dissection is carried out, exposing the 10th or 11th rib. The rib is

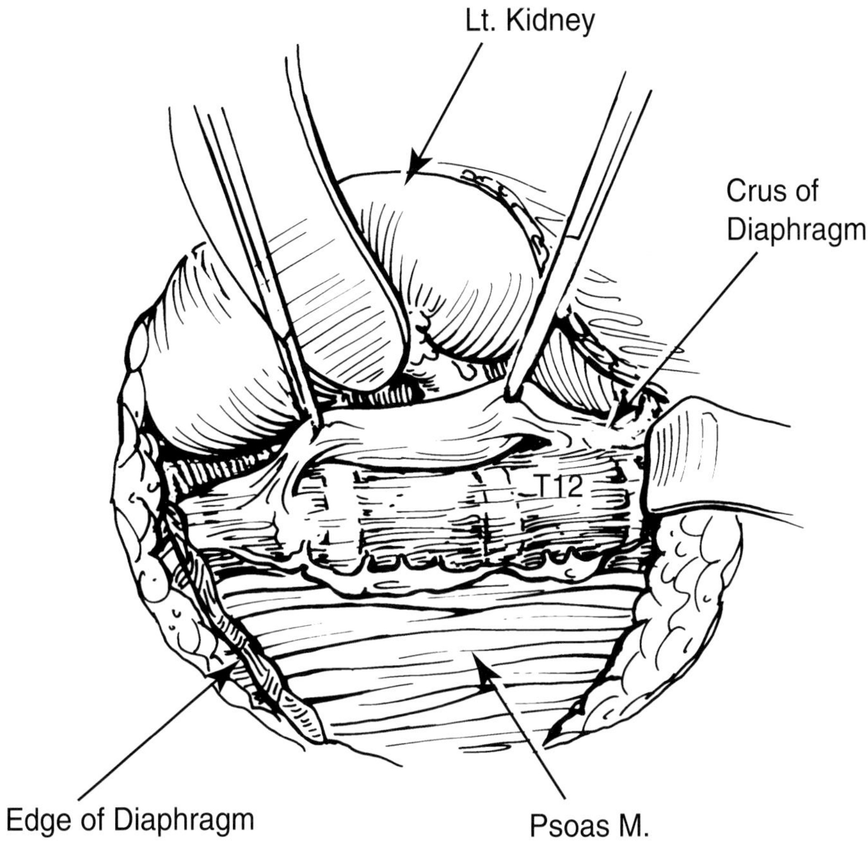

Figure 15. Soft tissue structures have been stripped away from the thoracolumbar spine, thus achieving a ventrolateral exposure via the ventrolateral transdiaphragmatic approach.

then cut approximately 4 cm from the rib head. The endothoracic fascia and pleura are carefully stripped from the inner surface of the rib to minimize the actual pleural opening. The opening is gradually dilated with a crank retractor. Using blunt dissection, the diaphragm is kept under tension and a circumferential incision is made in the medial portion of the diaphragm adjacent to the costal margin. This allows exposure of the upper retroperitoneal space, which is gradually developed by blunt dissection. The spleen, kidney, and stomach are retracted medially and caudally using a broad malleable retractor. The ventral surface of the thoracolumbar junction, the vertebral bodies, and the aorta can now be visualized (Figure 14). Again, following selective division of the segmental vessels near the aorta, the aorta may be mobilized. The crus of the diaphragm is stripped from the anterior longitudinal ligament using a periosteal elevator. The arcuate ligament is divided at its point of insertion into the lumbar transverse process at the 12th rib. The anterior longitudinal ligament and the ventrolateral surface of the vertebral bodies are carefully stripped of all soft tissue and exposed for appropriate resection (Figure 15). Following completion of the operation, the diaphragm is reattached to its costal margin, and the wound is closed in the usual fashion.

References

1. Cauchoix J, Binet J: Anterior surgical approaches to the spine. **Ann R Coll Surg Engl 27:** 234-243, 1957

2. Dwyer AF, Newton NC, Sherwood AA: An anterior approach to scoliosis. A preliminary report. **Clin Orthop 62:**192-202, 1969

3. Harrington KD: The use of methylmethacrylate for vertebral-body replacement and anterior stabilization of pathological fracture-dislocations of the spine due to metastatic malignant disease. **J Bone Joint Surg (Am) 63:**36-46, 1981

4. Heitmiller RF: The left thoracoabdominal incision. **Ann Thorac Surg 46:**250-253, 1988

5. Hodgson AR, Stock FE: Anterior spinal fusion. A preliminary communication on the radical treatment of Pott's disease and Pott's paraplegia. **Br J Surg 44:**266-275, 1956

6. Hodgson AR, Stock FE, Fang HSY, et al: Anterior spinal fusion. The operative approach and pathological findings in 412 patients with Pott's disease of the spine. **Br J Surg 48:**272-278, 1960

7. Lesoin F, Thomas CE III, Autricque A, et al: A transsternal biclavicular approach to the upper anterior thoracic spine. **Surg Neurol 26:**253-256, 1986

8. Leventhal MR: Spinal anatomy and surgical approaches, in Crenshaw AH (ed): **Campbell's Operative Orthopaedics.** St. Louis: Mosby Year Book, 1992, pp 3493-3516

9. Nanson EM: The anterior approach to upper dorsal sympathectomy. **Surg Gynecol Obstet 104:**118-120, 1957

10. Perot PL Jr, Munro DD: Transthoracic removal of midline thoracic disc protrusions causing spinal cord compression. **J Neurosurg 31:**452-458, 1969

11. Sundaresan N, Shah J, Foley KM, et al: An anterior surgical approach to the upper thoracic vertebrae. **J Neurosurg 61:**686-690, 1984

Chapter 8

Ventral Exposures of the Lumbar Spine

Edward C. Benzel, MD, FACS

The surgical approaches to the lumbar spine for decompression, fusion, and instrumentation vary widely. The massive vertebrae and the unique anatomical confines of this region provide significant challenges. A ventral or ventrolateral approach to the spine provides an appropriate and commonly utilized exposure of the dural sac. Multiple variations of this general approach have been employed. Each of these is addressed separately in this chapter.

Surgical Indications

Many indications for the surgical exposure of the ventral lumbar region exist, including tumor, trauma, degenerative disease, and infectious involvement of the ventral or ventrolateral aspect of the spinal column or dural sac. Adequate access for total vertebrectomy or limited decompression can usually be achieved with a ventral or ventrolateral approach. In addition to the role that the pathological process plays in the dictation of the surgical approach, the plans regarding spinal instrumentation also play a role. Ventral instrumentation constructs can be placed via the ventral exposures, whereas patient repositioning and a separate incision are required for dorsal instrumentation construct placement. Therefore, the choice of a ventral operation for lumbar pathology should be carefully considered.

Ventral surgical exposure of the thoracolumbar and upper lumbar spine can be formidable undertakings and are unquestionably invasive. The morbidity associated with these procedures should not be taken lightly. This is particularly true for transdiaphragmatic exposures where the pleural, retroperitoneal, and peritoneal cavities, as well as the diaphragm, are all violated. With this in mind, surgical approaches that involve only one body cavity and that preserve the integrity of the diaphragm should be performed, when possible. In this vein, the ventrolateral retroperitoneal approaches offer a decided advantage over their transthoracic-transdiaphragmatic counterparts and a minimal advantage over transperitoneal approaches.

Regional Anatomy

A clear understanding of the anatomy of the retroperitoneum and the thoracoabdominal junction is critical for the surgeon to appro-

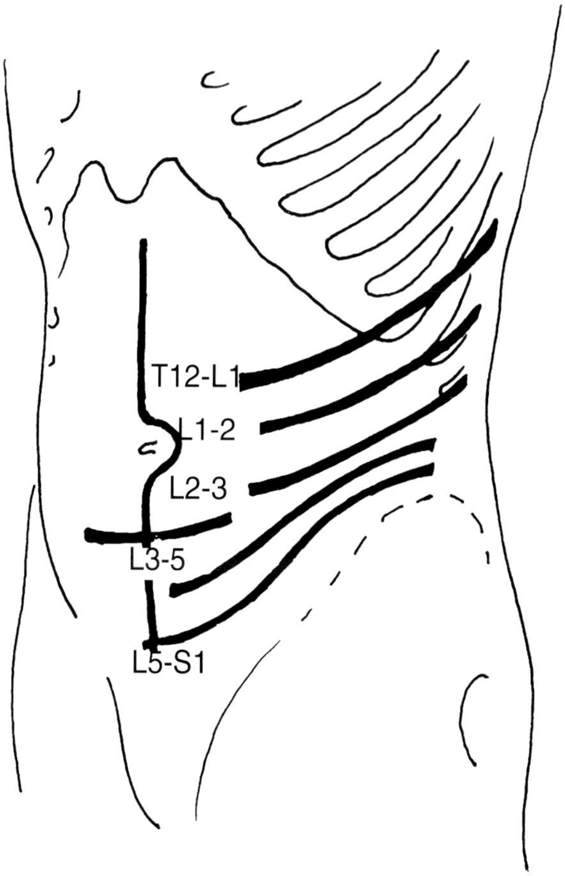

Figure 1. The determination of the appropriate location for the incision and the appropriate rib to resect for upper lumbar exposures is dictated by the rule of thumb used for transthoracic exposure. The optimal rib to be resected or the level of the skin incision is determined by the spinal level defined at the midaxillary region. For mid-to-low lumbar exposures, the approximate locations for the incision are as depicted.

priately and safely operate in this region. Several anatomical considerations are of significant importance.

The Level of the Approach

First, the orientation of the ribs is critical regarding the surgical access to the upper lumbar spine. As with surgical exposures in the thoracic region proper, the accurate selection of the level of approach is paramount. The intraoperative disadvantage of an exposure that is either too rostral or too caudal may be significant. The rule of thumb regarding the appropriate level of the approach for ventrolateral surgical exposure in the thoracolumbar and upper lumbar region is the same as that in the thoracic spine proper, i.e., the optimal rib to be resected is the rib that is at the level of the surgical pathology in the midaxillary region. For pathological processes located rostral to the T12 vertebral body, a transthoracic approach is most appropriate when a ventral dural sac exposure is indicated. For lumbar exposures, the incision varies in accordance with the spinal level and the surgical indication (Figure 1).

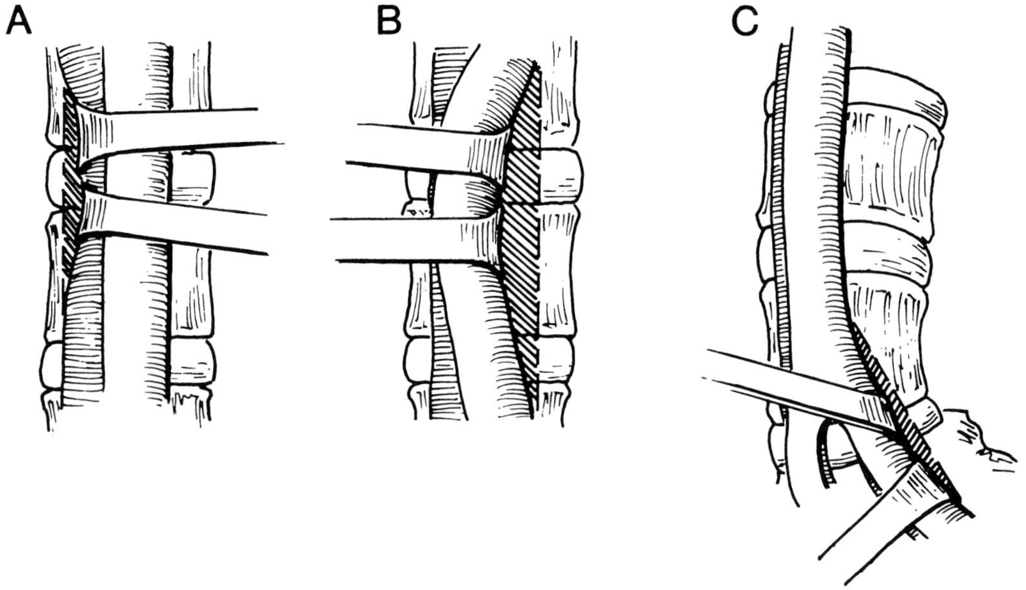

Figure 2. Ventral spinal vascular anatomy. **A** and **B)** Mobilization and retraction of the vena cava (right to left) and aorta (left to right). **C)** Mobilization and retraction of the iliac vein and artery for exposure underneath these structures, via a more lateral view. *Shaded areas* show exposure gained by retraction.

Side of Exposure

Second, the optimum side of exposure is determined predominantly by the anatomical confines dictated by vascular and other visceral structures. Vena cava mobilization is often difficult and dangerous due to its friability and location. Aorta mobilization provides a safer and more substantial ventral vertebral body exposure (Figure 2A and B). This is similarly true for the iliac vessels (Figure 2C). The liver, because of its mass and location, is more difficult to retract and mobilize than the spleen (Figure 3). Excessive splenic retraction, however, may result in injury to this organ.[11] An exposure from the left side is, thus, usually preferred. The vascular supply of the spinal cord is worthy of consideration in this regard.

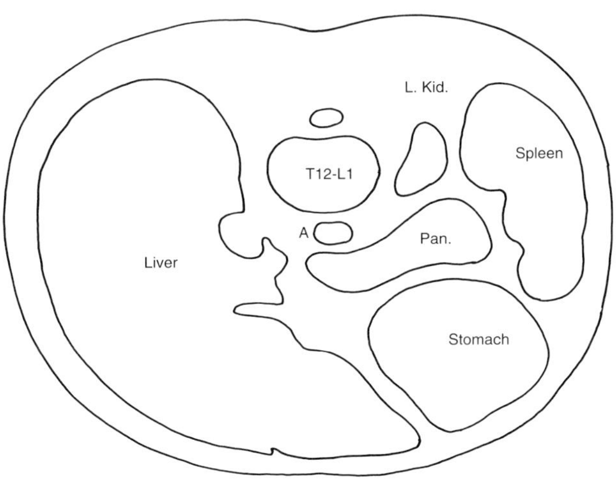

Figure 3. The liver and spleen provide obstacles to the surgical exposure of the spine. The liver, being the largest, provides the most substantial obstacle, whereas the spleen, because of its potential for injury, exposes the patient to a risk for a retraction-related injury.[11] These structures are illustrated from a caudal view at the T12-L1 level.

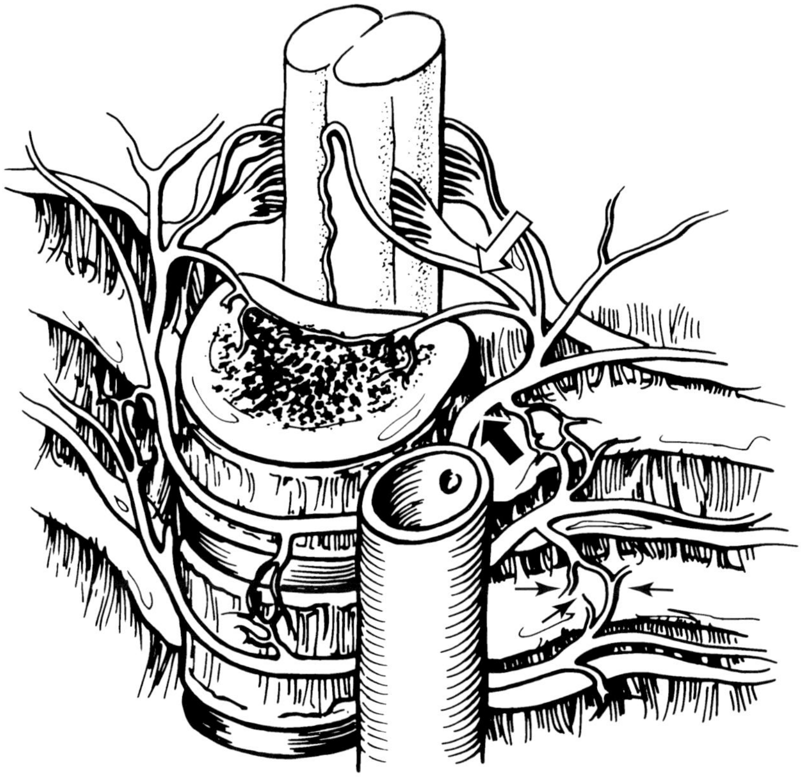

Figure 4. The radiculomedullary artery of Adamkiewicz is a critical provider of spinal cord blood flow. It is a terminal artery, and therefore its interruption may cause spinal cord ischemia. Because it arises directly or indirectly from segmental thoracic or lumbar aortic branches *(solid arrow),* its interruption has varying ischemia-producing effects, depending on the location of the interruption. Interruption at the level of the neuroforamina results in terminal artery disruption and a high risk of ischemic complications *(large open arrow).* A more proximal interruption (i.e., that which occurs with most ventrolateral approaches) interrupts the artery proximal to the collateral branches *(thin arrows),* and thus flow to the spinal cord is not interrupted and spinal cord ischemia does not result.[2]

Radicular Spinal Cord Blood Supply

The most common location of entrance of the radiculomedullary artery of Adamkiewicz into the spinal canal is in the mid-to-low thoracic region on the left side. Its presence may, thus, dictate the use of a contralateral or alternative surgical approach in some cases. The location of terminal arteries and collateral arterial supply are important to determine the significance of radicular spinal cord blood supply.[2] The ventrolateral approach is not, in general, affected by the location of radiculomedullary arteries, because the angle of approach does not violate terminal arteries. If, however, the approach disrupts the soft tissues at the level of the neuroforamina, terminal arterial supply to the spinal cord is endangered (Figure 4). An alternate approach should possibly be considered under these circumstances.

The Diaphragm

The diaphragm is a key anatomical obstacle to the ventral thoracolumbar and proximal lumbar region (Figure 5). The dome of the diaphragm extends rostrally to the midthoracic level. It is circumferentially attached to

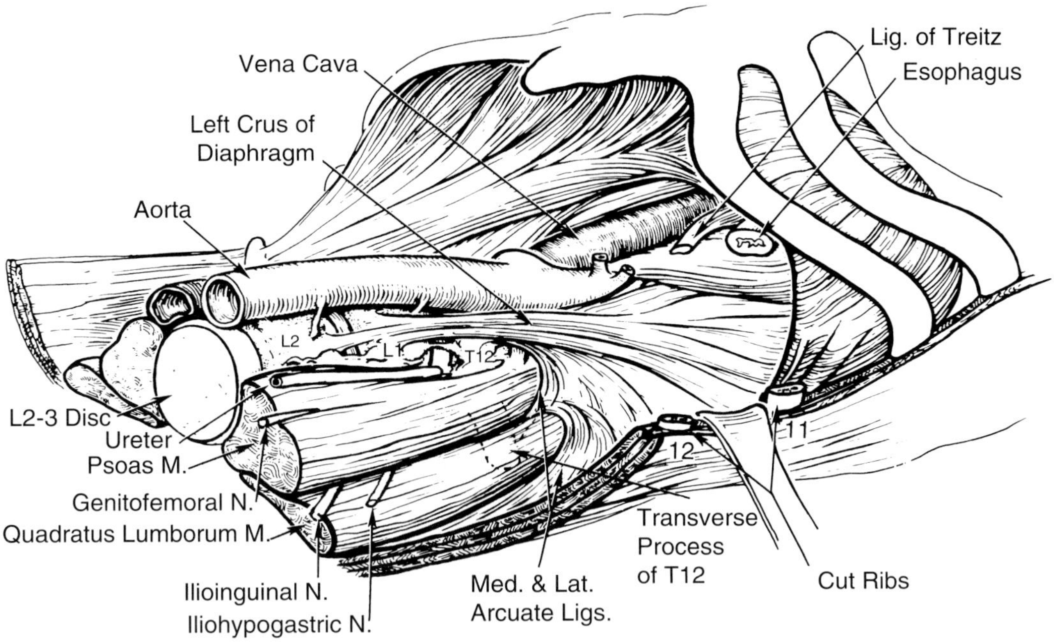

Figure 5. A wide-angle view illustrating the anatomical structures exposed via a ventral approach to the retroperitoneum and the diaphragm. The visceral structures are not depicted in order to optimize the appreciation of the critical anatomy. The ventral aspects of the 11th and 12th ribs have been resected in order to gain a "view" of the thoracolumbar region. Note the attachment of the crus of the diaphragm and the medial arcuate ligament attachments to the vertebral bodies of T12-L2. An approach to these spinal levels dictates the resection of these attachments.

the inferior costal margins, the xyphoid process, the medial and lateral arcuate ligaments, and the L1 transverse process and vertebral body. The medial arcuate ligament attaches medially at the crus of the diaphragm and L1 vertebral body, and laterally on the ventral surface of the L1 transverse process. It extends from its medial attachments in a lateral direction over the rostral aspect of the psoas muscle; thus, when combined with the L1 vertebral body and transverse process, it encompasses the rostral aspect of the psoas muscle. The lateral arcuate ligament begins where its medial counterpart leaves off, i.e., the L1 transverse process. It extends laterally over the quadratus lumborum muscle to the tip of the 12th rib. Ventrally, the diaphragm attaches to the xyphoid process and the costal margins of the lower six ribs. Dorsally, its point of attachment to the upper lumbar vertebrae (L1-3) is via the right and left crura of the diaphragm. More laterally, it is attached to the arcuate ligaments and the caudal aspect of the 12th rib.

Diaphragm innervation (phrenic nerve) originates centrally.[18] Therefore, diaphragm dissection should begin peripherally and extend in a circumferential manner (approximately 2 cm from its lateral-most extent), thus preserving the radially oriented innervation pattern, while allowing for enough peripheral diaphragm remnant to achieve suture at the time of closure.

Adjuncts to Surgery

For ventrolateral surgical exposures, the patient is usually placed in the supine position. Anatomical access is enhanced by elevating the side of surgery with a kidney rest or log roll. For thoracoabdominal approaches, however, a lateral decubitus posi-

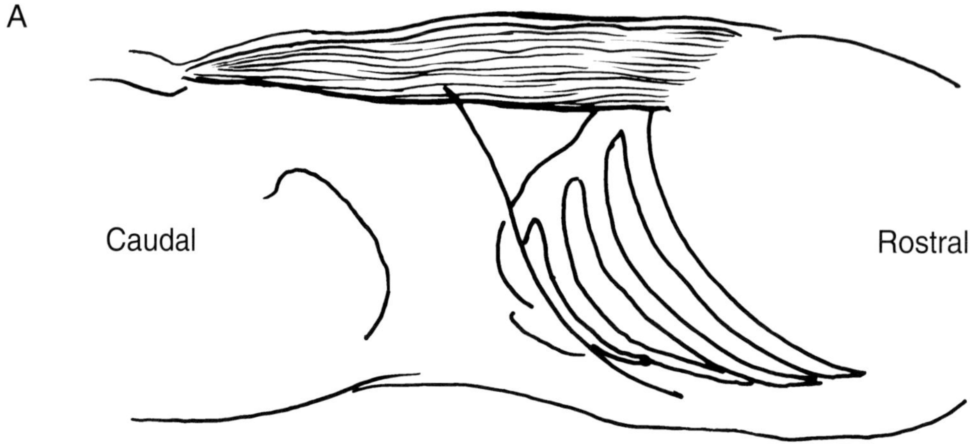

Figure 6A. See caption on page 105.

tion is recommended. The exposure of the ventrolateral lumbar spine can be maintained intraoperatively by table-mounted or self-retaining retractor systems. Anesthetic management is via routine techniques.

The placement of spinal implants through the ventral surgical approach is potentially hazardous. An augmentation of stability via the placement of ventral instrumentation is obviously of benefit if placed with minimal risk. In general, ventral spinal implants provide less structural support than their dorsal counterparts, due to their relatively short length, the low cortical:medullary bone ratio in the vertebral bodies (as compared to the pedicles), and the absence of the strong lamina, facet, and transverse process points of fixation. The inability to adequately toe-in (cross) the screws results in a tendency of the pathological segment to rotate.

Description of Operations

The surgical approaches to the ventral aspect of the lumbar spine are dictated by the anatomical confines of the particular region of the spine to be surgically approached.[7,14,17,19,20] The surgical exposure can be varied by approaching the spine through different intercostal spaces, directly through the retroperitoneum, over the pelvic brim, or transperitoneally. Each of these approaches is discussed and illustrated separately.

Ventrolateral Retroperitoneal Approach to the Upper Lumbar Spine

In a majority of cases, either a supra- or infradiaphragmatic exposure will gain access to the appropriate level of thoracolumbar spine pathology. Regarding infradiaphragmatic (retroperitoneal) exposure, subperiosteal dissection of the crus of the diaphragm from its vertebral attachments, beginning in a rostral or caudal position, aids in this process. Both the T11 and T12 vertebrae, however, can be approached from above or below the diaphragm.

The ventrolateral subdiaphragmatic approaches to the upper lumbar spine vary depending on the spinal segment(s) involved. Exposures involving the resection of 11th or 12th ribs may be used to gain access to the thoracolumbar and upper lumbar spine (Figure 6).[3,9,12] Although the initial exposure differs, the fundamental regional anatomical principles are the same. Therefore, if one understands the regional anatomy, the route chosen to reach the pathological process should not alter the definitive aspect of the operation (vertebral dissection).

The vertebral column is approached through the retroperitoneal space, followed by subperiosteal dissection along the vertebral body. This exposure is gained by approaching the vertebral body immediately ventral to the quadratus lumborum muscle.

B

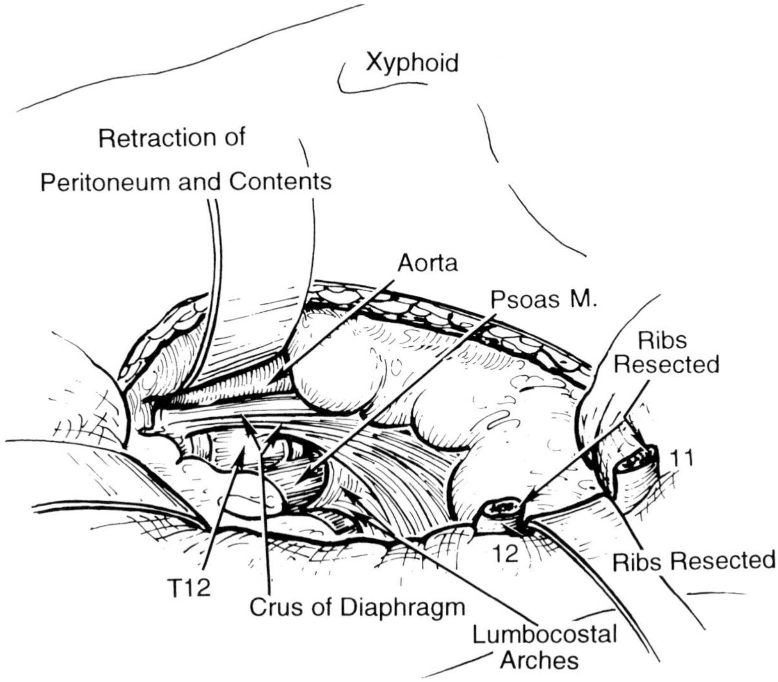

C

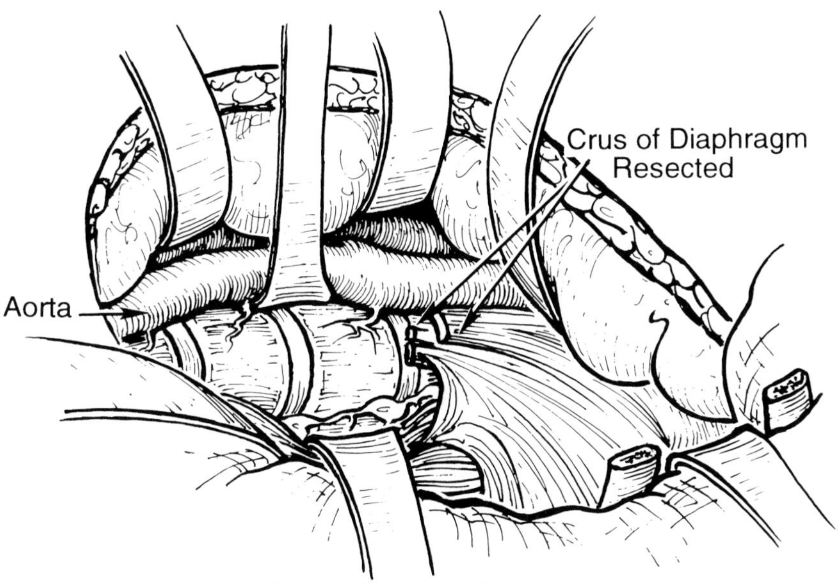

Figure 6. The ventrolateral subdiaphragmatic approach to the upper lumbar spine. The resection of the 11th and/or 12th rib gains access to the upper lumbar spine and to the retroperitoneal space. Further dissection along the visceral face of the ribs and along the quadratus lumborum muscle exposes the lateral aspect of the vertebral body and crus of the diaphragm **(A** and **B).** Incision of the crus of the diaphragm's attachment to the anterior longitudinal ligament and the arcuate ligament attachments to the transverse process of L1 allows the extension of the exposure rostrally to the lower aspect of T12 **(C).** This rostral exposure, however, is limited.

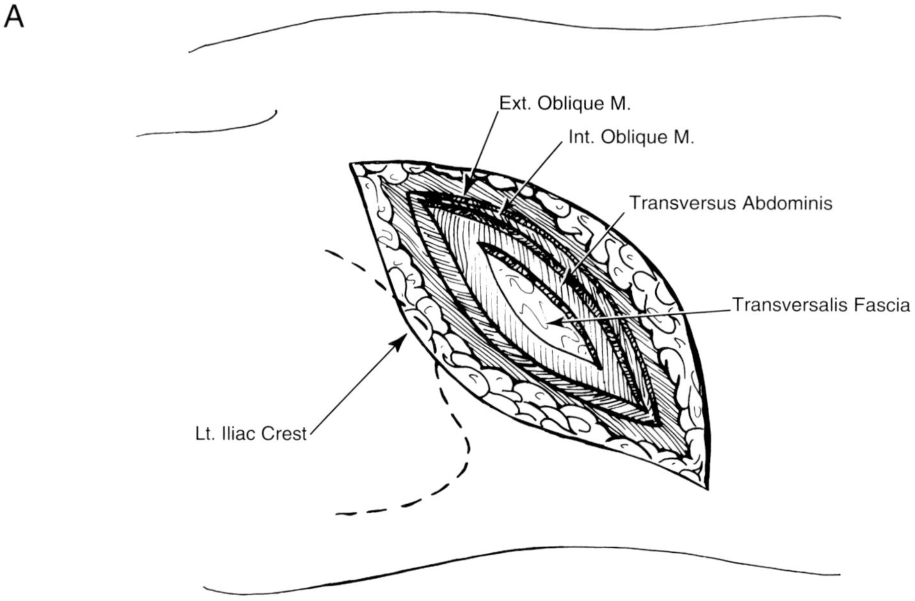

Figure 7A. A depiction of the ventrolateral retroperitoneal approach to the mid- and low lumbar spine. The skin incision and splitting of the external oblique muscle fibers gain access to the underlying internal oblique muscle layer. The internal oblique muscle layer is incised across its fibers. The transversus abdominis muscle is incised and the transversalis fascia exposed.

Detachment of the crus of the diaphragm from the anterior longitudinal ligament is necessary in upper lumbar exposures. Segmental arterial branches are ligated, thus gaining access to the ventral spine, potentially over multiple lumbar segments (Figure 6). The spinal canal can then be approached, following resection of the involved intervertebral discs.

Ventrolateral Retroperitoneal Approach to the Mid- and Low Lumbar Spine

The ventrolateral retroperitoneal approach to the midlumbar spine is essentially the same approach used to gain access to the sympathetic chain in the lumbar paravertebral region, i.e., a caudal extension of the approach described above. This exposure allows access to the ventrolateral spinal canal from L2 to below the pelvic brim; with greater difficulty, the upper lumbar spine can also be exposed. The dissection proceeds in an anatomical manner by splitting through the external oblique, internal oblique, and transversus abdominus muscles along the muscle fibers of each muscle layer, except the internal oblique muscle layer. The incision continues into the retroperitoneal space and then to the spine. The internal oblique muscle layer may be transected (across its muscle fibers). If this is not done, the width of the exposure is significantly limited. Furthermore, the morbidity of this maneuver is minimal. The sympathetic chain can be visualized in the groove between the psoas muscle and the vertebral body (Figure 7).

The advantages of this approach include the straightforward nature of the exposure which is familiar to most spine and vascular surgeons. It, however, provides a disappointingly narrow longitudinal exposure. This exposure is limited rostrally by the crus of the diaphragm and caudally by the pelvic brim. Through this approach, it is difficult to expose the neuroforamina without psoas muscle retraction or psoas muscle excision or incision (Figure 7E).

B

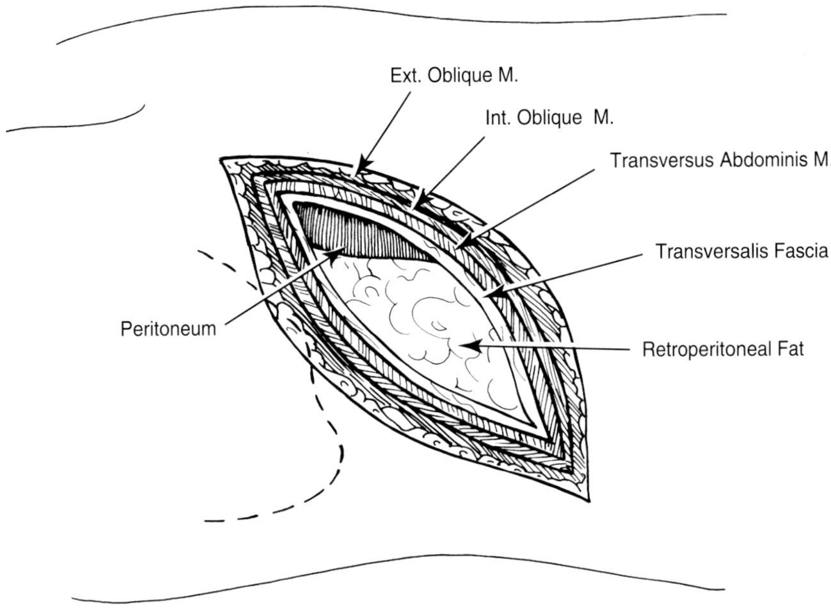

C

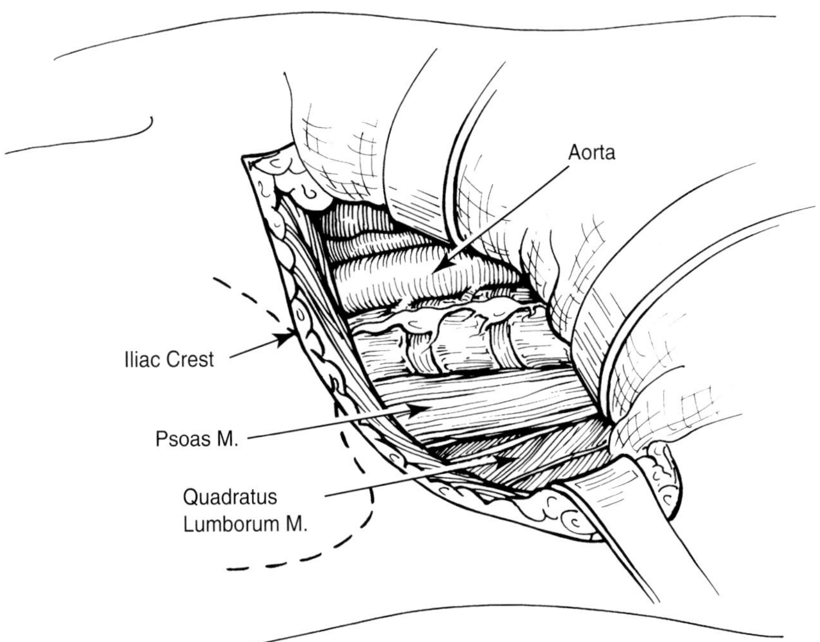

Figure 7B-C. The retroperitoneum is entered following the incision of the of the transversalis fascia **(B).** The sweeping of the retroperitoneum medially and ventrally, with care taken to avoid injury to the urogenital structures and the spleen, provides access to the ventrolateral lumbar spine **(C).**

D

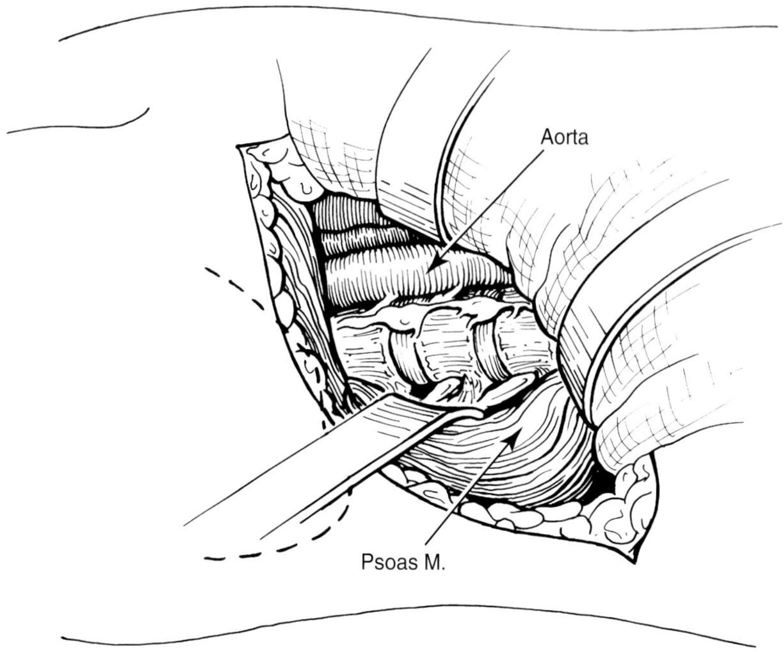

E

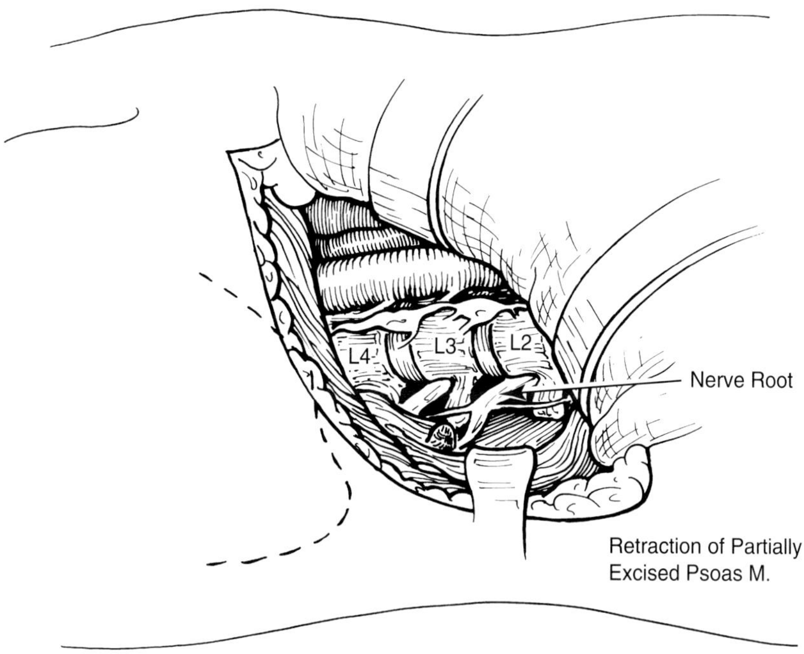

Figure 7D-E. Dissection along the vertebral body in a subperiosteal manner gains an exposure of the proximal exiting nerve roots **(D).** This may require stripping of the psoas muscle from the vertebral bodies. Care must be taken to avoid injury to the exiting nerve roots during this maneuver. In extreme cases, an incision of the psoas muscle may be required **(E).**

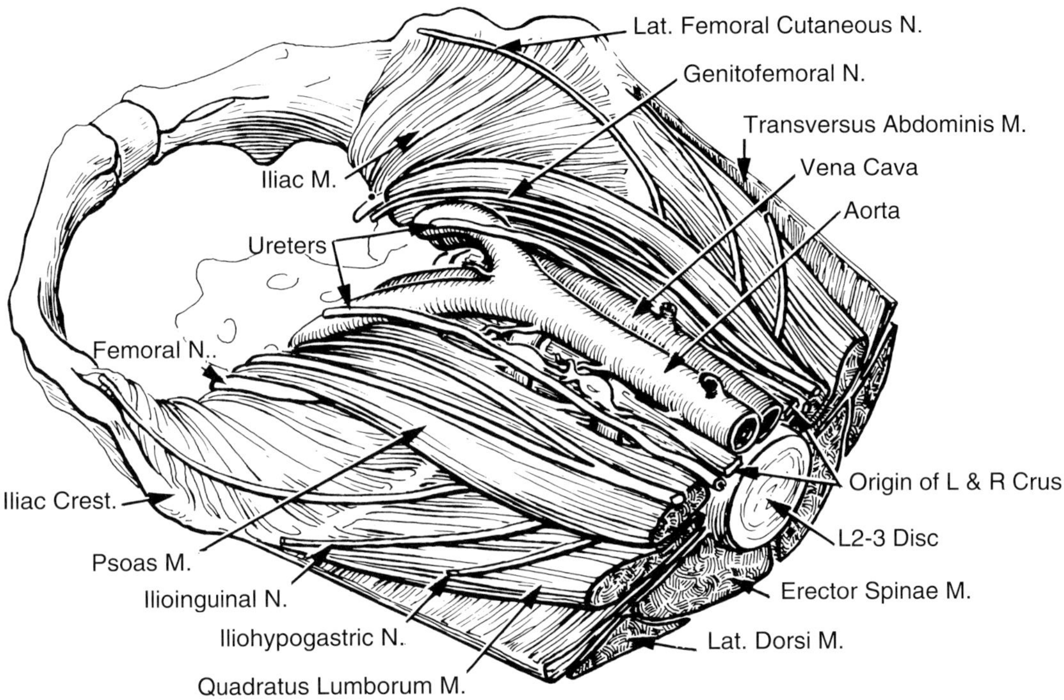

Figure 8. A wide-angle depiction of the anatomical structures exposed via a ventrolateral approach to the retroperitoneum in the pelvic region.

Pelvic Brim Retroperitoneal Approach to the Low Lumbar and Lumbosacral Spine

The approach to the intrapelvic portion of the lumbosacral spine (Figure 8) is challenging. To gain low lumbar exposure, an incision beginning lateral to and slightly above the anterior superior iliac spine can be carried medially and caudally, parallel and rostral to the iliac crest and inguinal ligament. This gains access to the muscular plane below this level. An incision along the external oblique

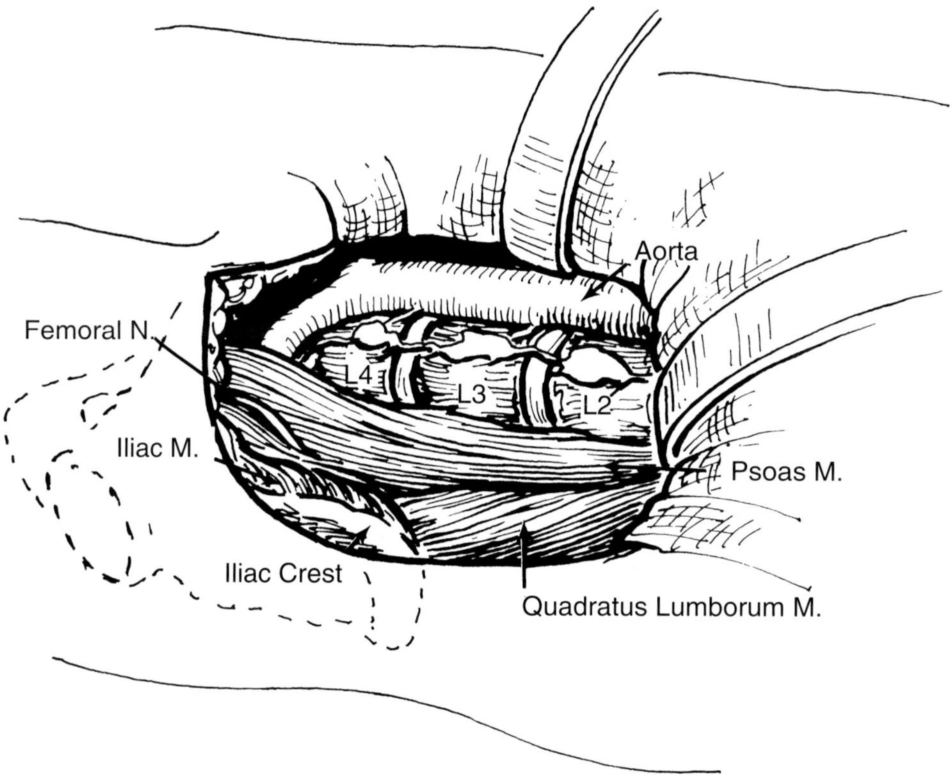

Figure 9. A depiction of the pelvic brim retroperitoneal approach to the low lumbar and lumbosacral spine. An incision beginning lateral to and slightly above the anterior superior iliac spine (as depicted in Figure 1) is carried medially and rostrally, parallel and rostral to the iliac crest and inguinal ligament. This gains access to the muscular plane below this level. Separating the obliquus externus muscle and incising the obliquus internus muscle exposes the underlying retroperitoneum (infraperitoneum). Sweeping the peritoneum medially and ventrally along the iliac and psoas muscles exposes the iliac veins and arteries and the underlying vertebral bodies. Further exposure dorsal to the iliac vessels gains access to the low lumbar and rostral sacral spine, whereas a more ventral exposure gains access to the midline aspect of the sacral promontory.

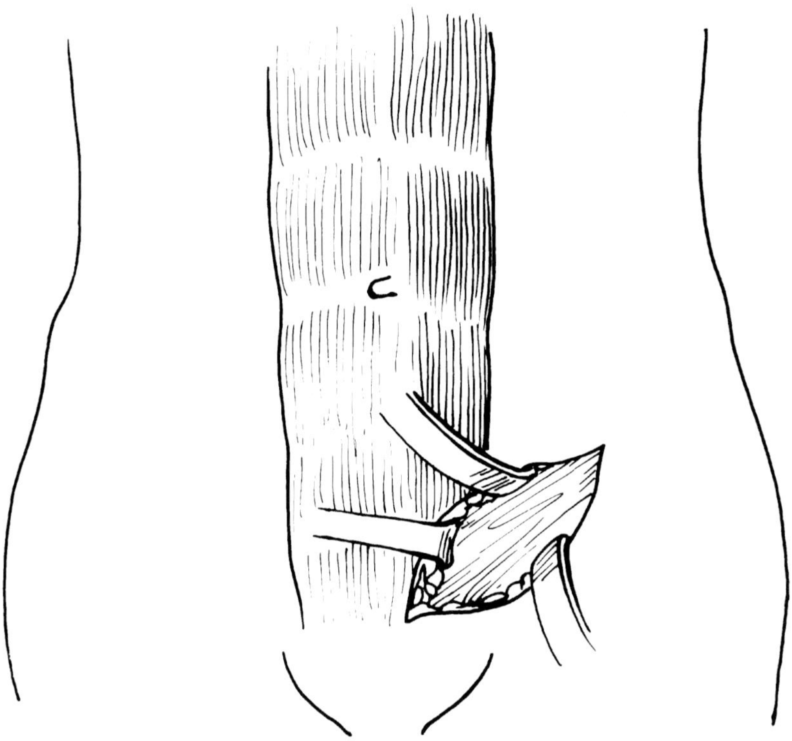

Figure 10. A limited low lumbar exposure via the Pfannenstiel incision is depicted. A horizontal incision through the ventral rectus sheath, followed by medial retraction of the rectus abdominis muscle and incision of the posterior rectus sheath and the medial aspect of the confluens of the lateral three ventral abdominal layers gains access to the low retroperitoneum. The psoas muscle is approached and the retroperitoneal structures retracted medially to expose the upper sacrum and low lumbar spine. Note the more direct angle of view, compared to the ventrolateral approaches (e.g., Figures 7 and 9). Further retraction can gain access to the sacral promontory between the iliac vessels via the retroperitoneal route.

muscle fibers and across the internal oblique and transversus abdominis muscle fibers, in turn, gains access to the extraperitoneal pelvic structures. The peritoneum and renal fascia are swept medially, taking care to prevent injury to the retroperitoneal nerves and ureter. The vertebrae under the aorta and iliac arteries are thus exposed (Figure 9).

A Pfannenstiel incision can be used for a narrow exposure of the low lumbar and lumbosacral region via an infraperitoneal approach (Figure 10). This incision is horizontal through the anterior rectus sheath. The rectus abdominis muscle is then retracted medially. Following the incision of the posterior rectus sheath, the retroperitoneum is exposed.[1,10]

A

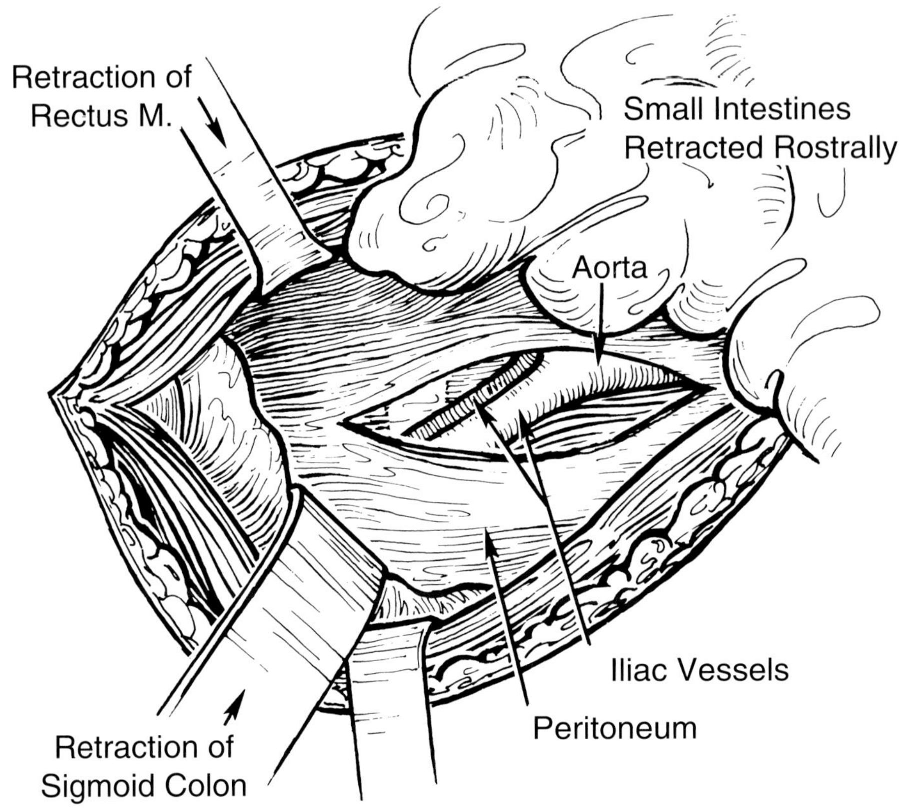

Figure 11. A depiction of the transperitoneal approach to the low lumbar and lumbosacral spine. A standard midline or horizontal subumbilical laparatomy incision is used to enter the peritoneal cavity. The sigmoid colon is retracted laterally. A longitudinal incision is made in the dorsal peritoneum, gaining access to the same exposure gained by the ventral version of the pelvic brim and the Pfannenstiel approaches (Figures 9 and 10) **(A).** Retraction of the aorta to the left provides a view of the low lumbar spine **(B).** Note the ventral angle of view. A lower exposure, involving the lateral and rostral retraction of the iliac vessels, exposes the L5-S1 region **(C).** The superior hypogastric plexus is clearly visualized overlying the iliac vessels and sacral promontary. A high exposure between the iliac vessels is both difficult and potentially dangerous.

Transperitoneal Approach to the Low Lumbar and Lumbosacral Spine

Much of the exposure achieved by the two previously described techniques may be gained via the transperitoneal approach.[1,5,8,16] Following the performance of a standard midline or horizontal subumbilical laparotomy incision and entry into the peritoneal cavity, the small intestine is packed in the upper abdomen and retracted to the right. The sigmoid colon is retracted laterally and a longitudinal incision is made in the dorsal peritoneum in the midline to expose the desired aspect of the retroperitoneal space (Figure 11). Care should be taken to avoid injury to the ureter. The sacral promontory is a consistent, easily identifiable landmark that should be utilized to identify the L5-S1 interspace.

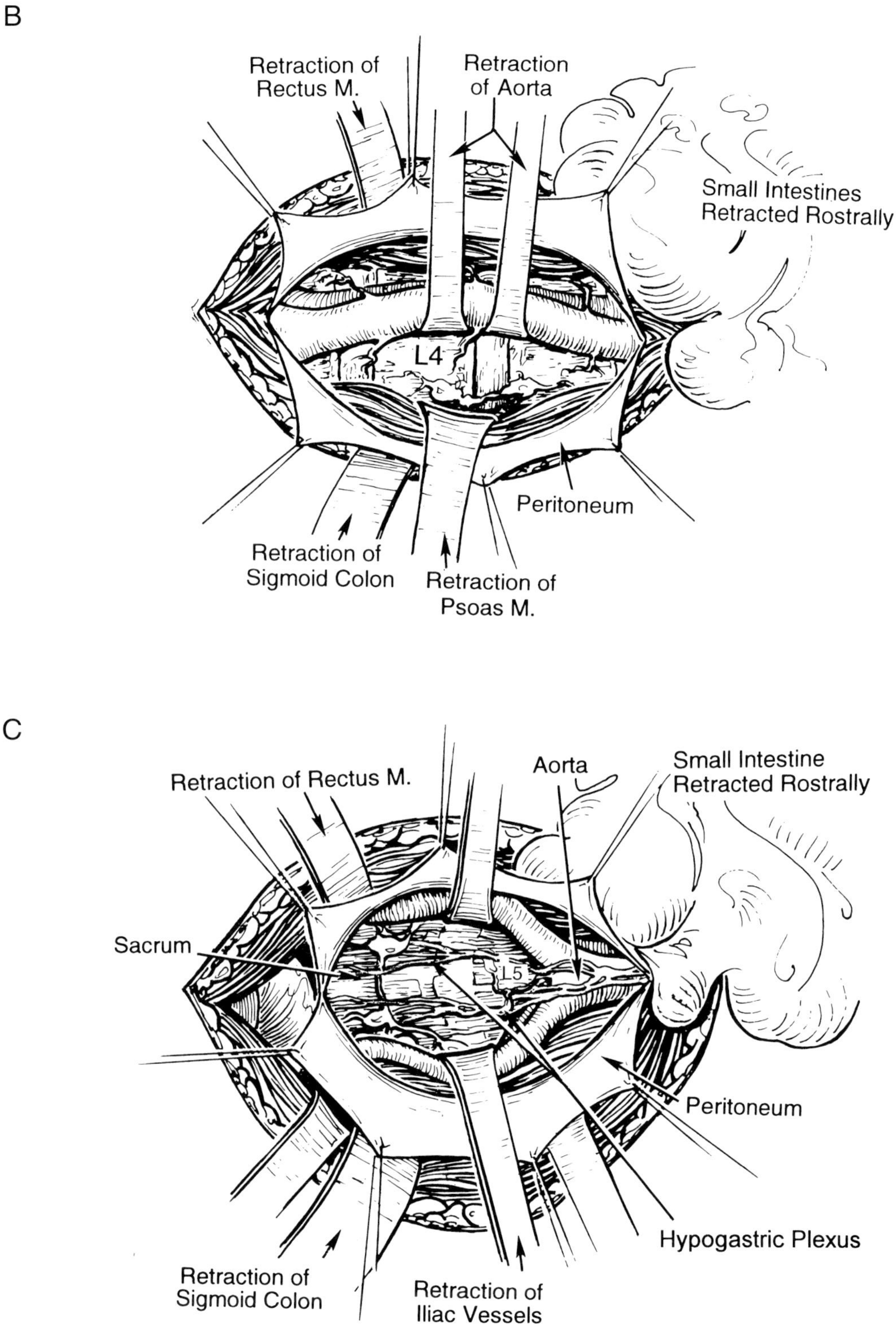

Figure 11B-C. See caption on page 112.

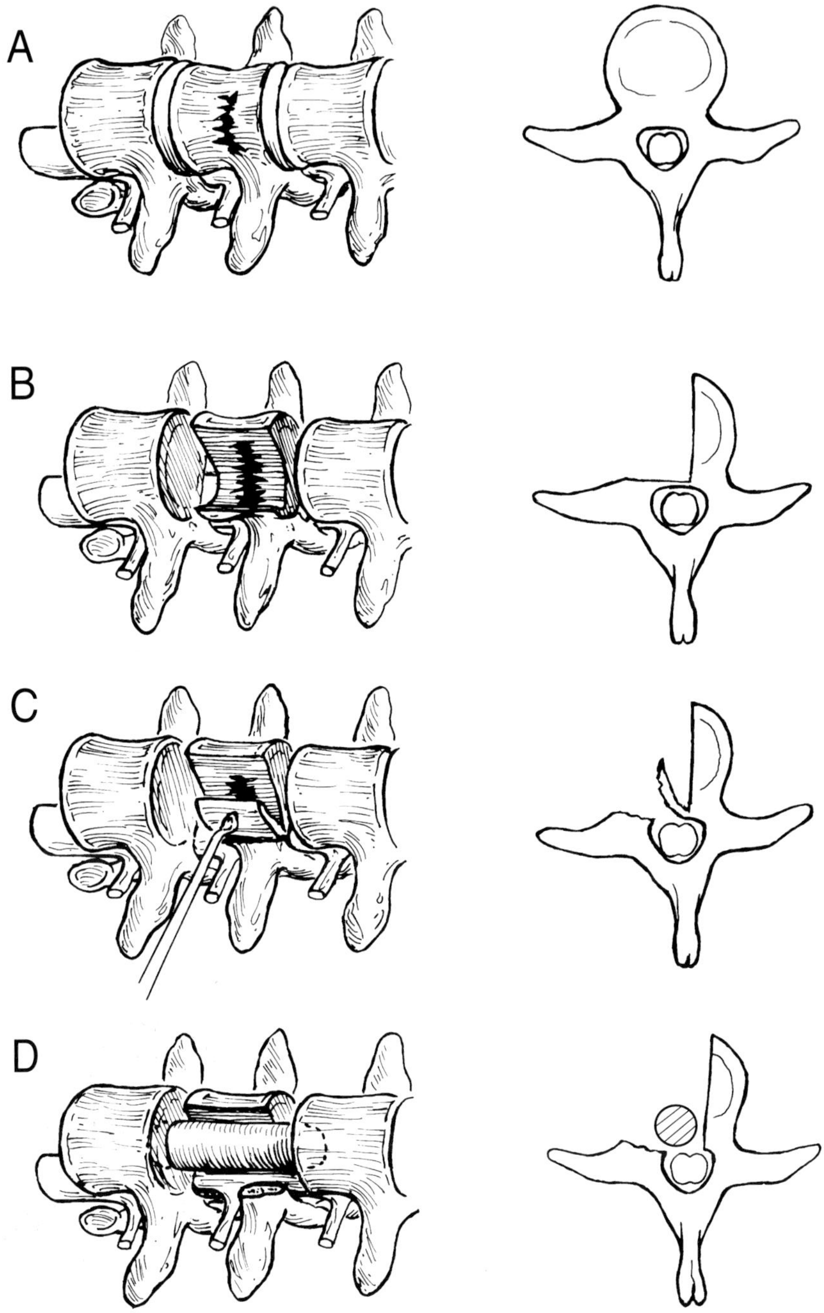

Figure 12. A depiction of vertebral body exposure and dissection. The ventrolateral exposure of the vertebral body **(A).** A rectangular window in the annulus fibrosus is made in two consecutive discs, followed by disc evacuation using a pituitary rongeur. The vertebral body located between two resected discs (pathological level) is resected with the use of a high-speed burr **(B).** The dural sac and nerve root are exposed by completing the resection of the offending vertebral body **(C).** Following the completion of the vertebrectomy and neural decompression, a ventral interbody strut graft is placed **(D).** It is emphasized that the entire vertebral body does not usually need to be removed. Note that only the offending components of the vertebral body and that aspect of the vertebral body required to gain access to the offending pathology are missing.

An excellent exposure of the retroperitoneal space is achieved through the transperitoneal approach. Lower retroperitoneal structures are easily visualized (especially those on the right, due to the limitations created by the presence of the sigmoid colon). The disadvantages are the requirement for a laparotomy and the potential for neural and vascular injury. This approach, however, is very useful when a wide exposure is required.[1] Of note is the true ventral exposure of the lumbosacral spine. Access above the L5 vertebral body through this "interiliac" approach is impeded significantly by the anatomical obstacles of the iliac vessels.

Disc and Vertebral Body Dissection

Regardless of the approach taken to the vertebral body, once it has been exposed, the bone dissection varies little. The usual angle of view is ventrolateral, although the ventral transperitoneal approach provides a relatively pure ventral angle of view. Disc material can be removed by first resecting a rectangular window in the exposed annulus fibrosus of the disc. This is followed by removal of disc material using a pituitary rongeur. If a vertebrectomy is planned, the discs on either side are so treated. The vertebral body can then be resected, usually by using a high-speed burr. Following adequate decompression of the dural sac and nerve roots, an interbody bone graft can be placed (Figure 12). A ventral instrumentation construct may then be placed, if indicated.

Of note is that foraminal and nerve root exposure is difficult prior to vertebral body and disc resection via ventral and ventrolateral approaches. The confines of the psoas muscle limits the lateral exposure of the vertebral body and the exit points of the nerve roots.

Complications and Avoidance of Pitfalls

Iatrogenic vascular and urological injuries may befall the unwary and inexperienced. In order to prevent their occurrence, an understanding of retroperitoneal anatomy is imperative. The chances for the occurrence of intraoperative soft tissue injuries are increased by the use of high-speed bone dissecting tools. The high angular velocity of commonly used bone dissecting tools encourages the movement of soft tissue into the cutting region, resulting in disruption of its integrity.

The ureter can be difficult to identify, particularly in cases where the anatomy is obscured, i.e., metastatic cancer. In these circumstances, the preoperative placement of a ureteral stent can provide tactile input to the surgeon regarding the location of the ureter.

The obvious morbidity associated with ventrolateral thoracoabdominal surgical approaches may dictate the use of the slightly suboptimal exposure gained by retroperitoneal approaches. For example, if only the L1-2 disc interspace is to be surgically approached (as opposed to an L1 vertebrectomy), a subcostal extrapleural T12 rib resection approach could be considered. This eliminates the need for diaphragm take-down. It, however, provides a slightly suboptimal angle of view of the disc interspace. Excessive left-sided retraction may result in splenic injury.[11]

If a long ventral longitudinal exposure of the thoracolumbar region is required, a transdiaphragmatic exposure is suggested. An incision of the diaphragm around its periphery is extended dorsally through the lateral arcuate ligament. The medial and lateral arcuate ligament attachment sites to the L1 transverse process are then incised. This opens up the diaphragm dorsally, thus connecting the supra- and infradiaphragmatic components of the operative field (see Chapter 3).

A special consideration should be given to the superior hypogastric plexus located ventral to the aorta, vena cava, and the iliac vessels in the lumbosacral region. Its injury can result in sexual dysfunction.[4,6,13,15]

References

1. Benzel EC: Surgical exposure of the lumbosacral plexus and proximal sciatic nerve, in Benzel EC (ed): **Practical Approaches to Peripheral Nerve Surgery.** Park Ridge, IL: American Association of Neurological Surgeons, 1992, pp 153-169

2. Champlin AM, Rael J, Benzel EC, et al: Spinal angiography in pre-operative evaluation for lateral extra-cavitary approach to thoracic and lumbar spine pathology. **AJNR** (In press)

3. Digby KH: The twelfth rib incision as an approach to the kidney. **Surg Gynecol Obstet 73:**84-85, 1941

4. Duncan HMM, Jonck LM: The presacral plexus in anterior lumbar fusion of the lumbar spine. **S Afr J S 3:**93-96, 1965

5. Flynn JC, Hogue A: Anterior fusion of the lumbar spine. End-result study with long-term follow-up. **J Bone Joint Surg (Am) 61:**1143-1150, 1979

6. Flynn JC, Price CT: Sexual complications of anterior fusion of the lumbar spine. **Spine 9:** 489-492, 1984

7. Found EM, Weinstein JN: Surgical approaches to the lumbar spine, in Frymoyer JW (ed): **The Adult Spine: Principles and Practice.** New York: Raven Press, 1991, pp 1523-1534

8. Freebody D, Bendall R, Taylor RD: Anterior transperitoneal lumbar fusion. **J Bone Joint Surg (Br) 53:**617-627, 1971

9. Harmon PH: Anterior excision and vertebral bone fusion operation for intervertebral disk syndromes of the lower lumbar spine: three- to five-year results in 244 cases. **Clin Orthop 26:**107-127, 1963

10. Harmon PH: A simplified surgical technic for anterior lumbar diskectomy and fusion; avoidance of complications; anatomy of the retroperitoneal veins. **Clin Orthop 37:**130-144, 1964

11. Hodge WA, DeWald RL: Splenic injury complicating the anterior thoracoabdominal surgical approach for scoliosis. A report of two cases. **J Bone Joint Surg (Am) 65:**396-397, 1983

12. Hodgson AR, Wong SK: A description of a technic and evaluation of results in anterior spinal fusion for deranged intervertebral disk and spondylolisthesis. **Clin Orthop 56:**133-162, 1968

13. Johnson RM, McGuire EJ: Urogenital complications of anterior approaches to the lumbar spine. **Clin Orthop 154:**114-118, 1981

14. Johnson RM, Southwick WO: Surgical approaches to the spine, in Rothman RH, Simeone FA (eds): **The Spine.** Philadelphia: WB Saunders, 1992, Vol 2, pp 1607-1738

15. LaBate JS: The surgical anatomy of the superior hypogastric plexus—"Pre-sacral nerve." **Surg Gynecol Obstet 67:**199-211, 1938

16. Lane JD Jr, Moore ES Jr: Transperitoneal approach to the intervertebral disc in the lumbar area. **Ann Surg 127:**537-551, 1948

17. Riseborough EJ: The anterior approach to the spine for correction of deformities of the axial skeleton. **Clin Orthop 93:**207-214, 1973

18. Scott R: Innervation of the diaphragm and its practical aspects in surgery. **Thorax 20:**357-361, 1965

19. Southwick WO, Robinson RA: Surgical approaches to the vertebral bodies in the cervical and lumbar regions. **J Bone Joint Surg (Am) 39:**631-643, 1957

20. Watkins RG (ed): **Surgical Approaches to the Spine.** New York: Springer-Verlag, 1983

Chapter 9

Lateral Exposures of the Thoracic and Lumbar Spine

Edward C. Benzel, MD, FACS

The surgical decompression of the thoracic and lumbar spinal cord and cauda equina continues to undergo a significant metamorphosis.[8,12,14,15] With good reason, ventral dural sac decompression has become increasingly popular.[5,9,10,11,13,16] Improving neurological outcome has been rewarding.[3,5] Deficiencies with respect to ventral approaches are, however, apparent. These include the inability to stabilize the spine ventrally, and the necessity to complement a ventral decompression and fusion procedure with a dorsal instrumentation procedure. This frequent need negates some of the advantages of the ventral decompression and fusion operation by obligating the surgeon to another equally lengthy procedure.

Furthermore, the combination of a ventral and dorsal operative exposure (360° operation) requires two separate incisions and two separate operative exposures. Most often these are performed sequentially. The sequential nature of these components of the overall operation, however, is not optimal. Usually, the most appropriate first step is dural sac decompression. With ventral procedures, most often the bone graft is placed after the decompression is performed. The ventral wound is then closed. This is followed by dorsal spinal implant insertion, with construct adjustment by applying distraction, compression, or bending moment application. These adjustments, by their nature, alter the relationship of the bone graft bed with the interbody bone graft. This can be used to an advantage by applying the desired force to the graft. On the other hand, these force applications can be detrimental. A previously placed bone graft's purchase may be loosened or overcompressed by construct manipulation.

If the operation is performed in two separate steps (as is the case with a ventral decompression and fusion followed by a dorsal implant placement), this adverse relationship between the bone graft and its acceptance bed could easily happen. In fact, it may occur unbeknownst to the surgeon, who is oblivious of the relationship between the bone graft and the interfacing vertebral bodies by virtue of the fact that the wound has already been closed. The surgeon should be afforded the option to alter this relationship and to meticulously adjust it, if necessary.

Surgeons have two options to manage this dilemma. They may choose to perform a ventral decompression operation, followed by fusion and the placement of a ventral implant. The efficacy of this approach is not known, but early reports are promising. Gross circumferential instability, however, is probably not optimally managed via this approach. The other option is to approach the spine from a lateral vantage, which allows for the performance of ventral decompression, followed by the placement of a dorsal spinal implant (if required). An interbody bone graft may then be placed and the implant adjusted to acquire the appropriate or desired amount of force application to the bone graft. This latter option can be achieved via the more popular lateral extracavitary approach or through a lateral transcavitary approach. Both are described here.

Lateral Extracavitary Exposure of the Thoracic and Lumbar Spine

Rationale for the Lateral Extracavitary Approach

If dorsal instrumentation and ventral decompression make up the desired management scheme, a ventral decompression via the lateral extracavitary approach, followed by the placement of a dorsal spinal implant (with precise adjustment of the forces applied to the spine) allows for the subsequent optimal placement of the bone graft. The appropriate, or desired, configuration of the spine can also be achieved. Similarly, appropriate, or desired, forces may be applied to the bone graft through force application via the rostral and caudal vertebral bodies. For this reason alone, the lateral extracavitary approach will persist as a viable option for the management of a variety of ventral thoracic and lumbar pathologies.[2,4]

The lateral extracavitary approach to the thoracic and lumbar spine was introduced by Capener (originally termed a "lateral rhachotomy")[6] and popularized by Larson et al.[10,11] Although the technique has been modified over the years,[2] it remains a formidable operation. Blood loss from decompressed epidural veins and bleeding bone may present significant intraoperative challenges. In addition, the approach requires the often excessive manipulation of lumbar nerve roots. Frequently, a poor angle of view of the ventral lumbar dural sac is achieved. Therefore, the lateral extracavitary approach is often a suboptimal approach for ventral lumbar lesions (below the L2 level). Furthermore, it is an operation that is usually performed in toto by the spine surgeon without the assistance of a general or thoracic surgeon. With ventral approaches, general or cardiovascular surgeons may assist with the exposure and closure. Finally, it is a difficult operation that is not easily mastered.

Nevertheless, the lateral extracavitary approach to the ventral thoracic and lumbar spine often allows for the optimization of surgical efficacy and efficiency. It, therefore, should be in the armamentarium of those who expect to manage complex surgical problems of the thoracic and lumbar spine.

Surgical Indications

As is the case with other operations that approach the thoracic and lumbar spine from a ventral orientation, the surgical indications include tumor, trauma, degenerative disease, and infectious involvement of the ventral or ventrolateral aspect of the spinal column or dural sac. More laterally located pathology may be ideally addressed via this approach. In that vein, thoracic disc herniations may be resected via a limited extracavitary approach. An interbody bone graft is easily placed, using the short segment of rib removed for access acquisition.

The lateral extracavitary surgical approach may be indicated in the thoracolumbar junction region where the ventral transdiaphragmatic approach is otherwise required for ventral decompression. The morbidity associated with the latter operation, requiring the violation of two body cavities and the retroperitoneum, may be unwarranted in most clinical situations.

Regional Anatomy and the Level of Approach

As with any surgical exposure, a clear understanding of the regional anatomy is imperative. For the lateral extracavitary approach, the paravertebral and dorsal retroperitoneal anatomy is of particular interest, and the location of the thoracodorsal fascia and its association with the erector spinae and quadratus lumborum muscles and the dorsal rib cage is important. Essentially, the thoracodorsal fascia invests the erector spinae muscles circumferentially and forms the dorsal fascial layer of the quadratus lumborum muscle, thus providing the latter's dorsal border. As such, it provides an avenue for dissection to the transverse processes in the lumbar region.

A review of the dorsal upper thoracic musculature is appropriate prior to upper thoracic lateral extracavitary surgical approaches. An in-depth knowledge of the ventrolateral thoracolumbar retroperitoneal anatomy (including the region of the diaphragm) is not necessary, because the lateral extracavitary exposure avoids this region entirely.

Side of Exposure

The lateral extracavitary operative approach to the thoracic and lumbar spine can be made from either side. Regional anatomical nuances and the side of the pathology predominantly dictate the side of the surgical exposure. Care must be taken to avoid the disruption of critical collateral blood flow to the spinal cord, particularly via the radiculomedullary artery of Adamkiewicz.[7] Although clearly not universally necessary, the avoidance of substantial anterior spinal artery collateral vessels seems prudent. Therefore, preoperative spinal angiography is appropriate in patients who have spinal cord function at risk (incomplete or no myelopathy) and in whom a lateral extracavitary approach to the spine is planned (between T2 and L3).

It is emphasized that the lateral extracavitary approach is the only approach that consistently violates the radiculomedullary artery of Adamkiewicz distal to all collateral connections and proximal to its anterior spinal artery anastomosis site. Therefore, it is perhaps the only operation that should be included in the group of dural sac decompression operations that should routinely be preceded by spinal angiography. Ventrolateral exposures, for example, do not require preoperative angiography, as they violate the radiculomedullary artery of Adamkiewicz proximal to collateral intersegmental arterial connections.[7]

The angiographic identification of a substantial radiculomedullary anastomosis with the anterior spinal artery that is located within the operative field (the segment level[s] of the pathology and two levels rostral and caudal to the pathology) theoretically obligates an approach from the opposite side or an alternative ventral or dorsal approach.

Adjuncts to Surgery

Anesthesia is induced with the patient on a transport cart. The patient is then placed in the prone (on log rolls or a specialized spine table or frame) or the three-quarter prone position (Figure 1).[1,2] X-ray localization, if appropriate, is then accomplished in order to precisely define the pathological level.

The Operation

Skin Incisions

A variety of incision options are available. One option is a long midline incision (Figure 2a). This approach requires an excessively long incision and mandates a significant subcutaneous dissection in order to acquire adequate lateral exposure. The healing of midline incisions is aggravated by underlying bony or instrumentation-derived skin pressure. At least in very thin or medically compromised patients, in whom wound healing is of concern, the decision to use a midline incision should, perhaps, be considered carefully. A hockey stick incision[10,11] allows the use of a shorter incision, but still employs a midline component and requires the performance of a significant subcutaneous flap (Figure 2b).

Semilunar skin incisions avoid the midline component of the incision, but obligate the use of a relatively large subcutaneous flap (Figure 2c). A straight paramedian skin incision requires minimal subcutaneous dissection because of its intermediate location between the lateral (ventral decompression)

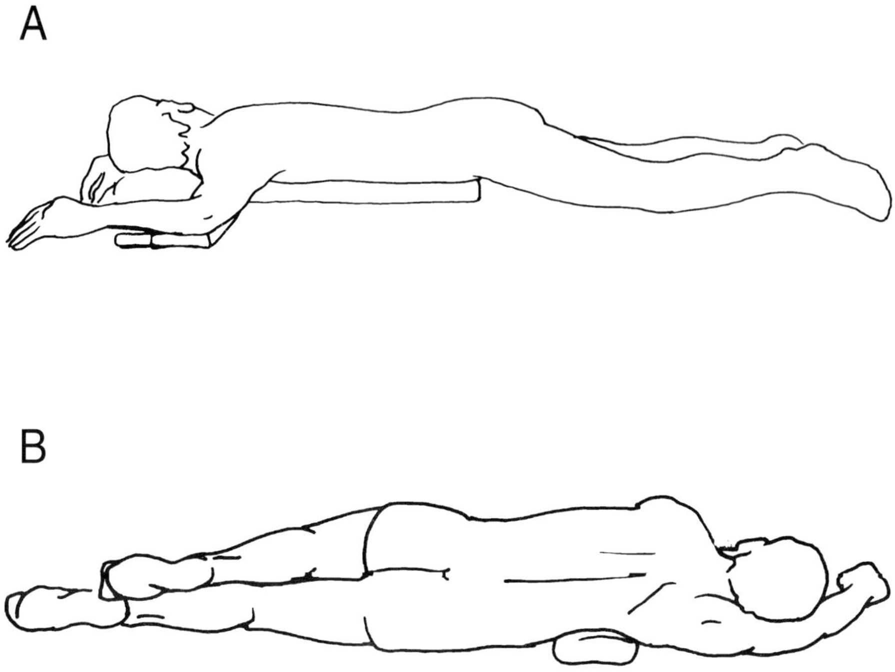

Figure 1. Patient positioning: the prone position **(A)** and the three-quarter prone position **(B).** Care is taken with both positions to minimize the abdominal pressure.

and medial (midline dissection for dorsal implant placement) margins of the exposure (usually about 6 cm from midline) (Figure 2d). A longer incision than usual is required and the nonmidline nature of the incision is distasteful to some.

The Fascia and Muscles

After performing the most appropriate skin incision, retraction with self-retaining retractors provides an excellent exposure of the operative field. Next, the thoracodorsal fascia is incised. This incision may take the shape of a T (Figure 2e) or a paramedian straight incision (Figure 2f). In the thoracic region, the dorsal upper back musculature (trapezius, latissimus dorsi, and rhomboid muscles, etc.) is flapped from the midline or split along its fibers in order to gain access to the underlying dorsal rib cage in the paramedian region (Figure 3).

The erector spinae muscles, which lie immediately under the thoracodorsal fascia, are then retracted medially (Figures 4 and 5). The dissection proceeds from lateral to medial, underneath the erector spinae muscles. In the thoracic region, these muscles overlie the rib cage (Figure 4), whereas in the lumbar region, they overlie the quadratus lumborum muscle (Figure 5). When the erector spinae muscles are extremely bulky, a vertical muscle-splitting incision is necessitated by the desire to eliminate excessive muscle retraction. This, however, provides less of a ventral (lateral) view of the dural sac.

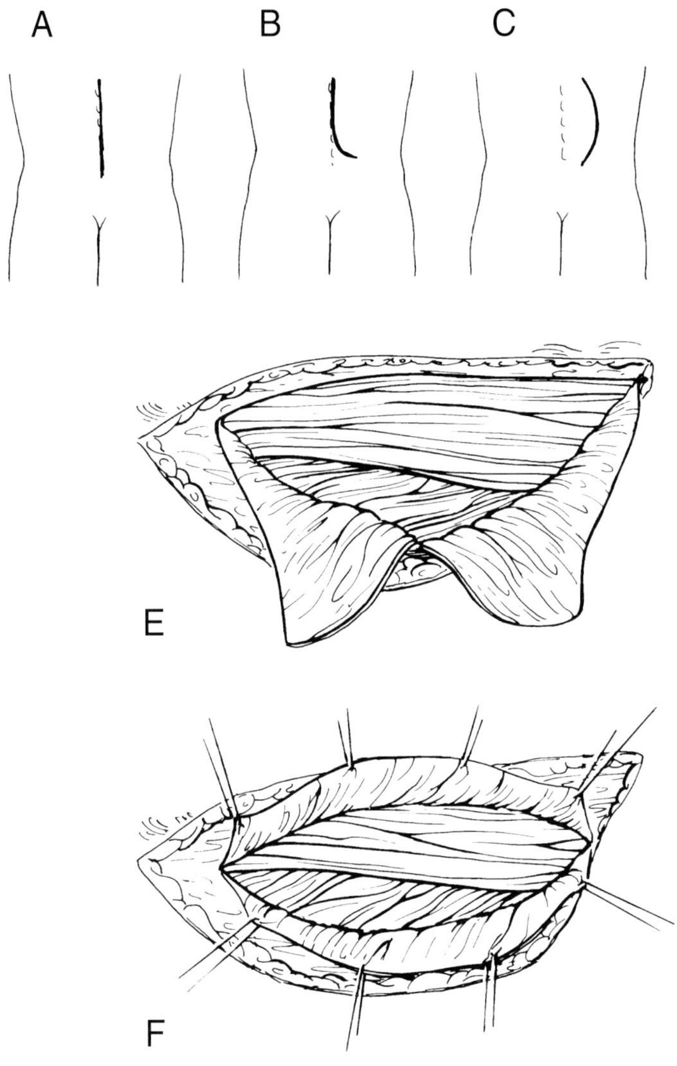

Figure 2. Skin incisions: the long midline **(A),** the hockey stick **(B),** the semilunar **(C),** and the straight paramedian **(D)** skin incisions may be used for the lateral extracavitary exposure of the thoracic or lumbar spine. Fascial incisions: a T-shaped **(E)** or a paramedian straight **(F)** fascial incision may be used to transgress the thoracodorsal fascia.

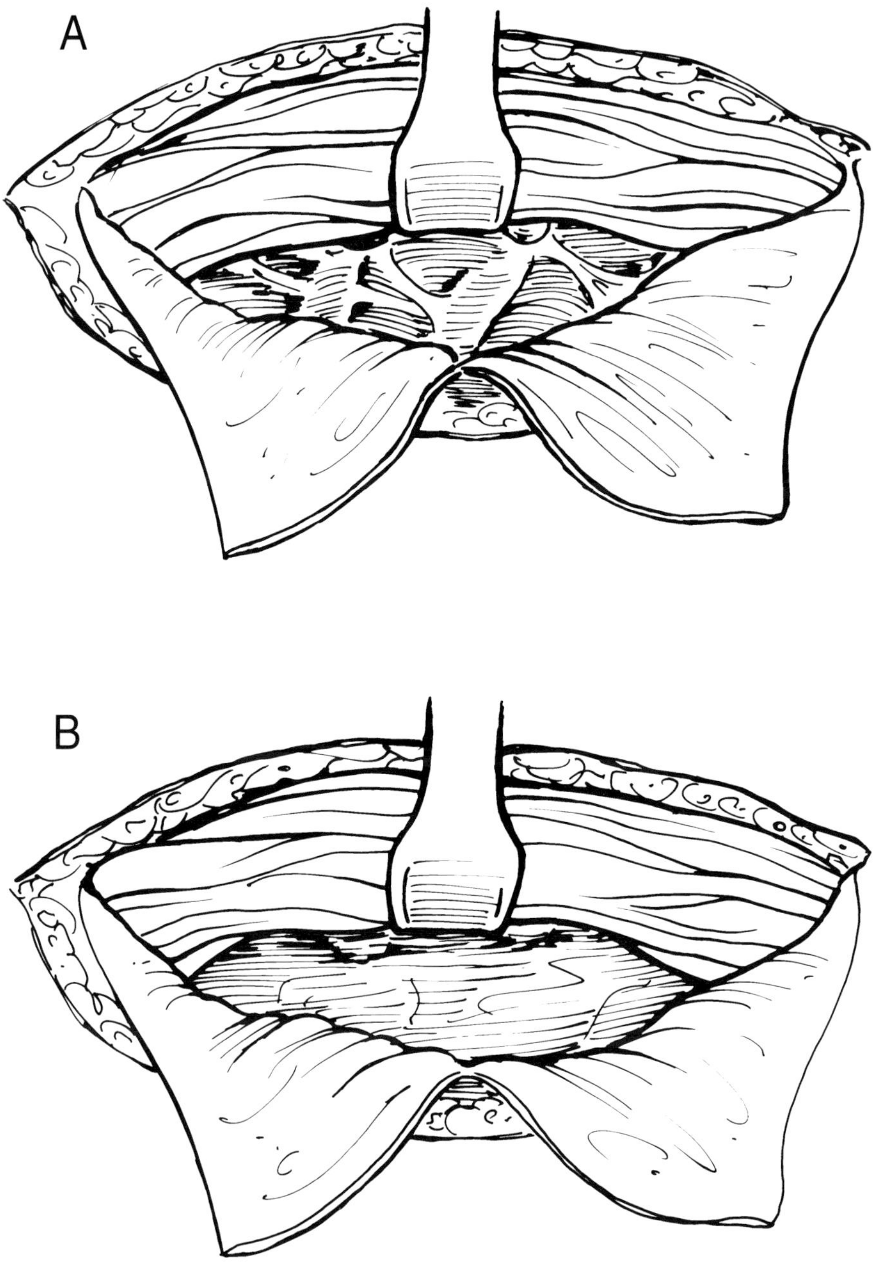

Figure 3. Incision of the thoracodorsal fascia gains access to the lateral aspect of the erector spinae muscle in the thoracic **(A)** or the lumbar **(B)** regions, depending on the level of the pathology.

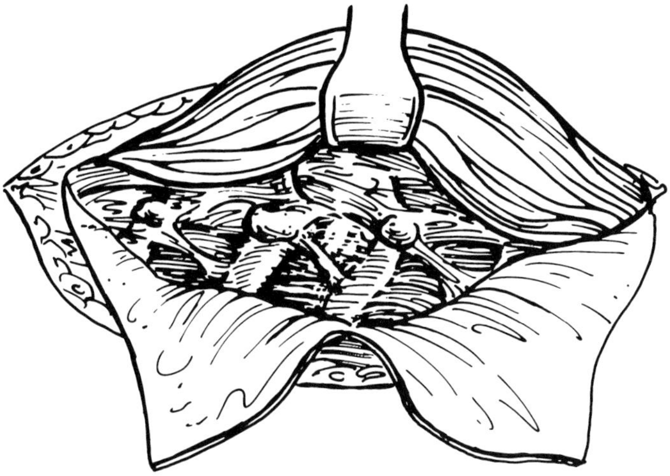

Figure 4. Retraction of the thoracic erector spinae muscles medially begins to expose the underlying ribs, as depicted.

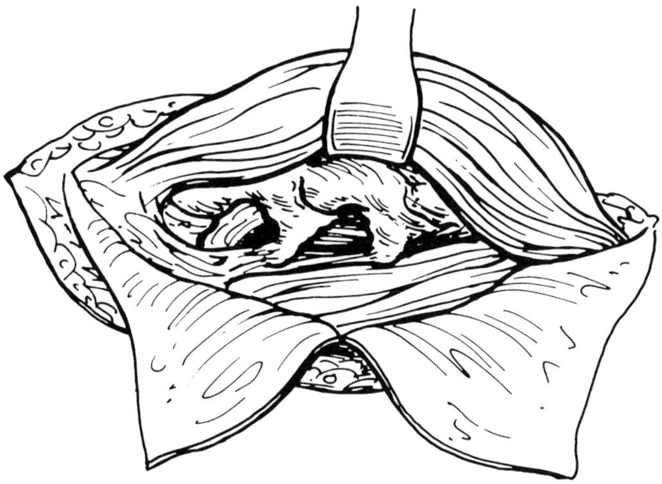

Figure 5. Medial retraction of the lumbar erector spinae muscles provides exposure of the quadratus lumborum muscle.

A

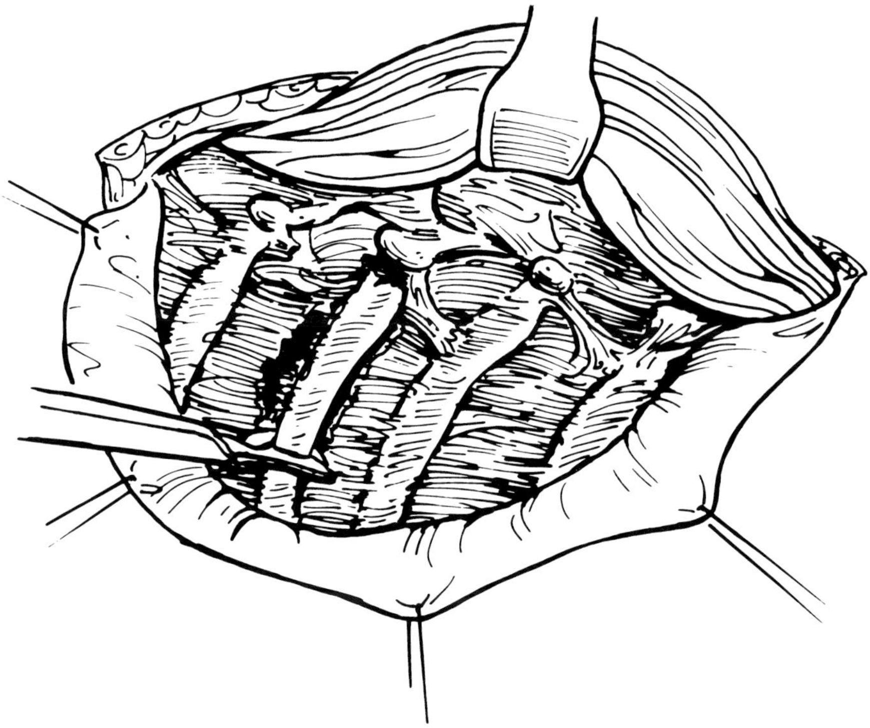

Figure 6A. In the thoracic region, the medial 6 to 10 cm of the ribs are resected.

Exposure of the Lateral Aspect of the Spine

In the thoracic region, the medial 6 to 12 cm of one to three ribs are resected (Figure 6a). They are first dissected free of the surrounding soft tissues (including the neurovascular bundle) in a subperiosteal manner. A Doyne rib dissector is helpful for this dissection. A rib cutter is used to incise the ribs laterally. Medially, the costotransverse and costovertebral joints are disarticulated by careful, sharp dissection and manipulation. Care must be taken to aggressively dissect the parietal pleura off the undersurface of the ribs, the costovertebral joints, and the lateral aspect of the vertebral bodies in order to minimize the chance of acquiring a pleural tear during the disarticulation. During the subperiosteal dissection, care is taken to avoid injury to the subcostal neurovascular bundle. The rib is saved for bone grafting.

In the lumbar region, the transverse processes are reached by following the plane between the erector spinae and the quadratus lumborum muscles medially to the transverse processes (Figure 6b). The appropriate transverse processes are sharply freed from the surrounding soft tissues. A subperiosteal dissection is then performed along the underside of the transverse processes, the lateral aspect of the pedicles, and the lateral aspect of the vertebral bodies (Figure 6c). The exiting nerve roots are located within the muscles juxtaposed to the vertebral bodies and take off at a minimal angle from the vertical (10°-15°).

In the thoracic region, the nerve roots are incised distally and tagged with a suture. Following the completion of the operation, intercostal nerves are sacrificed and tied or coagulated proximal to the dorsal root ganglion in order to prevent symptomatic

B

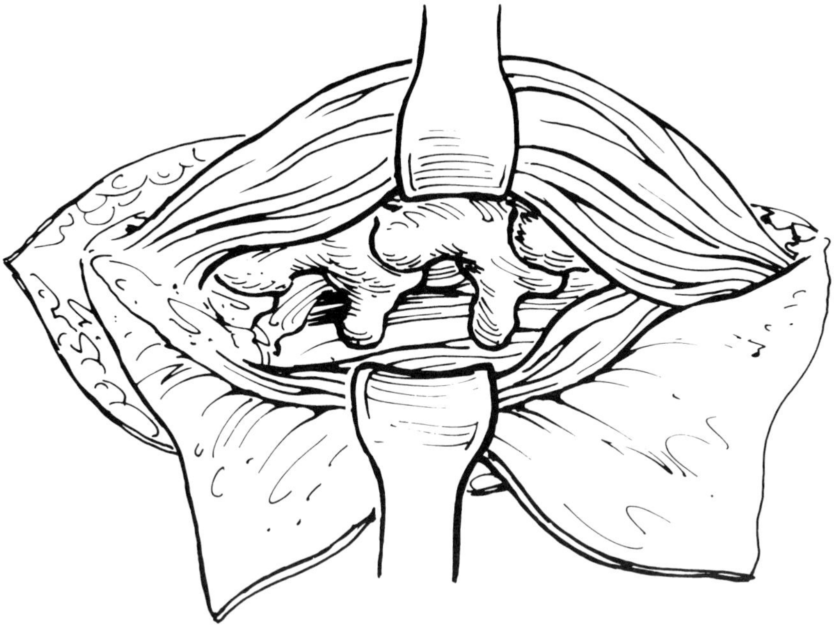

Figure 6B. In the lumbar region, the transverse processes are accessed via the plane between the quadratus lumborum and erector spinae muscles.

C

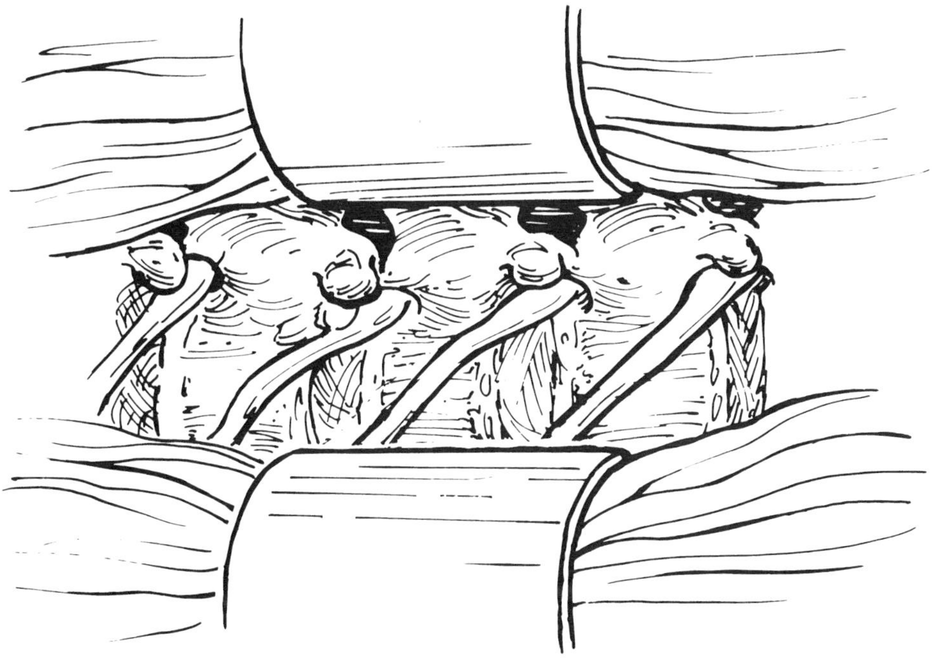

Figure 6C. Further subperiosteal dissection along the undersurface of the ribs, pedicles, and vertebral bodies gains access to the lateral aspect of the spinal column .

neuroma formation. The nerve roots cannot be sacrificed in the lumbar region due to their eloquence. As mentioned previously, this significantly complicates the lateral extracavitary exposure in the lumbar region below the L2 level.

Dural Sac Decompression

The nerve roots are followed medially to their respective neuroforamina and the pleura is retracted ventrally with a padded wide retraction blade. After dissection of the nerve roots to the medial aspect of the pedicle, the pedicle of the pathological vertebral body is removed with rongeurs. This exposes the lateral aspect of the dural sac and a lateral view of the relationship between the dural sac and the ventrally positioned compressive pathology (Figure 7a).

The affected intervertebral discs are then incised and removed, usually with pituitary rongeurs. The offending portion of the vertebral body is removed with a high-speed burr by first creating a trough just ventral to the dorsal vertebral body cortex. This trough may extend from just rostral to the upper disc to just caudal to the lower disc (Figure 7b). The layer of bone left in place should be thin so that the spinal decompression can ultimately be achieved by simply pushing the shelf forward, usually with a reversed-angle curette (Figure 7c).

Bone Graft Insertion

After an adequate decompression of the neural elements and the insertion of dorsal spinal implants (if needed), slots are made in the caudal aspect of the rostral vertebral body and the rostral aspect of the caudal vertebral body. Rib or other suitable grafting material is then fashioned and inserted into the slots, like a bookshelf into its slots (Figure 7d). A ventral plate, as an alternative to dorsal instrumentation, may be placed after insertion of the bone graft, if deemed appropriate.

Several ribs may be inserted. If several bone grafts are indeed used, an absorbable suture (e.g., 0 polyglactin) may be positioned around the first graft and then wrapped around the last graft, inserted, and tied. This minimizes the chance of the most lateral bone graft from dislodging and displacing laterally (Figure 8).

Following the establishment of hemostasis, the wound is closed in multiple layers. A tube thoracostomy is placed if a pleural tear is encountered and cannot be readily or confidently repaired, or a bronchopleural fistula was created.

Lateral Transcavitary Exposure of the Thoracic Spine

The lateral extracavitary exposure of the thoracic spine is often associated with the relative obscurement of the lateral pedicle and vertebral body anatomy. The stripping of the parietal pleura away from these structures via subperiosteal dissection causes bleeding surfaces and often lessens the clarity of the margins between the pathology and normal tissue, the disc and vertebral body, and the orientation of the adjacent costovertebral joints, etc. Furthermore, the extrapleural dissection obligates a slightly lesser lateral view than might be achieved via an intrapleural dissection. Therefore, one may choose another option, the lateral transcavitary approach. Similar to the lateral extracavitary approach, the transcavitary approach gains access to the lateral aspect of the spine. It, however, differs in several respects. A single rib is usually removed. The incision is made medial to the level of the costotransverse joint (with the transverse process) at the level of the pathology and continues further laterally than is usually the case with the extracavitary approach. The parietal pleura is then incised. The spreading of the ribs provides a view as depicted in Figure 9a.

The nerve root may be followed to the neuroforamen to clearly localize the adjacent pedicles and their well-defined relationships with the pathology and the vertebral body. Segmental arteries and veins are readily visualized via this approach as they course around the vertebral body. Similarly, the

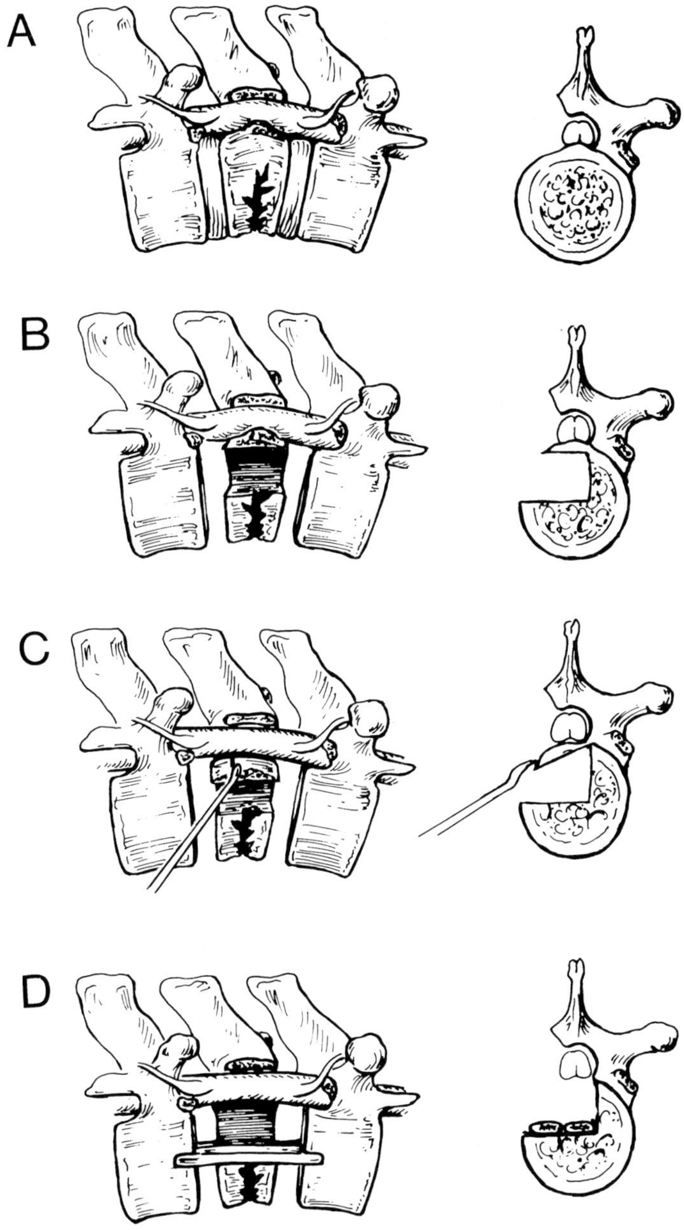

Figure 7. The appropriate pedicle is removed, and visualization of the lateral aspect of the dural sac, as well as its relationship between the ventrally situated compressive pathology, is attained **(A)**. A trough is made just ventral to the dorsal aspect of the vertebral body with a high-speed burr and/or curved curette **(B).** The trough is thinned to facilitate the ventral displacement of the remaining shelf of bone away from the dural sac via a reversed angle curette **(C)**. A rib or other suitable graft is impacted into slots fashioned in the caudal aspect of the rostral vertebral body and rostral aspect of the caudal vertebral body **(D).**

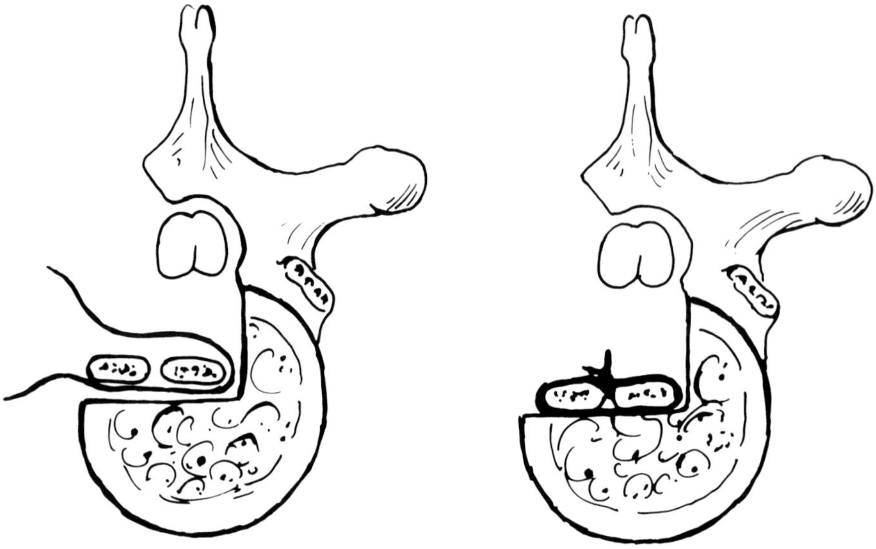

Figure 8. If several grafts (usually ribs) are positioned into the slots created, they may be tied together by encircling the first graft with a suture prior to insertion. Encompassing all the grafts and tying the suture following adequate placement of the last bone graft helps secure the grafts, as depicted.

A

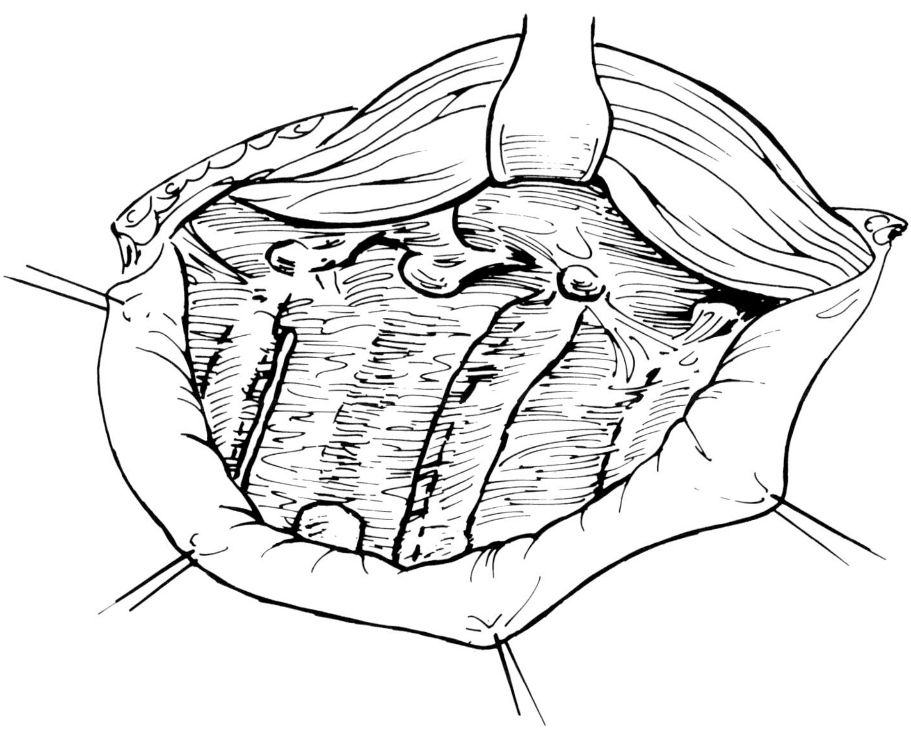

Figure 9A. The lateral transcavitary approach. The dissection and incision of a single rib more laterally than is normally the case for the lateral extracavitary approach, followed by its incision at the level of the costotransverse joint, provide access to the underlying fascia and parietal pleura.

B

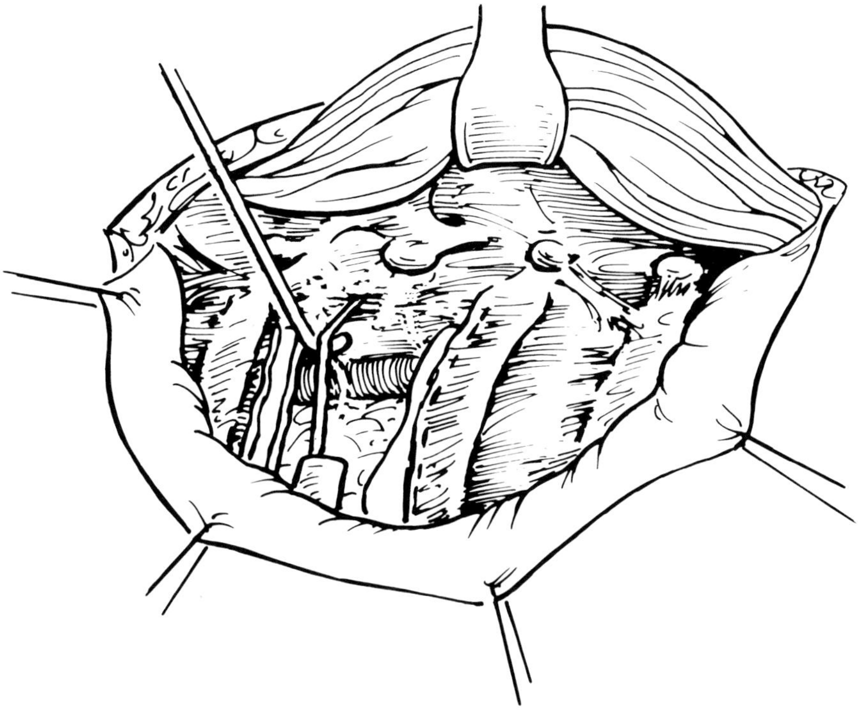

Figure 9B. The parietal pleura is then incised and the ribs spread with a self-retaining rib retractor. The intercostal nerve is followed to the neuroforamen. A clear view of the pathology and the relationships between the pathology and normal structures is achieved.

C

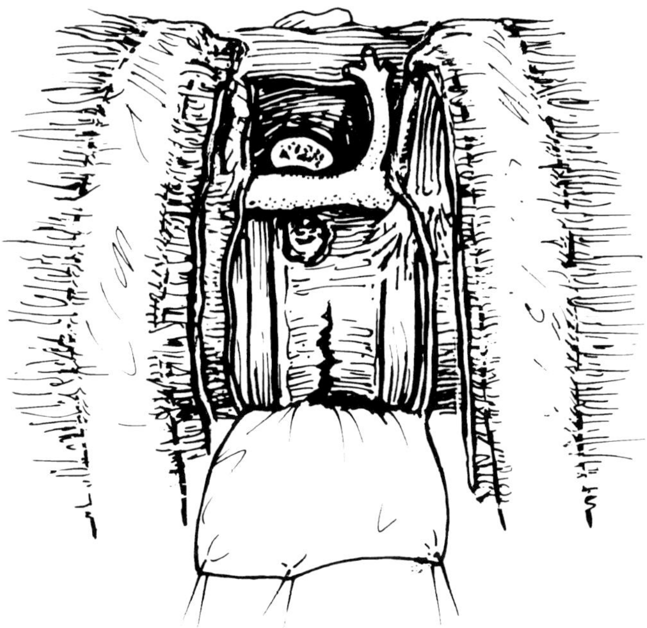

Figure 9C. A parietal pleura flap is then created by dissection in a subperiosteal fashion, providing visualization of the underlying pathology and normal tissue.

pathology and its relationship to the adjacent normal structures is defined clearly (Figure 9b).

Dissection of the parietal pleura from the lateral aspect of the spine in a flap-like manner gains access to the pathology (Figure 9c). The operation then proceeds as with the lateral extracavitary approach described previously in this chapter.

The wound is closed routinely. The ribs are approximated as they are for the ventrolateral transthoracic approaches (described in detail in Chapter 7). A tube thoracostomy is employed for several days.

Complications and Avoidance of Pitfalls

The degree of difficulty of the lateral extracavitary and lateral transcavitary exposures of the thoracic and lumbar spine should not be underestimated. Adequate surgical experience is required for the operation to be performed with facility. A working knowledge of the dorsal retroperitoneal anatomy is imperative.

Surgeon endurance is also necessary, because the operation may last 4 to 8 hours. Blood loss, particularly from epidural veins located in the recently decompressed ventral dural sac region and from bleeding medullary bone, can be excessive. Therefore, great care should be taken to minimize abdominal pressure during surgery by appropriate operative positioning.

References

1. Ausman JI, Malik GM, Dujovny M, et al: Three-quarter prone approach to the pineal-tentorial region. **Surg Neurol 29:**298-306, 1988

2. Benzel EC: The lateral extracavitary approach to the spine using the three-quarter prone position. **J Neurosurg 71:**837-841, 1989

3. Benzel EC, Larson SJ: Functional recovery after decompressive operation for thoracic and lumbar spine fractures. **Neurosurgery 19:**772-778, 1986

4. Benzel EC, Larson SJ: Operative stabilization of the posttraumatic thoracic and lumbar spine: a comparative analysis of the Harrington distraction rod and the modified Weiss spring. **Neurosurgery 19:**378-385, 1986

5. Bohlman HH, Eismont FJ: Surgical techniques of anterior decompression and fusion for spinal cord injuries. **Clin Orthop 154:**57-67, 1981

6. Capener N: The evolution of lateral rhachotomy. **J Bone Joint Surg (Br) 36:**173-179, 1954

7. Champlin AM, Rael J, Benzel EC, et al: Preoperative spinal angiography for lateral extracavitary approach to thoracic and lumbar spine. **AJNR 15:**73-74, 1994

8. Clark WK: Spinal cord decompression in spinal cord injury. **Clin Orthop 154:**9-13, 1981

9. Erickson DL, Leider LL, Brown WE: One-stage decompression-stabilization for thoracolumbar fractures. **Spine 2:**53-56, 1977

10. Larson SJ: Unstable thoracic fractures: treatment alternatives and the role of the neurosurgeon. **Clin Neurosurg 27:**624-640, 1980

11. Larson SJ, Holst RA, Hemmy DC, et al: Lateral extracavitary approach to traumatic lesions of the thoracic and lumbar spine. **J Neurosurg 45:**628-637, 1976

12. Morgan TH, Wharton GW, Austin GN, et al: The results of laminectomy in patients with incomplete spinal cord injuries. **Paraplegia 9:**14-23, 1971

13. Schmidek HH, Gomes FB, Seligson D, et al: Management of acute unstable thoracolumbar (T-11-L-1) fractures with and without neurological deficit. **Neurosurgery 7:**30-35, 1980

14. Schneider RC: Surgical indications and contraindications in spine and spinal cord trauma. **Clin Neurosurg 8:**157-184, 1962

15. Wagner FC Jr, Chehrazi B: Spinal cord injury: indications for operative intervention. **Surg Clin North Am 60:**1049-1054, 1980

16. Whitesides TE Jr, Alshah SGA: On the management of unstable fractures of the thoracolumbar spine. Rationale for use of anterior decompression and fusion and posterior stabilization. **Spine 1:**99-107, 1976

Chapter 10

Dorsal Exposures of the Thoracic and Lumbar Spine

Nevan G. Baldwin, MD

The dorsal approaches to the spine are the most commonly employed techniques. They are also the techniques with which nearly all spine surgeons are the most familiar. In this chapter, dorsal approaches are considered to be those operations performed between or through the erector spinae muscle columns. The various dorsal spine approaches include the standard midline dissection (such as for laminectomy), the transpedicular approach, costotransversectomy, and lateral approaches to the far lateral disc. A broad range of pathology can be addressed via these approaches, and they are perhaps the most technically simple methods (Figure 1).

Early spine surgery consisted of predominantly dorsal exposures of the spine. With technical advances, most importantly in the areas of spinal instrumentation and anesthesia, the range of conditions treated with these approaches has continued to broaden. Dorsal techniques are suitable for use in cases of trauma, degenerative or neoplastic diseases, vascular disorders, congenital deformities, and the treatment of painful conditions and spasticity. Dorsal spine exposures are so simple and so familiar that the surgeon should probably view the decision-making process in terms of the question, "When should I not use a dorsal approach?"

Anatomy

While the general anatomy of the dorsal spine is familiar to all spine surgeons, certain nuances warrant emphasis. The blood supply of the thoracic and lumbar spine arises from segmental branches of the aorta to the L4 level. The sacrum and the L5 vertebra usually derive their blood supply from branches of the sacroiliolumbar system, which arises from branches of the internal iliac arteries.[8,9]

Arterial Anatomy

As they proceed dorsally, the segmental arteries divide into dorsal and lateral components. The dorsal branches pass lateral to the intervertebral foramen where they give rise to a spinal branch that passes through the foramen into the spinal canal. This spinal branch often consists of multiple small trunks that follow a parallel course into the foramen. The dorsal branch continues along the lateral aspect of the spine, providing blood supply to the pars inter-

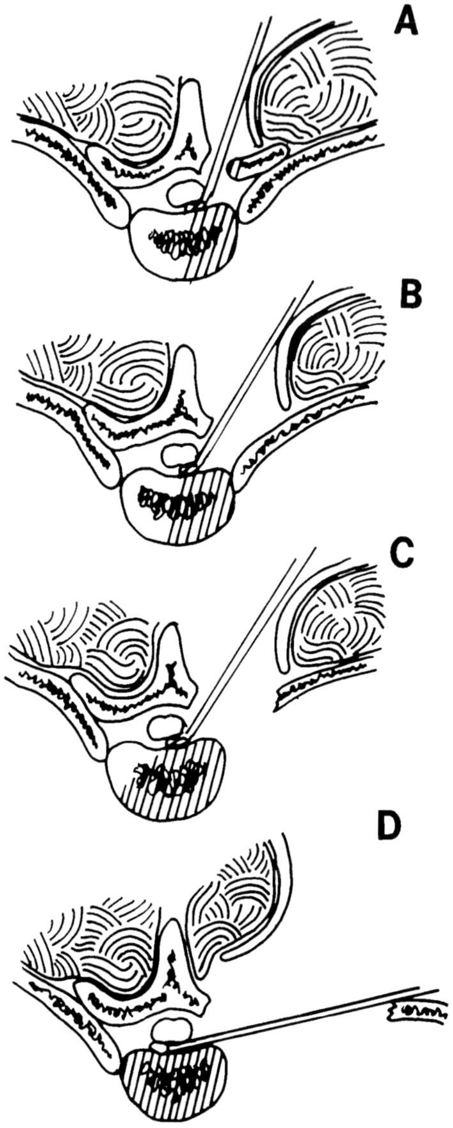

Figure 1. A variety of dorsal spinal approaches are useful to address pathology of the dorsal spinal elements as well as the vertebral body. Laminectomy allows access to a portion of the vertebral body **(A).** The transpedicular approach can be used to access more of the vertebra **(B)** and still more can be addressed with a costotransversectomy **(C).** If necessary, essentially the entire vertebral body is accessible with conversion to a lateral extracavitary approach **(D).** This is accomplished by simply mobilizing the erector spinae musculature and reflecting these muscles medially.

articularis, the facets, and the lamina. An anastomotic vascular network lies outside the neuroforamina (Figure 2A) and a second network is found in the extradural space within the spinal canal (Figure 2B). If sacrifice of the segmental vessels is required, dividing them as closely as possible to the aorta leaves the anastomotic network intact. In these cases, the use of a more ventral approach helps minimize the incidence of complications.

The richest blood supply of the spinal

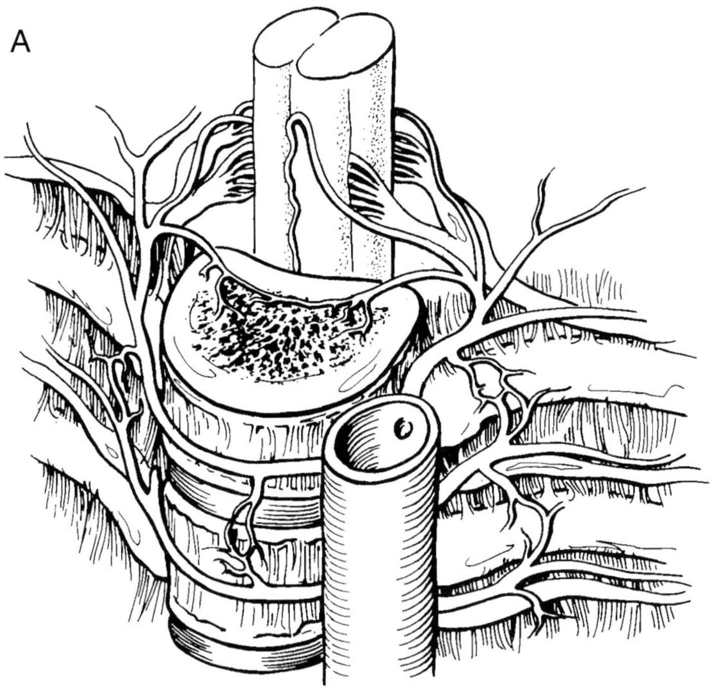

Figure 2A. The arterial supply to the spinal column and the spinal cord arises from the paired intersegmental branches of the aorta. An anastomotic network among these arteries is located proximal to their passage through the neuroforamina. If arterial vessels must be sacrificed during surgery, they should be taken as close to the aorta as possible to avoid disrupting this vascular network.

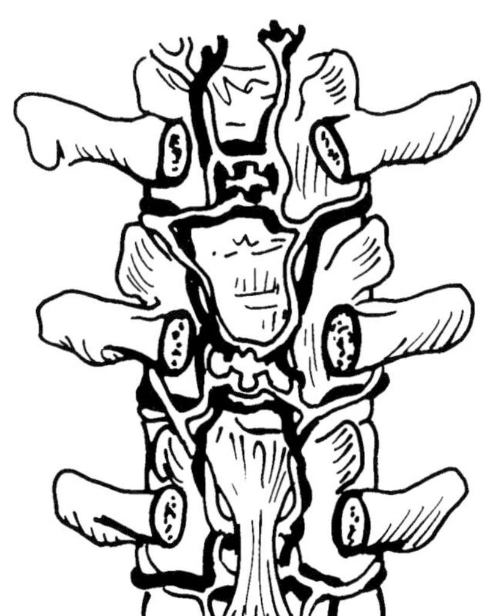

Figure 2B. The anastomotic network of arterial feeding vessels to the spine *(arteries shown in white)* also has an intracanalicular portion. The intracanalicular vessels are shown from a dorsal view with the facet joints and laminae removed. Batson's venous plexus *(veins shown in black)* is a rich anastomotic network of valveless veins draining blood from all spinal components, including the spinal cord, bony elements, and soft tissues.

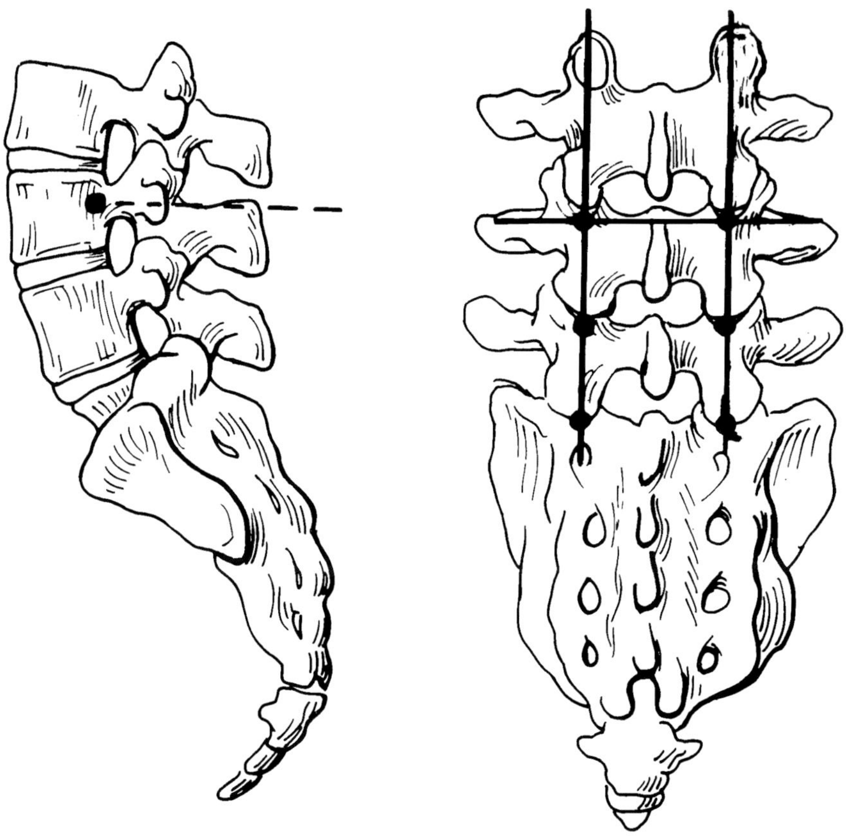

Figure 3. In the lumbar spine, the position of the pedicle is indicated by the intersection of lines drawn through the central axis of the transverse process and the long axis of the superior articular process. In most instances, the pedicle can be reliably localized using these landmarks.

column is in the cervical and lumbar regions, whereas the poorest supply is usually found between the T4 and T9 levels. A large radiculomedullary artery, the artery of Adamkiewicz, is often observed in the region of T9-11, usually arising on the left side.[6] While preservation of this artery is critical in surgical procedures, its patency does not guarantee that adequate spinal cord blood flow will be maintained. If a transpedicular approach is planned adjacent to this vessel, the soft tissues in the foramina must be protected as the pedicle is isolated and the drilling begun. Similarly, if a costotransversectomy is performed, the rib must be dissected free of all surrounding soft tissues before removal. This prevents inadvertent stretching and possible injury to the artery as the rib is disarticulated. The minimization of the disruption of the vessels and prevention of hypotension during surgery are the best methods of minimizing vascular complications.

Venous Anatomy

The venous drainage of the spinal cord flows into Batson's plexus, which consists of a group of veins extending from the occiput to the coccyx. These veins are nonvalved

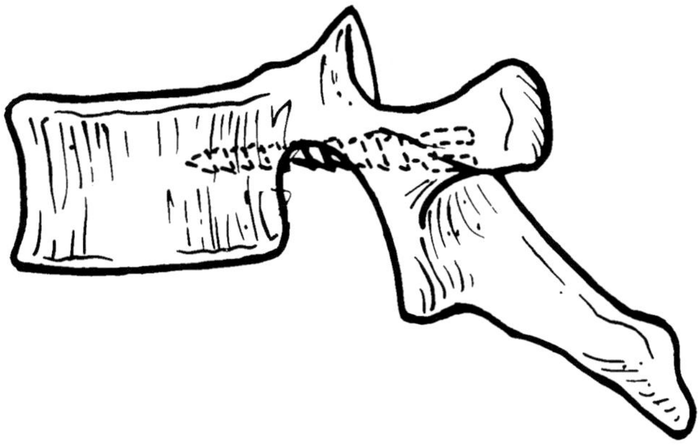

Figure 4. In the thoracic spine, the transverse process commonly does not align directly with the pedicle in the axial plane. In the vertebra depicted, the transverse process more closely aligns with the neuroforamen than with the pedicle, making the usual anatomical landmarks for screw insertion unsafe for that purpose.

and communicate directly with the azygos and vena cava systems (Figure 2B).[6] The three contributing portions of Batson's plexus include: the extradural vertebral veins, an extravertebral venous plexus (segmental veins of the neck, chest, lumbar region, pelvis, inferior vena cava), and the veins draining the bony elements of the spinal column. Because of this rich anastomotic network of venous drainage, venous insufficiency is seldom observed in spinal surgery, except in the case of vascular malformations.

Bony Anatomy

In the lumbar spine, the bony anatomy is relatively constant. The pedicles are broad in both their sagittal and coronal diameters. The pedicles are also located consistently at the intersection of the vertical line drawn through the superior articular process of a vertebra and the "horizontal" through the middle of the transverse process (Figure 3). These landmarks are commonly used in the placement of spinal instrumentation. The transverse processes are, however, occasionally found in an anomalous position, either more rostral or caudal to their usual location. If the surgical plan involves the use of these landmarks for instrumentation placement, inspection of plain x-rays should always be carried out preoperatively because the anteroposterior view will readily identify an anomalous transverse process.

The bony anatomy of the thoracic spine varies considerably from that of the lumbar region. The pedicles of the thoracic spine have broad sagittal diameters, but are much thinner in the coronal dimension than their lumbar counterparts. Whereas the long axis of the lumbar pedicles projects (in the sagittal plane) parallel to the vertebral body endplate, the thoracic pedicles vary in their angular relationship to the endplate. The sagittal angle of the thoracic pedicle varies throughout the thoracic spine, and there is significant variability among patients as well.

The position of the transverse processes of the thoracic spine does not reliably indicate the position of the vertebral pedicle. In portions of this spinal region, alignment of the pedicle and the transverse process shifts such that the middle of the transverse process can actually align more closely with the foramen than with the pedicle. Therefore, the relationship of the transverse process and pedicles cannot be safely used for the placement of spinal instrumentation (Figure 4).

The spinal musculature encountered with the dorsal spine approaches consists predominantly of the erector spinae muscle

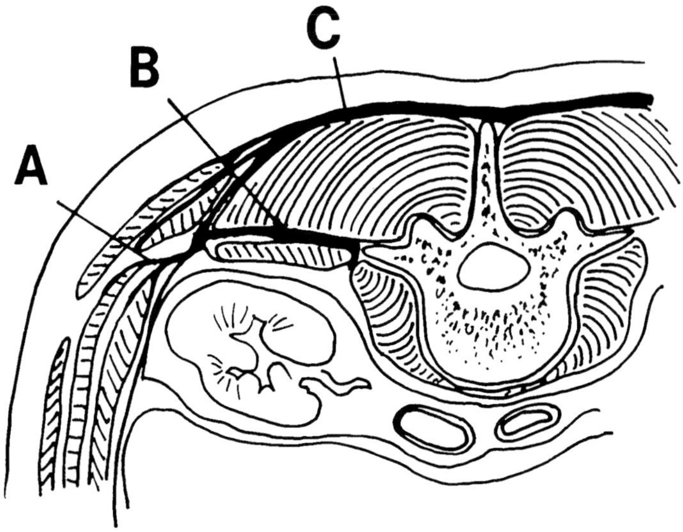

Figure 5. The aponeurosis of the abdominal muscles (A) fuses into the ventral (B) and dorsal (C) layers of the investing fascia surrounding the erector spinae musculature. These fascial planes allow the erector spinae muscle group to be mobilized from either medial to lateral or lateral to medial, as needed for surgical exposure.

column. This muscle column is invested by fascia, both ventrally and dorsally (Figure 5). The dorsal layer constitutes the thoracolumbar or thoracodorsal fascia. It is thin in the thoracic region, but becomes thicker in the lumbar region. Laterally, the thoracodorsal fascia fuses with the aponeurosis of the transversus abdominis muscle; caudally, it attaches to the iliac crest and the lateral crest of the sacrum. The ventral layer of the fascia surrounding the erector spinae muscle column is attached medially to the transverse processes of the spine and fuses laterally with the aponeurosis of the transversus abdominis muscle. This layer thickens between the 12th rib and the L1 vertebra to become the posterior lumbocostal ligament.[12]

Nerve Root Anatomy

The nerve roots coursing out of the lumbar spine pass immediately ventral to the transverse processes of the next lower spinal level. The intertransversarii muscle and its aponeurosis form a bridge between each adjacent pair of transverse processes. Therefore, dissection to expose the transverse processes carries very little risk of injury to the nerve roots if the plane of dissection is maintained dorsal to this muscle layer.

Additional risk may be posed to the nerve roots during dissection to expose the transverse processes in the patient with a scoliotic curvature. In this patient, the biomechanical principle of spinal motion coupling dictates that if there is lateral bending deformity, there must also be a component of axial plane rotation.[11] In the lumbar region, the transverse processes on the concave side of the curve are rotated ventrally. A resultant dorsal displacement of the nerve roots can therefore exist. Laxity of the intertransversarii muscles can allow the nerve roots to course more superficially in the space between adjacent transverse processes (Figure 6). The roots may also occupy a more lateral position in these patients, passing lateral to the tip of the transverse process. In such situations, dissection to expose the transverse process can more readily result in neural injury.

In the thoracic spine, the articulation of the rib varies with regard to its relationship to the transverse process. In the upper thoracic region, the rib aligns directly with the transverse process. In the mid- and low thoracic

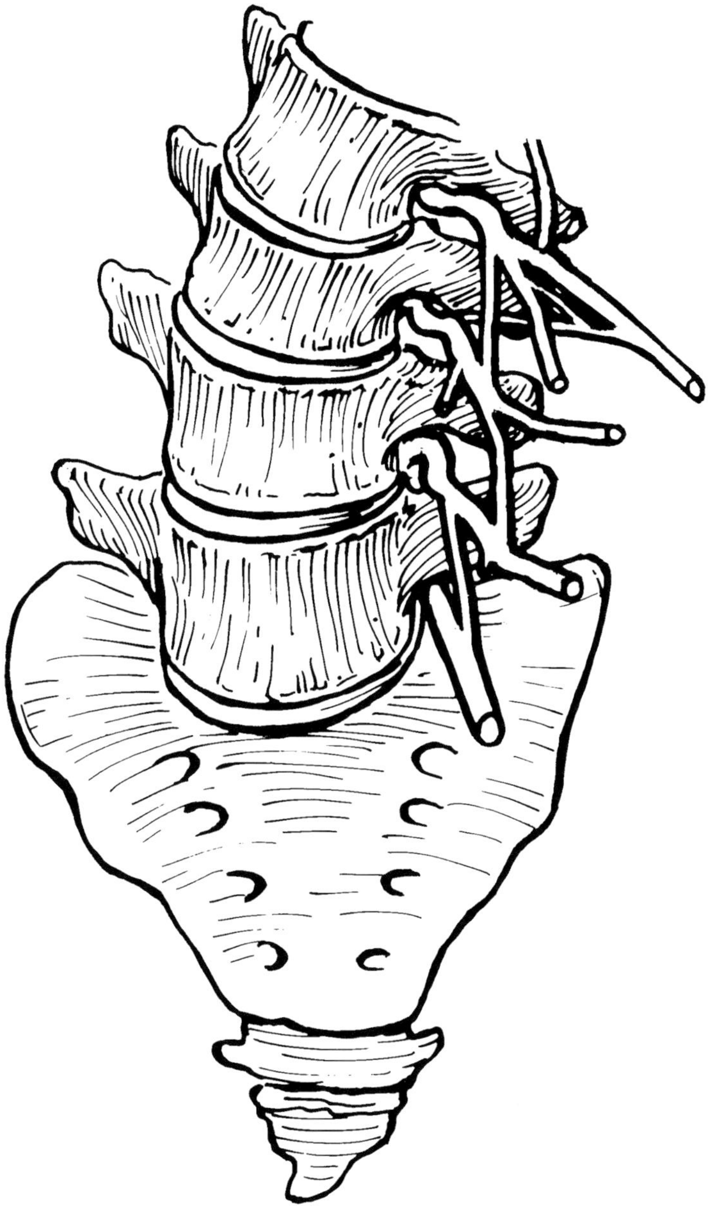

Figure 6. Each nerve root coursing out of the lumbar and lower thoracic spine normally passes ventral to the transverse process of the next caudal segment. When scoliotic deformities are present, there is also axial plane rotation of the vertebrae. Rotation of the transverse processes ventrally causes the nerves to be more superficial in the intertransverse spaces, thereby rendering the nerve roots more susceptible to injury during dissection to expose the transverse processes.

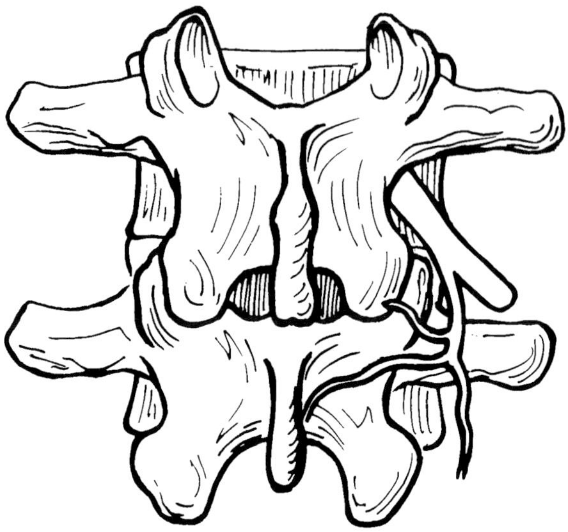

Figure 7. Facet joint innervation arises from the dorsal branch of the nerve root at the foramen. The dorsal branch of the exiting nerve root gives off an articular branch, which passes along the rostral portion of the transverse process and the lateral aspect of the superior articular process to reach the facet joint.

regions, the ribs articulate slightly more rostrally, passing along the ventrorostral surface of the transverse processes. The sympathetic chain is located immediately ventral to the transverse processes, between the pleura and the spine. When the pleura is reflected ventrally during surgery, the sympathetic ganglia are often found on the pleural surface, rather than on the spine.

The innervation of the facet joints is provided by dorsal branches of the nerve roots as they exit the foramina. The dorsal branch of a given nerve root passes through the caudal aspect of the foramen, where it turns dorsally, piercing the intertransverse ligament. It then branches, and the articular branch passes along the lateral aspect of the superior articular process and into the facet joint capsule at the lateral and caudal surfaces of the joint (Figure 7).[4] The remainder of the dorsal branch passes further dorsally to innervate the deep and medial paraspinous musculature. A small area of skin receives sensory innervation from the dorsal branches of the L1, L2, and L3 nerve roots.[4]

Techniques of Dorsal Spinal Exposures

The direct dorsal midline approach is the most commonly used exposure in spinal surgery. The details of this technique are familiar to all spine surgeons and, therefore, are not covered here. One caveat, though, is associated with dissection in the presence of bony destruction by tumor, trauma, infection, or intrinsic bone disease: blunt dissection with periosteal elevators should be avoided. Pressure placed on an unstable spine or poor quality bone during dissection can result in catastrophic neural injury. In such patients, electrocautery or sharp dissection should be employed.

Transpedicular Approach

Indications

The indications for use of the transpedicular approach include: tumor or infection of the pedicle and/or vertebral body, vertebral body fractures having dorsally displaced fragments with spinal canal compromise, or a herniated disc. It can be used for the entire thoracic region and down to the L2 level. Below the level of the conus medullaris, the thecal sac can be safely retracted. Therefore, in the lumbar region, this approach is needed only in instances where the pedicles are involved by the pathology.

This approach has limited usefulness for thoracic disc surgery because of the limited angle of view ventral to the thecal sac. It is useful, however, in the case of a disc that is eccentric to one side and that does not appear to be significantly calcified. Discs that are calcified often have eroded the dura mater and subsequently become adherent to it by scar formation. With a limited ventral view, manipulation of disc fragments is dangerous and an alternative approach is preferable. If the artery of Adamkiewicz is located at the foramen involved by the disc herniation, this approach may be ideal because the risk of vascular injury is less than that of a more lateral approach. The pedicle through which a disc should be approached is that of the vertebral body caudal to the herniation.

Technique

The operative preparation of the patient for the transpedicular approach includes placement of a Foley catheter, anti-embolic stockings, and prone positioning. For patients with spinal instability, placement on chest rolls or a spinal surgery frame that maintains the neutral position is required. Attention should be given to the need for intraoperative x-rays. Devices that limit the radiographic view should be avoided. In the patient with no instability, a frame that allows flexion may be preferable. Securing the patient's position with tape is also advisable, since rotation of the table during surgery may improve the surgeon's view of the pathology. Confirmation of the correct spinal level is accomplished with x-ray as the exposure proceeds.

The pedicle can be entered directly by drilling through the dorsal aspect of the pars interarticularis at its junction with the superior articular process. For those having less experience with this approach or in instances where the anatomy is obscured by the pathology, performing a laminectomy or laminotomy will help to readily locate the pedicle. Remnants of the ligamentum flavum are removed to more fully expose the lateral margin of the thecal sac, the nerve roots, and the pedicle. The pars interarticularis and its associated superior facet are removed using either a high-speed air drill or rongeurs. As the neuroforamen is exposed, caution must be exercised to prevent injury to neural or vascular structures. The pedicle is then carefully drilled away. Drilling the internal portion of the pedicle first and later removing the outer cortical part provide a margin of safety regarding the prevention of injury to nearby structures. After thinning the cortical bone from the inner cancellous surface, pituitary forceps or curettes can be used to remove the remainder of the pedicle. Following removal of the pedicle, the vertebral body or the adjacent disc are easily entered. If no arteries are present in the foramen, sacrifice of a thoracic nerve proximal to the dorsal root ganglion can be accomplished with no significant risk. This often affords a considerably improved view of the vertebral body and disc. Fractured bony fragments can be easily impacted ventrally using a reverse-angled curette or fragment impactors that are manufactured for this purpose. Biopsy or tumor resection can be performed with ease as well.

After addressing the pathology, the issue of stability also must be considered. If necessary, a bone graft can be placed via this type of exposure. For unilateral transpedicular approaches, unless a substantial portion of the vertebral body is resected or weakened by the disease process, the spine should be stable. If the approach is bilateral and/or aggressive resection of the vertebral body has been performed, stabilization may be required. Further discussion regarding issues of stability is found in any textbook on biomechanics. A particularly straightforward approach to this problem has been presented by Benzel.[1]

Costotransversectomy

Indications

Indications for a costotransversectomy are essentially the same as those for the transpedicular approach. The costotransversectomy can also be used for thoracic sympathectomy and is useful in many instances where the pathology extends along the lateral margin of the spine. For the purposes of this chapter, costotransversectomy is considered to be an approach performed medial to the erector spinae muscles. Although the costotransversectomy is sometimes described to include dissection lateral to these muscles,[10] the more lateral trajectory is considered to be in the realm of the lateral extracavitary approach discussed herein.

Technique

The positioning and preparation for the costotransversectomy approach is essentially the same as that for the transpedicular approach. Because this operation requires removal of a proximal rib segment, there is some risk of injury to small vessels near the spine. A preoperative spinal angiogram is recommended so that the artery of Adamkiewicz can be identified and preserved.

The incision can be made in the midline or a few centimeters lateral to midline. If a bilateral operation is planned, such as sympathectomies for hyperhidrosis, then a midline incision is optimal. For unilateral procedures, a vertical incision 3 cm lateral to the midline works well. An x-ray obtained at the time of positioning or the use of a marker placed preoperatively assists with proper placement of the incision.

After making the incision, dissection is carried medial to the erector spinae muscles along the spinous process and lamina. The rib of interest is exposed and the dissection continued one level above and one below this rib to reflect the erector spinae muscles laterally. An x-ray is obtained to identify the proper spinal level. The neurovascular bundle of this level is then located. The rib to be removed is stripped of periosteum by first using electrocautery along the dorsum to open the layer, followed by circumferentially stripping with periosteal elevators. The rib is then divided at the lateral extent of resection, using a rib cutter. For a sympathectomy, only a few centimeters of rib are removed. If broader exposure is needed, such as for a large tumor, a larger amount of rib should be resected. The costotransverse joint is sharply incised and the transverse process removed with rongeurs. The rib segment can be manipulated to open the joint as the incision is performed, allowing further removal of periosteum from the ventral surface of the rib at its proximal end. Removal of the rib segment is completed with rongeurs. Alternatively, the rib can be manually disarticulated, but this causes more blood loss than a piecemeal resection. Some bleeding always occurs as the rib is removed but this is easily controlled by packing with Gelfoam or Surgicel. The neurovascular bundle is followed medially to the neuroforamen, and the pedicle is then cleared of the remaining soft tissues in order to obtain a clear view of the local anatomy and a complete exposure of the relevant local landmarks.

The pathology can be addressed as needed following completion of this exposure. During a costotransversectomy, if the need for a more lateral view arises, the operation is easily converted to a lateral extracavitary approach by dissecting along the dorsum of the erector spinae musculature and then reflecting the muscles medially. Removal of a second rib will likewise provide the necessary exposure in some instances.

Approaches for the Lateral Herniated Disc

With the development of high-resolution computed tomography (CT) and magnetic resonance imaging (MRI), the diagnosis of lateral and far lateral disc herniation has been facilitated. Before the availability of these imaging methods, the diagnosis of lateral disc herniations rested solely on clinical, electromyographic, and nerve conduction findings.

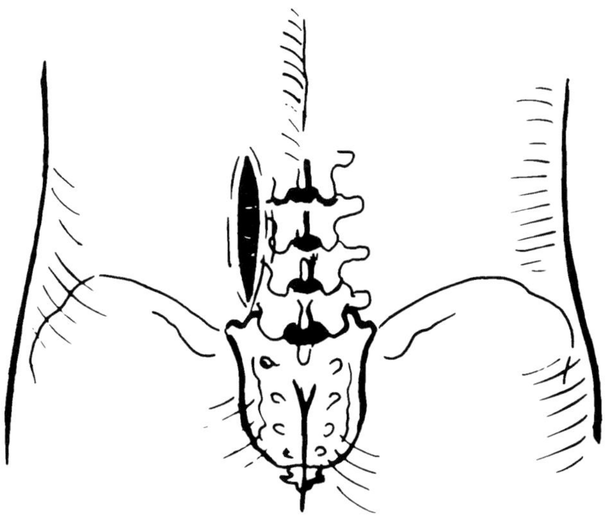

Figure 8. A far lateral disc herniation can be managed by use of a paramedian incision and a muscle-splitting approach through the erector spinae muscle column. This allows excellent visualization of the lateral aspect of the intervertebral disc and neuroforamen while minimizing the difficulty of exposure due to the ilium. At the L5 or L5-S1 levels, this is perhaps the optimal technique.

Myelography does not routinely demonstrate lateral disc herniations well because the pathology is beyond the lateral extent of the dural root sleeve. Maroon et al[7] have suggested that discography with postdiscography CT is the most sensitive diagnostic method for this condition. With more recent improvements in the quality of MRI, the most accurate diagnostic method at the present time is debatable. However, because MRI is noninvasive, it is the initial procedure of choice for most surgeons. Discography with CT should be reserved for cases in which the MRI is negative and strong clinical suspicion exists.

Surgery for lateral disc herniations can be performed using either a midline or lateral approach. With lateral approaches to the discs of the lumbosacral junction (L5-S1) or the last lumbar (L4-5) level, the iliac crest may pose a barrier to adequate exposure. To avoid this problem, the use of a paramedian incision only 4 cm from the midline along with a muscle-splitting dissection of the erector spinae muscle group maintains an angle of view medial to the iliac crest and provides excellent visualization of the disc lateral to the neuroforamen (Figure 8).[7]

An alternative technique of lateral discectomy is accomplished by using a transverse incision placed over the level of the herniated disc. Dissection in the plane between the erector spinae and the quadratus lumborum muscles exposes the transverse processes. A table-mounted retractor is used to reflect the erector spinae muscles medially and dorsally. The operating microscope may then be brought into the field. Firm retraction, best achieved with a table-mounted system, is a key to this approach. With adequate retraction, the angle of view is then essentially the same as that of the muscle-splitting technique. The nerve root is identified by dissection between the transverse processes and followed medially to the lateral aspect of the neuroforamen. Confirmation on x-ray of the appropriate level is obtained as the disc is cleared of overlying soft tissue. Discectomy is then performed in the routine fashion.

Jane and colleagues[3] have described another approach to a lateral disc herniation (Figure 9). This method starts with a midline

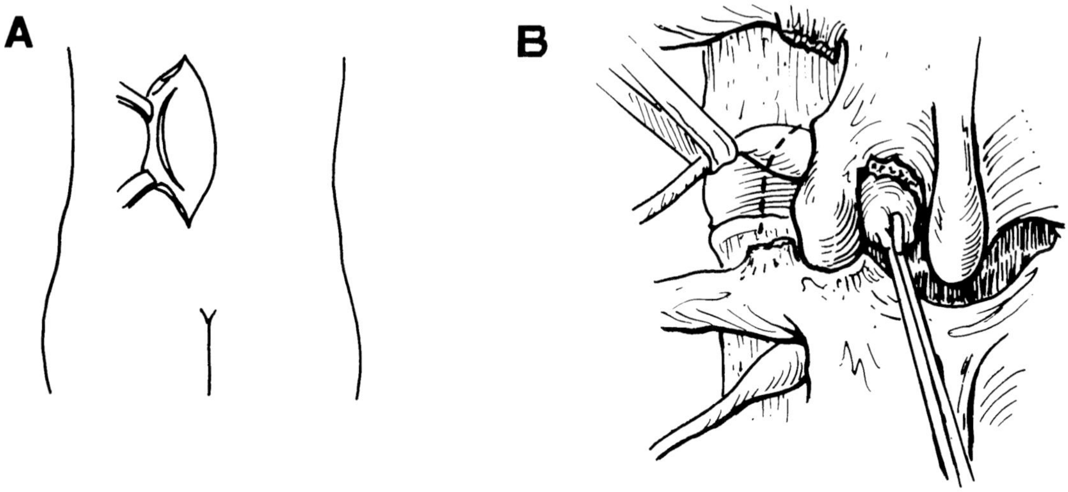

Figure 9. The combined medial and lateral approach described by Jane et al[3] begins with a midline dissection down to the lumbodorsal fascia. The fascia is incised in an arc **(A)**. The completed exposure **(B)** is shown, reflecting the paraspinous musculature, hemilaminotomy, removal of the lateral portion of the superior facet (*dashed line* represents original lateral border of the superior facet), and removal of the intertransversarii muscle. With this approach, the neuroforamen can be decompressed both medially and laterally.

skin incision, dissection to the fascia, and then the opening of the lumbodorsal fascia in a gentle arc away from the spinous processes. The musculature is dissected from the spinous processes and reflected laterally. The ligamentum flavum is opened while x-ray confirmation of dissection at the appropriate level is obtained. A small hemilaminotomy is made and the spinal musculature is reflected further laterally, exposing the transverse process rostral and caudal to the herniated disc. The lateral portion of the superior facet of the caudal vertebral body is removed to clearly visualize the foramen. The intertransversarii muscle is dissected from the transverse process rostral to the disc, thereby exposing the underlying nerve root. The root is then protected while discectomy is performed. This approach allows for removal of disc material from a lateral orientation, as well as medially through the laminotomy site. A significant advantage of this technique is that the foramen is easily explored from the medial and lateral aspect, thus ascertaining that the nerve root is free while the facet joint remains functionally intact.

In the patient with a lateral disc herniation, preoperative inspection of plain x-rays of the spine is particularly important. In some cases, particularly in patients with advanced degenerative changes of the spine, adequate decompression of the nerve root is difficult without resection of a substantial portion of the facet joint. It is therefore important to inspect x-ray films for the presence of a defect in the pars interarticularis, particularly on the side opposite to the disc herniation. If a contralateral pars defect is noted, the approach should be tailored to preserve the facet joint to the greatest extent possible. Alternatively, consideration should be given to the performance of an arthrodesis at the time of discectomy.

Summary

The variety of surgical approaches to the spine represent a continuum. The key to a better operation may, in some instances, be the conversion of one approach into another or the melding of two or more approaches to enhance the surgical exposure. When operating via a dorsal approach, conversion to a more lateral direction is usually a simple matter of lengthening the incision. Alternatively, the incision can be made into the shape of a T or a hockey stick.

As is the case with incisions, there are many ways to manage the erector spinae musculature in the surgical field. Perhaps the simplest method is to lengthen the dissection along the medial aspect of the muscles, thereby allowing lateral mobilization without undue retractor pressure. If this proves impractical, dissection can be carried along the dorsal aspect of the muscles out to their lateral margin. They can then be reflected medially. The muscle fibers can also be split longitudinally, or the muscle can be divided in a transverse direction and later reapproximated.[2,5,10]

A dorsal approach to the spine should be used in any case where it is felt that the pathology will be adequately addressed by this technique. In instances where one is not certain that a dorsal approach will suffice, it may often be reasonable to begin with a dorsal exposure and to convert to another technique if necessary.

References

1. Benzel EC: Destabilizing effects of spinal surgery, in Benzel EC (ed): **Biomechanics of Spine Stabilization: Principles and Clinical Practice**. New York: McGraw-Hill, 1995, pp 97-102
2. Chan DPK, Whitesides TE Jr, Spetzler RF: Surgical approaches to the spine and bone grafts in spinal surgery, in Evarts CM (ed): **Surgery of the Musculoskeletal System, ed 2.** New York: Churchill Livingstone, 1990, pp 1817-1856
3. Jane JA, Haworth CS, Broaddus WC, et al: A neurosurgical approach to far-lateral disc herniation. Technical note. **J Neurosurg 72**:143-144, 1990
4. Kennemore DE: Percutaneous radio-frequency denervation of spinal facets, in Wilkins RH, Rengachary SS (eds): **Neurosurgery**. New York: McGraw-Hill, 1985, pp 2427-2429
5. Larson SJ: The lateral extrapleural and extraperitoneal approaches to the thoracic and lumbar spine, in Ruge D, Wiltse LL (eds): **Spinal Disorders: Diagnosis and Treatment**. Philadelphia: Lea & Febiger, 1977, pp 137-141
6. Leventhal MR: Spinal anatomy and surgical approaches, in Crenshaw AH (ed): **Campbell's Operative Orthopaedics**. St. Louis: Mosby Year Book, 1992, pp 3493-3516
7. Maroon JC, Kopitnik TA, Schulhof LA, et al: Diagnosis and microsurgical approach to far-lateral disc herniation in the lumbar spine. **J Neurosurg 72**: 378-382, 1990
8. Parke WW: Applied anatomy of the spine, in Rothman RH, Simeone FA (eds): **The Spine, ed 3.** Philadelphia: WB Saunders, 1992, pp 35-88
9. Rengachary SS: Surgical anatomy of the sacrum, in Doty JR, Rengachary SS (eds): **Surgical Disorders of the Sacrum**. New York: Thieme Medical, 1994, pp 21-33
10. Simeone FA, Rashbaum R: Transthoracic disc excision, in Schmidek HH, Sweet WH (eds): **Operative Neurosurgical Techniques**. Philadelphia: WB Saunders, 1988, pp 1367-1374
11. White AA III, Panjabi MM: **Clinical Biomechanics of the Spine**. Philadelphia: JB Lippincott, 1990
12. Woodburne RT: **Essentials of Human Anatomy**. New York: Oxford University Press, 1978, pp 283-303

Chapter 11

Operative Positioning and Retraction

Charles L. Branch Jr, MD

For surgical exposure of the spine, positioning of the patient in the operating room and subsequent retraction of the tissues play extremely important roles in the ultimate success of the surgical procedure. Careful consideration of the positioning of the patient with the use of support devices not only may enhance or allow for certain exposures of the spine, but may contribute to or prevent associated injuries to peripheral nerves or other structures during the procedure. Knowledge of and appropriate selection of retraction devices is also key to the adequate exposure of the spinal structures involved, and may play a role in the prevention of injury to the associated structures.

After the surgeon has decided upon a particular approach to the spine, the following considerations should be addressed:

1. Are there special anesthesia requirements (fiberoptic nasal or oral intubation, an armored endotracheal tube, single lung ventilation)?
2. Is a specialized spine surgery table or support required?
3. Is intraoperative radiographic imaging planned and, if so, will this affect the choice of operating table or support?
4. Is the stability of the patient's spine such that special precautions are required during the transfer to the operating table from the patient's bed?
5. If a table-mounted retraction system is to be used, is the operating table compatible with this retraction system?

Such a review, performed 2 or 3 days prior to the proposed procedure, may prevent unnecessary delays or other problems. Therefore, a region- and operation-specific approach to retraction and positioning is undertaken here.

Transoral Exposure

The patient is positioned in the supine position, generally with the head fixed via a three-point fixation device in an extended position. A major consideration is the avoidance of extreme extension in the patient with an unstable cervical spine. On the other hand, adequate extension must be accom-

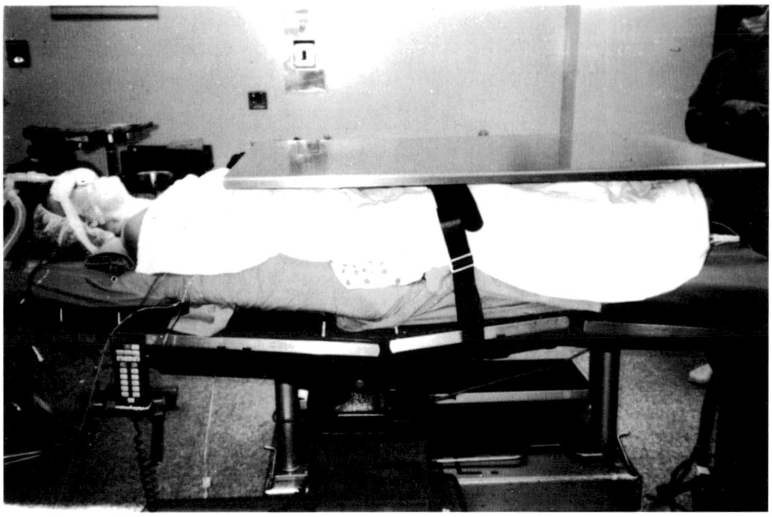

Figure 1. Operative positioning for the ventral exposure of the upper cervical spine. Note that the table is flexed at the back and at the knees.

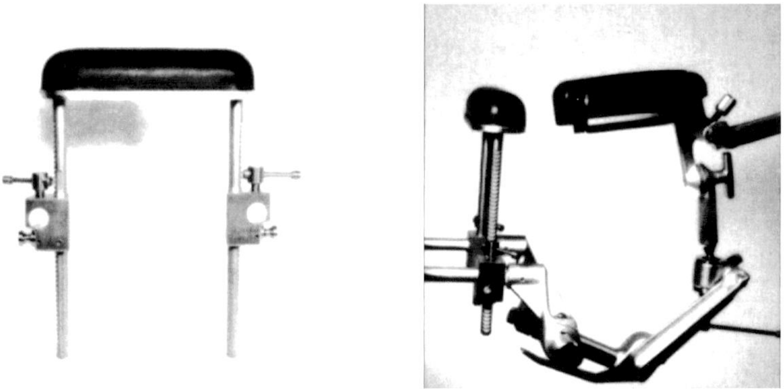

Figure 2. A dorsal cervical support, such as the Mayfield headrest system **(right)** with the P.C.S. **(left)**, may be utilized to provide midcervical spine stability intraoperatively. (Courtesy of Ohio Medical Instrument Company, Inc)

plished in order to facilitate visualization of the dorsal pharynx through this approach. The remainder of the operating table is flexed at the patient's back and knees. Since lateral intraoperative radiographic imaging is generally used for this approach, the fluoroscope is positioned at the beginning of the procedure and included in the draping of the field. If anteroposterior imaging is planned, consideration of the position and affect of the three-point fixation device upon radiographic imaging has to be addressed prior to the initiation of the procedure.

Two basic transoral retraction systems include the self-retaining retractor that is fixed on the upper and lower teeth or jaw with a ring, around which are fixed other palatal or lateral retraction blades. An example of this type of retractor is the Crockard transoral retractor (Codman Shurtleff, Inc,

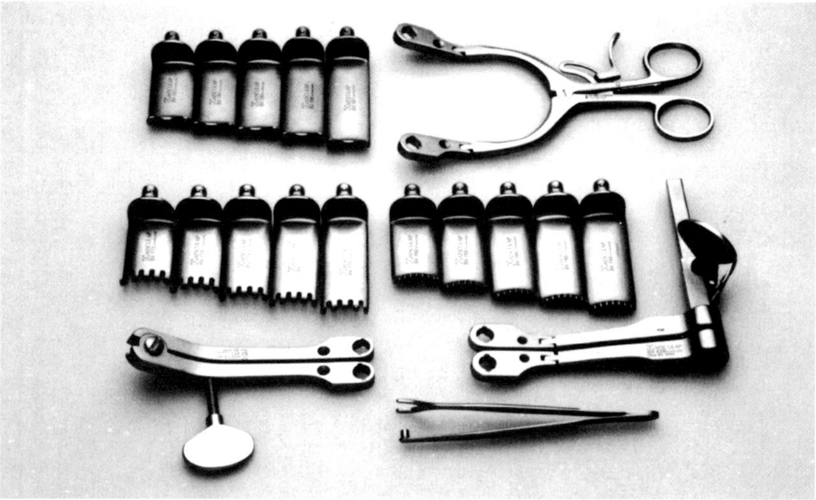

Figure 3. The Caspar cervical spine retractors. (Courtesy of Aesculap)

Randolph, Massachusetts). An alternative device is a table-mounted unit that uses a post attached to the operating table as the point of fixation from which the retractor blades are subsequently attached. The Sonntag transoral retractor (Aesculap, Burlingame, California) and the Farley retractor (Thompson Surgical Instruments, Traverse City, Michigan) are examples of this style of retractor.

Ventral Cervical Exposure

The ventral approach to the lower cervical spine (from C2 through the cervicothoracic junction), using either a transverse or longitudinal incision, is generally performed with the patient in the supine position (Figure 1). A bolster beneath the cervical spine may be created with a towel or by using a custom gel or inflatable pad. While for the majority of these cases no specialized apparatus is required, occasionally there are special requirements mandating the use of traction, a horseshoe headholder, and a specialized bolster. If the application of significant intraoperative cervical traction is anticipated and the patient requires the application of Gardner-Wells tongs or a halo ring, the procedure is best performed with a traction pulley attachment. An example of this is the Mayfield horseshoe headrest system with the Papadopoulos Cervical Spine Support (P.C.S.) (Ohio Medical Instrument Company, Inc, Cincinnati, Ohio) (Figure 2). A dorsal cervical support may then be elevated or lowered to support the dorsal aspect of the cervical spine during the fusion procedure. These components are not radiolucent and, therefore, if anteroposterior imaging is anticipated (such as with ventral screw fixation of the odontoid), then an attempt to visualize this region should be made prior to initiation of the surgical procedure.

The placement of a longitudinal bolster in the interscapular region that allows for dorsal movement of the scapula and humerus augments visualization of the C6 and C7 regions. Care should be taken to not place excessive stress on the brachial plexus if a bolster is used for this procedure. For this procedure and all procedures in the supine position, the table is flexed both at the patient's low back and knees to avoid a perfectly flat surface for an extended procedure.

Retraction systems fall into two categories: self-retaining and table-mounted. The most commonly used self-retaining retractors are the Caspar retractors (Aesculap) and the Cloward retractors (Codman). These retractors use a force against opposing tissue surfaces to maintain exposure (Figure 3).

A

B

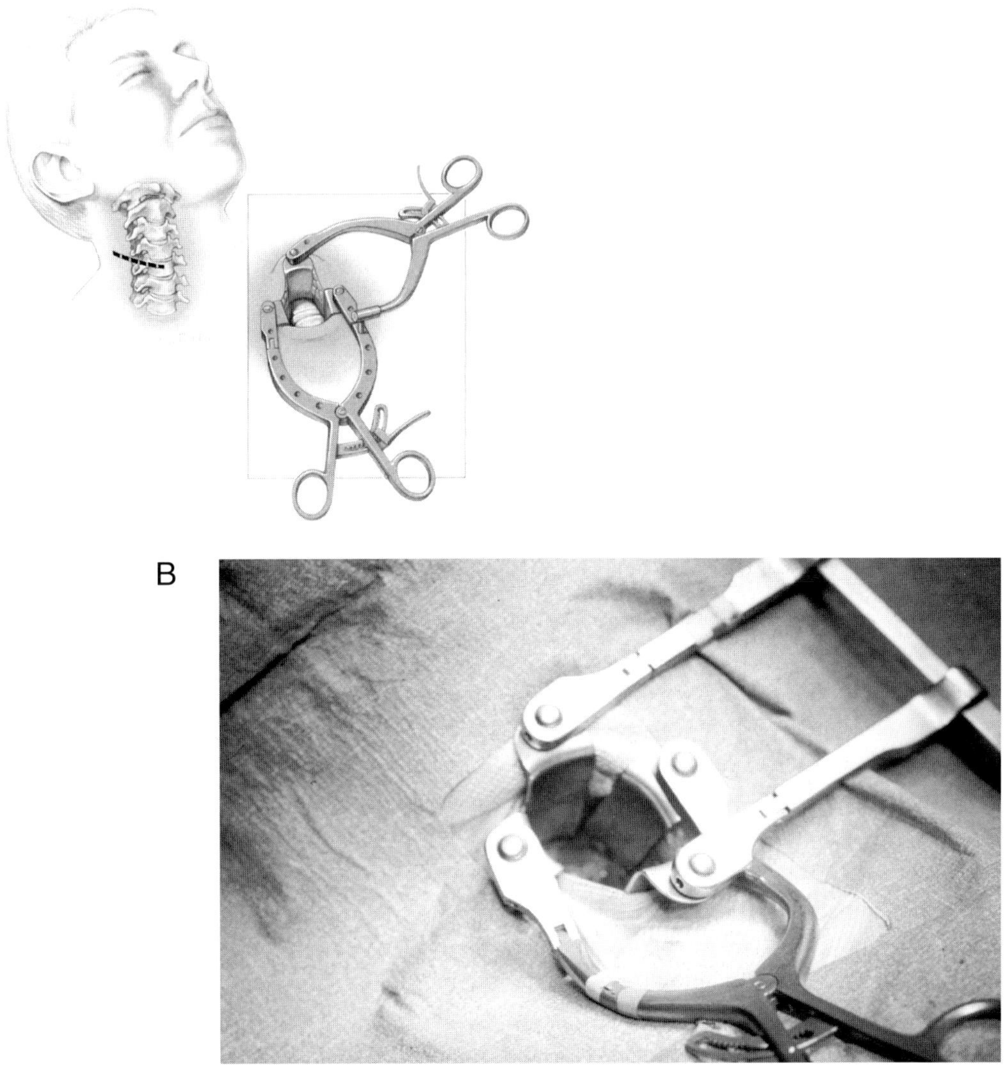

Figure 4. Drawing **(A)** and intraoperative photograph **(B)** of the Apfelbaum retractor system, used for ventral exposure of the upper cervical spine. (Courtesy of Aesculap)

They have toothed lateral blades that should be carefully placed into the longus colli muscles to avoid damage to the trachea and esophagus or the carotid sheath. The longitudinal retractor blades may be smooth. For the odontoid screw fixation technique, the Apfelbaum system (Aesculap) has specially modified retractor blades (Figure 4). The alternative is the table-mounted Farley system (Thompson Surgical Instruments) in which a post attached to the operating table is used to oppose tissue forces (Figure 5); variable placement of blades allows for the use of this retractor without toothed blades for both the conventional ventrocervical approaches and the ventral upper cervical approaches as well. With either system, significant tissue forces can be generated. Periodic release of the retractors is generally recommended, especially for extensive procedures.

A

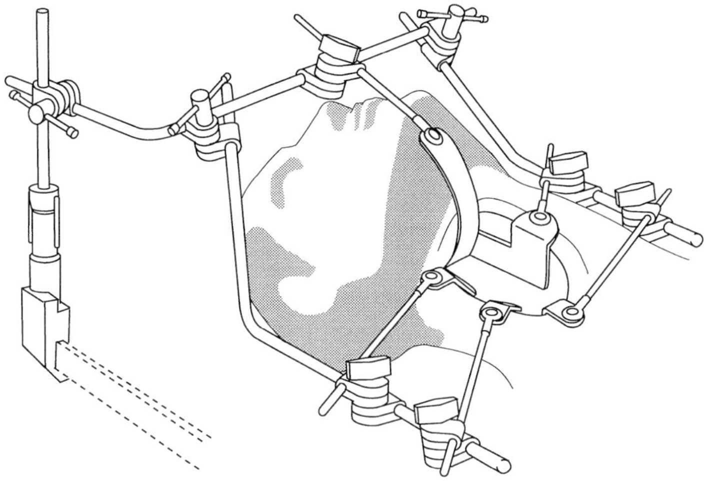

B

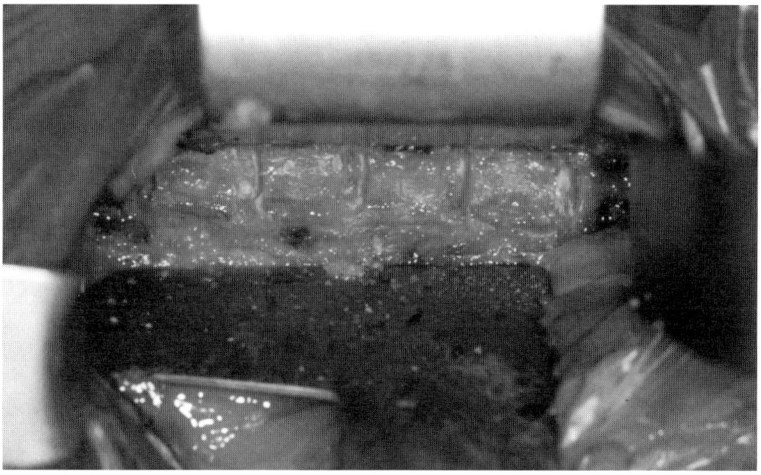

Figure 5. Drawing **(A)** and intraoperative photograph **(B)** of the table-mounted Farley system, used for ventral exposure of the cervical spine. (Courtesy of Thompson Surgical Instruments, Inc)

Ventral Thoracic Exposure

The ventral or ventrolateral approach to the thoracic spine is generally accomplished with the patient either in a lateral or semilateral position. The site of the approach is generally the surgeon's preference or related to the structures involved. After the patient is placed on the operating table in the lateral decubitus position, care is taken to avoid compression or distortion of the brachial plexus with use of a foam axillary roll. Care should also be taken to avoid compression of the ulnar nerve on either the dependent or rostral arm during positioning. In general, the operating table remains flat for this procedure, although occasionally it is extended beneath the area of interest to facilitate retraction of the rib cage. If radiographic imaging with fluoroscopy in multiple planes

A

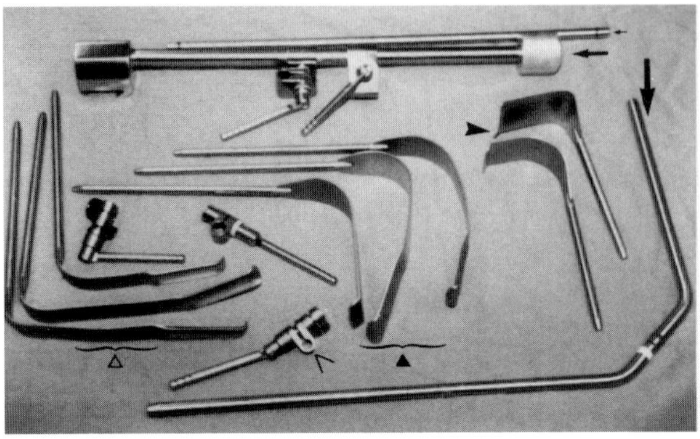

B

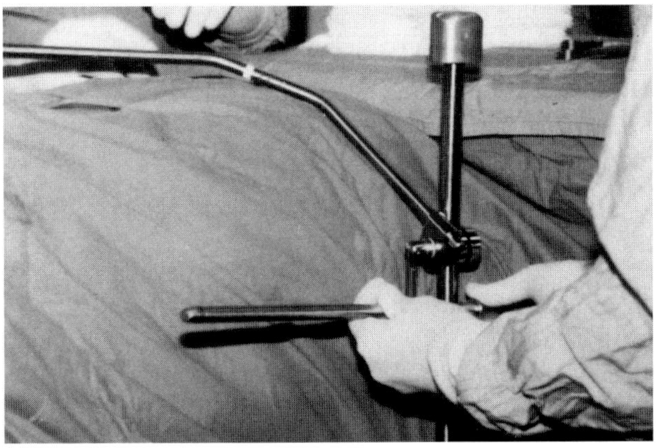

Figure 6A-B. A) The Omni-Tract Lateral Spine Retractor System: deep blades *(open triangle)*, intermediate retractor attachment device *(open arrowhead)*, intermediate blades *(solid triangle)*, superficial blades *(solid arrowhead)*, operating table attachment device *(small arrows)*, and interconnector *(large arrow)*. **B)** Photograph showing the system being attached to the table.

is anticipated, often the patient is placed backward on the table, allowing for through-the-table fluoroscopy.

Retraction is best obtained with a crank-type retractor that maintains adequate distraction of the rib cage. The Omni-Tract Modular Wishbone System (Omni-Tract Surgical, St. Paul, Minnesota) provides a table-mounted retraction system that not only allows for distraction of the ribs, but also includes a third arm to retract lung parenchyma. In the absence of the table-mounted system, maintenance of exposure with the crank retractor for the ribs and a hand-held Deaver or comparable retractor is adequate, but cumbersome for the surgical assistant.

Ventral Lumbar Exposure

Essentially, the same considerations are required for the intra- or extraperitoneal ventral lumbar approach as for thoracic approaches. The patient is best placed in the lateral decubitus or semisupine position, with the table either flat or slightly extended. The optimal retraction systems are the table-mounted systems (Omni-Tract Surgical, Thompson Surgical Instruments) that allow for different width and depth of blades to maintain exposure of the spine without the aid of a surgical assistant for that purpose. Care should be taken during placement of the blades so that the patient is firmly positioned on the table. This prevents sliding into

C

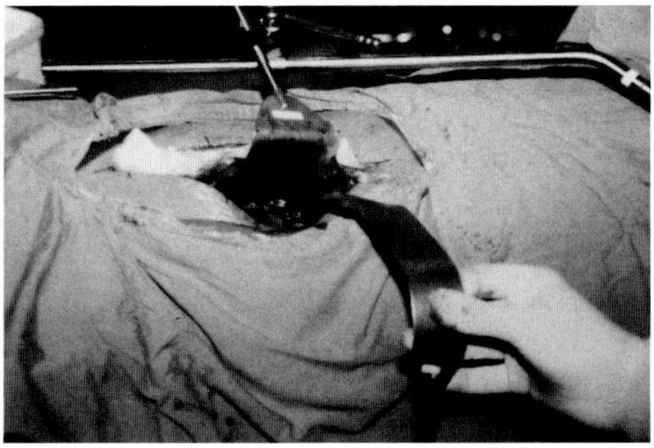

D

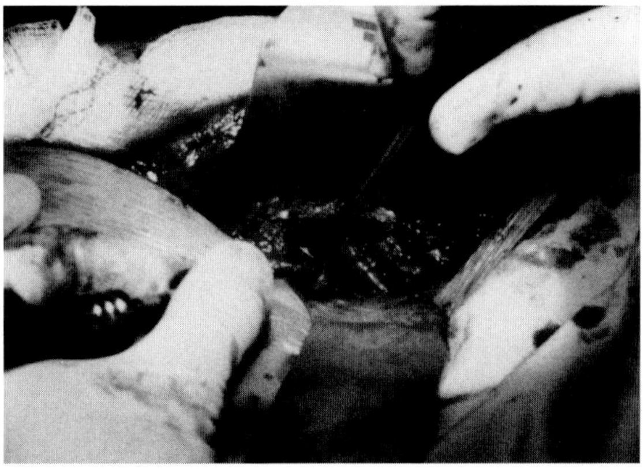

Figure 6C-D. C) Photograph of the Omni-Tract Lateral Spine Retractor System showing the blades during positioning. **D)** Intraoperative photograph showing deep lateral exposure of the dural sac achieved using the table-mounted retractor.

or under the table-mounted retractor systems, as these could cause injury to viscera or vessels because they are rigid and fixed to the table itself. Placing moistened laparotomy sponges or packs between the retractor blades and the viscera or peritoneum may add a measure of safety, but may consume space or encroach upon the surgical field.

Dorsolateral Thoracic and Lumbar Exposure

The dorsolateral approach or lateral extracavitary approach to the thoracic or lumbar spine requires the patient to be prone or near prone on the operating table. If the patient is placed on conventional chest rolls and firmly secured to the table, changing the angulation of the entire table facilitates the optimization of the angle of view. With this approach, a table-mounted system such as the Omni-Tract Lateral Spine Retractor System (Omni-Tract Surgical) allows for sturdy upward retraction of the paraspinous musculature with simultaneous downward displacement of the pleura or retroperitoneal structures (Figure 6). In general, the retractor base is attached to the siderail of the operating table and then the secondary arms are attached to this base post. As soon as the erector spinae muscles are dissected from the ribs or transverse processes, a 2-inch blade can be inserted and attached to the arm of the retractor to lift these muscles away from the spine, thus allowing for completion of the medial rib or transverse process

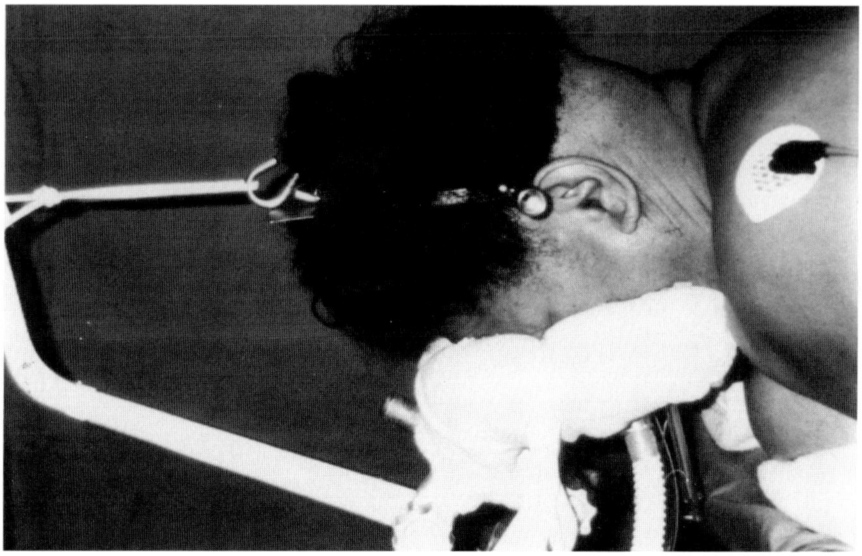

Figure 7. The horseshoe headholder, used with the application of cervical traction.

resection. Once this is accomplished, the second retractor blade is used to provide a downward force against the retroperitoneum or pleura to maintain the exposure channel to the lateral aspect of the spine.

While these retractors provide excellent exposure, they may be associated with an excessive force application that ultimately results in some injury to the surrounding tissues if care is not maintained to avoid this during the procedure. Various widths and lengths of retractor blades are available for use in the thoracic and lumbar regions.

Dorsal Cervical Exposure

The dorsal approach to the cervical spine may be accomplished via either a semisitting or a prone position. The potential hazards or risks of the sitting position have been extensively discussed and are not within the scope of this chapter. While the sitting position may be used for decompressive procedures, it is not recommended for procedures in which deformity correction is planned. For the sitting position, a three-point fixation device must be used. With the prone position, either a horseshoe or three-point fixation may be used.

Control of the head and cervical spine should be maintained during the induction of anesthesia, especially if significant instability is present. If the use of traction is anticipated, the traction device may be applied prior to induction of anesthesia so that anatomical alignment is maintained during intubation. Alignment should be carefully maintained until the patient is firmly fixed to the operating table in the prone position. As with ventral approaches, a flat operating table should be avoided.

When a horseshoe is used to support the head, special care must be taken to avoid compression of the eyes. An umbilical tape around the foam support of the horseshoe may be tightened after the patient is firmly affixed to the operating table and it is confirmed that there is no pressure on the eyes (Figure 7). The anesthesia team should periodically check this position during the surgical procedure, especially if traction is used to correct spinal deformity. Periodic movement of the patient's head will also prevent pressure sores on the forehead and cheeks. The halo traction ring, if positioned carefully on the horseshoe headholder, will allow for adequate traction and prevent ocular compression as well. A device is available for affixing the halo ring to the Mayfield fixation unit, but traction to correct deformity is limited or impossible. Therefore, a system using conventional weights hung over a traction bar may be utilized.

If intraoperative imaging with a C-arm image intensifier is planned, both lateral and anteroposterior views should be obtained prior to actually beginning the surgical procedure. The anteroposterior view may be impaired by the table or fixation apparatus and the lateral view of the lower cervical spine is often impaired by the shoulders. This view may be improved by adding supports between the chest bolsters and the shoulders or with gentle caudal traction on the arms. Using excessive traction on the arms and securing them with tape to maintain lower cervical spine visualization may be associated with brachial plexus injury and should be avoided.

Retraction with self-retaining retractors provides adequate exposure for most procedures using this approach. Conventional cerebellar retractors work well for deep exposures, and pediatric cerebellar retractors provide adequate exposure without interference from the knee of the retractor. The table-mounted retractor systems have been used effectively, especially if eccentric or more dorsolateral exposure is required. The retractor blade pulls against a fixed base instead of using opposing tissue force. The head should be firmly fixed to the operating table or the force of the table-mounted retractor may pull the head off to the side of the horseshoe headholder.

Dorsal Thoracic Exposure

The dorsal approach is accomplished with the patient prone on the operating table. When a conventional table is used, the approach to different levels or areas of the spine require different positioning considerations. For upper thoracic spine exposure, the patient's head is placed in a horseshoe headholder to maintain spine alignment. The arms are tucked by the sides and carefully secured to the operating table. Care should be taken to avoid nerve compression at the points where tape or other supports are used. When the mid- or low thoracic spine is approached, the head may be turned onto a foam pad and the arms flexed above the head. Care should be taken to avoid abducting the arm at the shoulder to greater than 90° so that the chance for brachial plexus stretch is minimized.

Conventional operating tables are adequate for the majority, if not all, of the thoracic and thoracolumbar exposures; however, if anteroposterior fluoroscopic imaging is required or if the patient's spine is so unstable that turning the patient onto the table increases the potential for neurological injury, a specialty table may be of benefit. The Jackson spinal surgery and imaging table (OSI, Hayward, California) is an example of this type of specialty table (Figure 8). The patient is transferred to the table in the supine position, after which time the contoured support cushions attached to a carbon fiber frame are positioned on the patient and the frame is secured to the table. The patient is then rotated into the prone position and the basetable removed. Patient rotation or Trendelenburg positioning may be accomplished intraoperatively, thus facilitating exposure and radiographic imaging. As with any positioning for a prolonged procedure, care must be taken to avoid pressure on neural structures.

Retraction for midline thoracic or thoracolumbar exposures generally does not warrant highly specialized retractors. The articulated or fixed-angle Weitlander retractors with straight retractors of varying lengths facilitate most exposures. A paramidline approach may be facilitated with the table-mounted retractors described earlier in this chapter. Table-mounted retractors

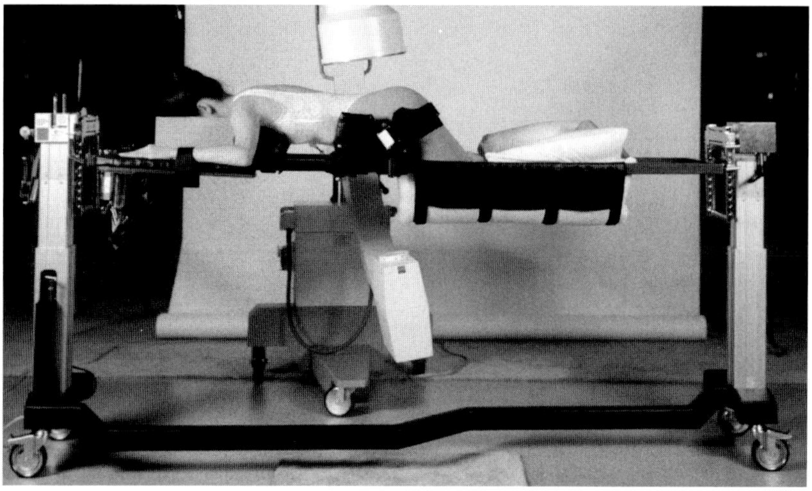

Figure 8. The Jackson spinal surgery imaging table. (Courtesy of OSI)

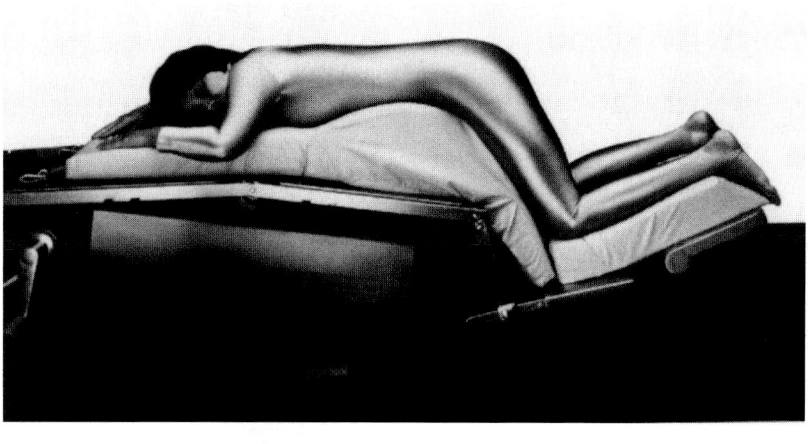

Figure 9. The Cloward surgical saddle. (Courtesy of Cloward Instrument Corp)

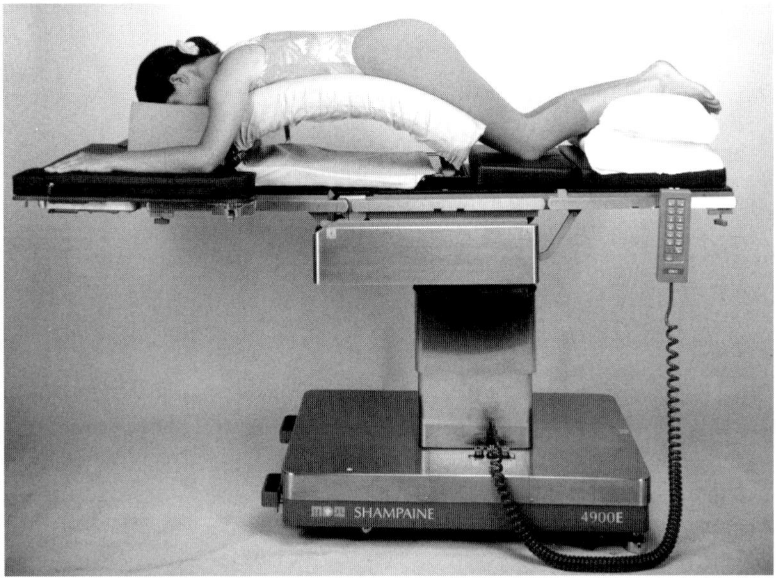

Figure 10. The Wilson frame. (Courtesy of OSI)

may not be compatible with some specialty tables, a factor that should be considered preoperatively.

Dorsal Lumbar Exposure

There are sporadic reports of performing a dorsal approach to the lumbar spine with the patient in the lateral position. Advantages include improved venous drainage and decreased blood loss, especially with the patient who is significantly overweight. Most experience, however, is with the patient in the prone position on bolsters or a specialty frame or table. The decision to use a specialty frame may be based upon the patient's size or weight, whether or not anteroposterior imaging is anticipated, the need for internal fixation or instrumentation, or the availability of a specialty frame. Essentially, all cases using this approach may be managed adequately on a conventional operating table with gel- or foam-filled bolsters. The table is flexed at the patient's back and knees as determined by the individual case.

Since epidural venous distention has an impact upon operative blood loss, and abdominal compression increases epidural venous pressure, several unique frames have been devised to position the patient to both minimize abdominal compression and avoid significant focal pressure on the iliac crest. The Cloward surgical saddle (Cloward Instrument Corp, Honolulu, Hawaii) is a customized foam cushion that is placed on the operating table (Figure 9) and contoured to prevent abdominal compression and to diffuse pressure points on the ribs and iliac crest. The Wilson frame (OSI) is a comparable device, which sits upon the conventional operating table and may be adjusted mechanically to accommodate patients of different girth or length (Figure 10). This device uses two adjustable bolsters that may be moved apart up to 10 inches or flexed. The Andrews spinal surgery table (OSI) is available commercially as both a frame that attaches to the operating table or as a specialty table itself; this table places the

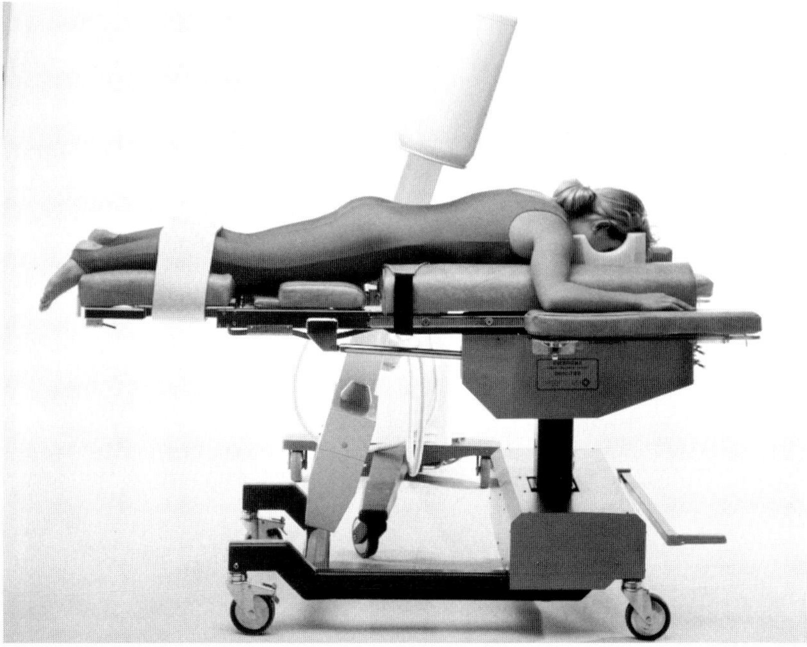

Figure 11. The Andrews spinal surgery frame. (Courtesy of OSI)

patient in a crouched or kneeling position (Figure 11). The advantage is absolute abdominal dependency with reduction in epidural venous pressure, whereas the disadvantage is that it is a cumbersome attachment to the table or an additional special table requiring meticulous attention to patient supports or restraints.

All of the aforementioned patient supports may be used for procedures requiring decompression, internal fixation, or both. Advocates of the specialty frames indicate that the potential decrease in blood loss during lengthy internal fixation cases make these devices especially useful for this indication.

Retraction for midline lumbar approaches is most commonly obtained with crank-type retractors with blades of varying widths and depths. Unilateral or hemilaminectomy reraction may be obtained with the Taylor blade, which anchors into the soft tissue just lateral to the facet joints, or a self-retaining unilateral blade retractor, such as the Williams retractor. If a paramedian approach is used for a far lateral disc herniation, table-mounted retractor systems provide optimal exposure, with blades that are 6 to 8 inches long and 1 to 2 inches wide.

Summary

Positioning of the patient for spinal surgery plays a significant role regarding the surgeon's ability to perform the desired procedure and the potential for or the avoidance of morbidity. The choice of retractors or retraction systems, like patient positioning, may make a significant contribution to the ease and safety of the proposed procedure.

There are a multitude of devices currently available. The spine surgeon performing the gamut of approaches or exposures both ventral and dorsal, transoral to lumbosacral, should have access to and be familiar with a dedicated transoral retractor system, ventral cervical system, a table-mounted system, a crank-type or self-opposing lumbar system, and a variety of conventional self-retaining retractors.

Chapter 12

Indications, Complications, and Comparison of Approaches

Eric J. Woodard, MD

A large variety of operative exposures is available for approaching spinal pathology at all levels of the vertebral column. The decision regarding the most appropriate approach to use for a particular clinical situation involves many factors. Regional anatomy, spinal pathology, the proposed goal of the surgery (e.g., decompression, total resection, arthrodesis, and/or instrumentation, technical experience), and the individual characteristics of the patient should all be considered when choosing the operative approach. In general, any level of the spine can be approached either ventrally or dorsally. Some of the most commonly used surgical approaches to the cervicothoracic, thoracic, lumbar, and lumbosacral regions are discussed, emphasizing major advantages, pitfalls, and salient technical points of each. Standard textbooks of spinal technique should be consulted for more specific surgical details.[11,12,17,22] Discussion of the upper and subaxial cervical regions are minimized in this chapter, because they have been vigorously addressed in previous chapters.

Cervicothoracic Region

The cervicothoracic region comprises the spinal levels between C7 and T2. This is a transitional zone between the lordotic cervical spine and the kyphotic thoracic spine.[9,20] Surgical exposure of this area is complicated by the constricting effect of the thoracic outlet, and the proximity of upper mediastinal vascular structures and lung apices.[11,21] The most common ventral and dorsal routes to the cervical and cervicothoracic regions are listed in Table 1.

Ventromedial Exposure

The ventromedial approach to the subaxial cervical spine has been well described by several authors.[5,6,11,19,22] It is the route commonly used for Smith-Robinson and Cloward fusion procedures in the midcervical region and is well known to most neurosurgeons.[5,18] In the cervicothoracic region, this technique is also useful for limited ventral access to the upper two thoracic vertebrae and the T1-2 disc space.[22]

Table 1. **Classification of Approaches**

Ventral Approach	Dorsal Approach
Cervicothoracic region	
ventromedial	dorsal midline
supraclavicular	transpedicular
transsternal	dorsolateral
transmanubrial	
transaxillary	
Thoracic and thoracolumbar regions	
transthoracic	dorsal midline
thoracoabdominal	transpedicular
retroperitoneal	dorsolateral
Lumbar region	
retroperitoneal	dorsal midline
transperitoneal	transpedicular
	paramedian (Wiltse et al[23])
	dorsolateral

The lordotic angle of T1 and T2, however, makes extensive ventral vertebral body resection and reconstruction by this approach technically difficult.[5,9,10]

The patient is positioned supine, in slight extension if possible. The skin incision may be placed either transversely just above the clavicle or obliquely along the medial aspect of the sternocleidomastoid muscle (Figure 1). The choice of incision is usually dictated by the degree of exposure required (Figure 1, *dashed line*). In general, when more than three vertebral bodies need complete exposure, an oblique incision is used. The underlying subcutaneous tissues and platysma muscle should be handled atraumatically to facilitate anatomical closure. Dissection is carried between the sternocleidomastoid muscle and carotid sheath laterally, and the trachea and esophagus medially in standard fashion.

Care should be taken to identify the recurrent laryngeal nerve between the trachea and esophagus when using a right-sided approach.[11,21] The right recurrent laryngeal nerve exits the carotid sheath at a variable level, coursing medially and entering the tracheoesophageal groove behind the upper pole of the thyroid gland. This variation increases the chance of stretch or direct nerve injury.[11,22] Similarly, with left-sided approaches, the thoracic duct must be identified as it enters the dorsal aspect of the subclavian vein. Injury to this structure may lead to chylothorax. Once recognized, the duct should be doubly ligated.[11,20,21]

The ventromedial exposure is indistinguishable from that used in the midcervical areas. Its advantages include: technical familiarity, low morbidity, and direct ventral access for ventral pathology. The major disadvantage is limited exposure. Patients with a foreshortened neck will have limited access to lower levels via this approach.[11] Similarly, care should be taken when retracting the upper mediastinal vascular structures and lung apices.

Supraclavicular Exposure

The supraclavicular approach is a variation of the ventromedial technique that was originally described as an exposure for upper thoracic sympathectomy.[15] This approach uses a transverse incision that is carried beyond the lateral border of the sternocleidomastoid muscle (Figure 2).[11,20,22]

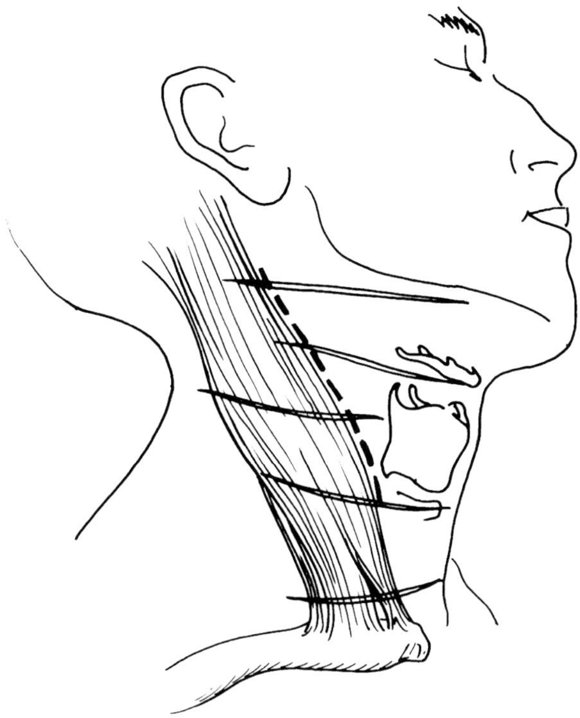

Figure 1. Skin incisions for accessing the mid and low cervical spine.

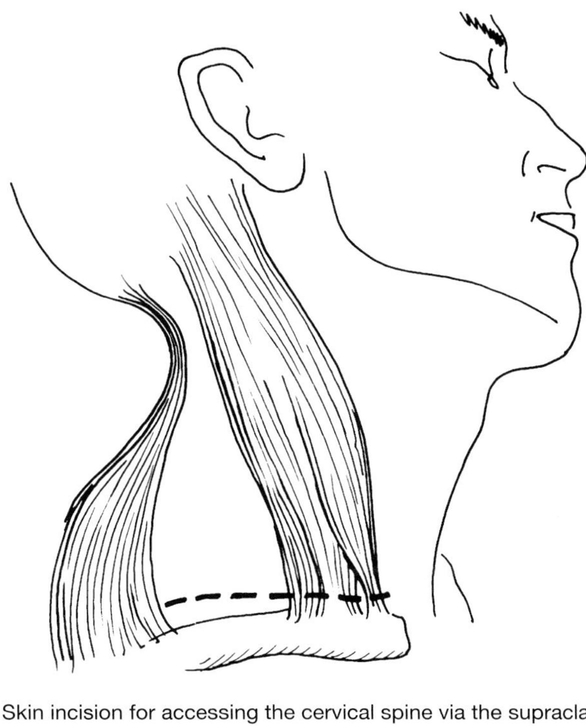

Figure 2. Skin incision for accessing the cervical spine via the supraclavicular route.

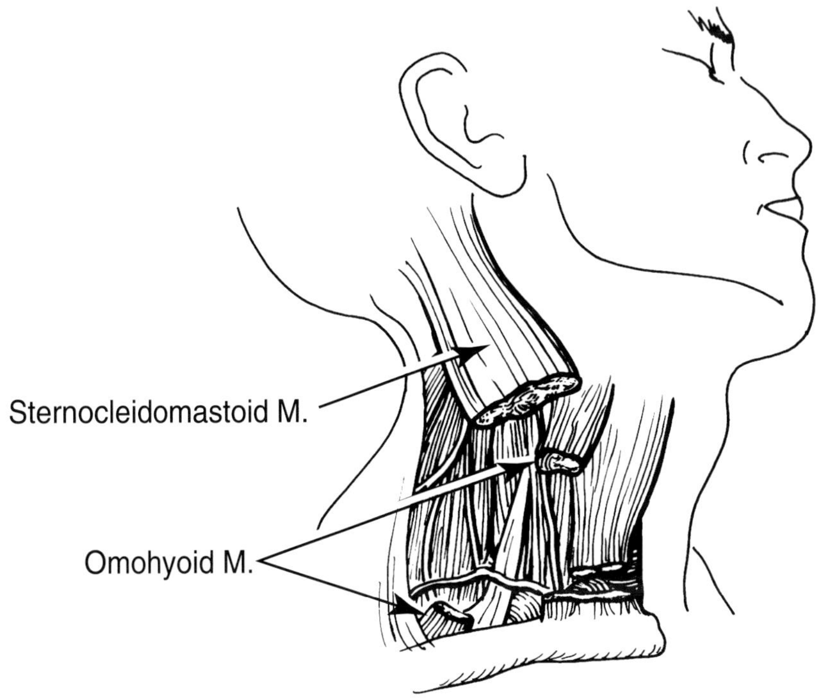

Figure 3. The surgical exposure of the spine via the supraclavicular route is facilitated by sternocleidomastoid and omohyoid muscle section.

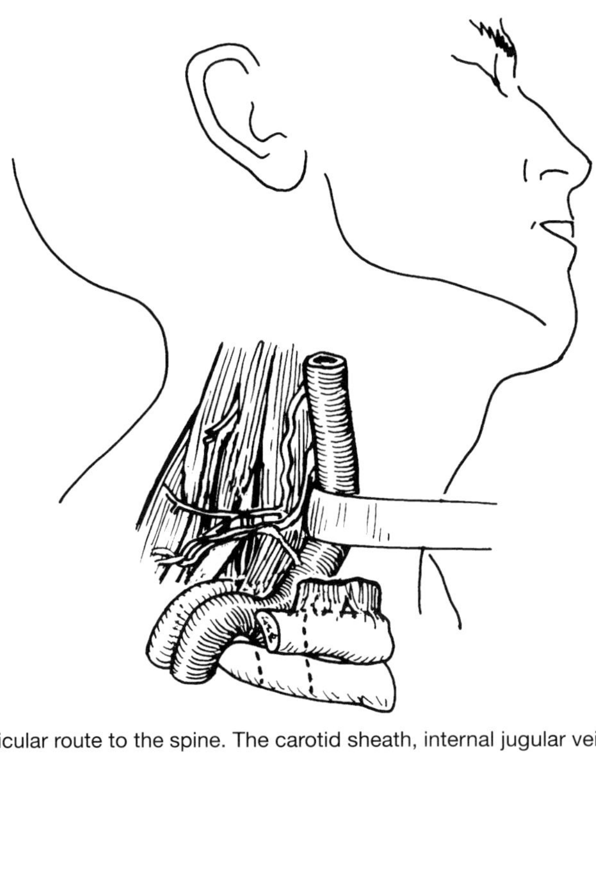

Figure 4. The supraclavicular route to the spine. The carotid sheath, internal jugular vein, and phrenic nerve are retracted medially.

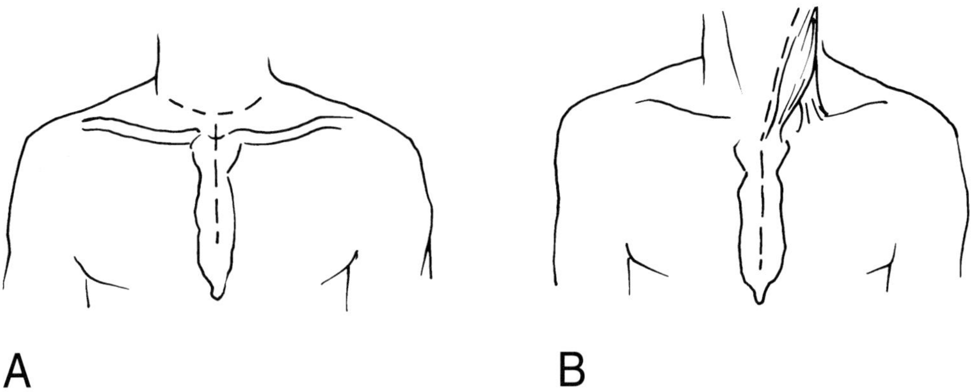

Figure 5. The T-shaped incision **(A)** and the medial sternocleidomastoid incision **(B)** for the transsternal exposure of the ventral cervicothoracic junction and the upper thoracic spine.

The sternocleidomastoid muscle is divided along with the underlying omohyoid and strap muscles, and the dissection is carried through the underlying intermediate cervical fascia (Figure 3). The thyrocervical trunk and its major branches should be identified and protected. The carotid sheath, internal jugular vein, and phrenic nerve are identified and mobilized medially, and the underlying anterior scalene muscle is retracted laterally or divided (Figure 4). Sibson's fascia, a fascial investment of the anterior scalene muscle, forms the floor of this area and is intimately associated with the pleura. Mobilization and caudal retraction affords protection of the lung apices. Continuing the dissection medially, Sibson's fascia becomes confluent with the prevertebral fascia, which is approached in a similar manner as the ventromedial technique.[11,20,22]

The supraclavicular approach offers a reasonable, but limited, exposure of the lateral aspect of C7. It is usually reserved for biopsy or limited spinal cord decompression, because exposure is inadequate for extensive vertebrectomy or reconstruction. Depending on the configuration of the patient's thoracic inlet, clavicles, and manubrium, the T1 and T2 vertebrae may additionally be approached by this route.[11,20,22]

Complications associated with the supraclavicular technique are similar to those of the ventromedial approach. Visceral (esophagus, trachea, and thyroid gland) injury, recurrent laryngeal nerve trauma, thoracic duct trauma, mediastinal vessel injury, and pleural tears are infrequent but potential problems.[21] Flooding the wound with saline under positive pressure ventilation can be used to identify pleural disruption. Primary repair should be attempted.

Transsternal Exposure

The transsternal approach provides a more direct ventral route to the upper thoracic vertebrae. This technique was originally described by Cauchoix and Binet[4] and used by Hodgson et al.[9,10] Direct ventral access (to as low as the T3 or T4 level) is possible in most normal individuals. This approach is performed with the patient in the supine position, with a slight degree of neck extension. Most authors recommend a left-sided technique to avoid recurrent laryngeal nerve injury.[11,20] Two incisions are commonly advocated: 1) a T-shaped incision with a transverse supraclavicular limb and vertical midsternal limb; and 2) a medial sternocleidomastoid incision (Figure 5).[10] The latter extends to the sternum, allowing extensive exposure of both the lower cervical region and the upper thoracic region.[20]

Regardless of the incision chosen, an appropriate superficial layer dissection is

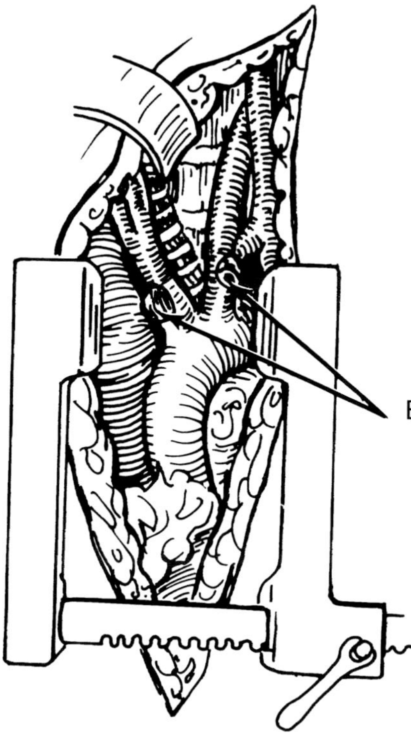

Figure 6. The plane of dissection provided by the transsternal technique.

carried out through the platysma muscle, and the anterior strap muscles are divided transversely above the manubrium. The manubrium and the entire longitudinal length of the sternum are exposed and divided using an oscillating saw. The sternum is retracted laterally, thus exposing the upper mediastinal structures. These are easily separated from the underside of the sternum with blunt finger dissection.[10] The pleura is separated from the thymus along the left side, allowing the latter to be retracted to the right. The brachiocephalic vein may be divided or retracted caudally to facilitate exposure.[20] A plane is developed between the left carotid artery and the brachiocephalic trunk, thus exposing the trachea and esophagus. These are retracted to one side (Figure 6). In most individuals, the transsternal technique provides full ventral access to the thoracic vertebral bodies to as low as the T3 or T4 level.[10,20]

Although the transsternal approach is the most direct and extensive ventral route to the upper thoracic vertebrae, it does require working in a "deep bloody hole" in proximity to important mediastinal structures.[9] Potential serious complications include disfiguring scars, sternal infection, pseudoarthrosis, chest deformity, arm swelling, chylothorax, great vessel injury, visceral injury, or death.[20] Although somewhat dated, Hodgson et al[9] reported a 40% perioperative mortality rate.

Transmanubrial Exposure

A variation of the transsternal approach to the upper thoracic levels has been recently reported by Sundaresan and DiGiancinto,[20] a transmanubrial approach. They recommend a T-shaped incision, as described by Hodgson and Yau.[10] After exposure of the manubrium and medial one-third of the clavicle, the clav-

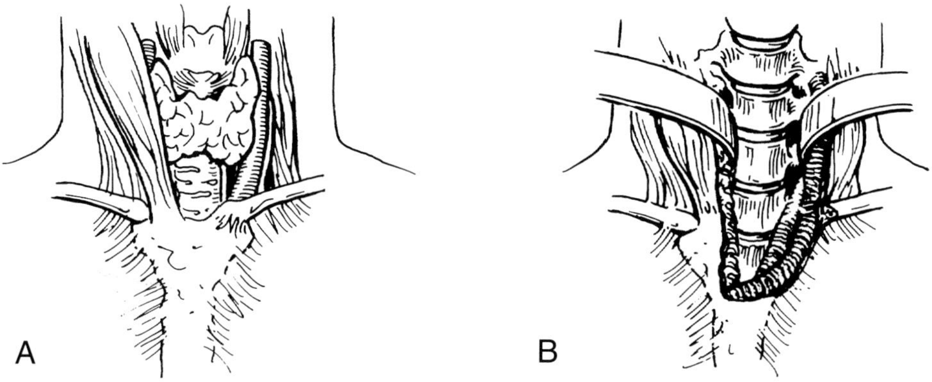

Figure 7. Resection of the manubrium (transmanubrial exposure) provides access to the upper thoracic spine via a similar, but slightly more limited, approach than that provided by the transsternal technique.

icle is divided and disarticulated from the sternoclavicular joint. A manubrial "window" is created with a high-speed burr, and the dorsal cortical margin is removed with curettes and rongeurs. Dissection of the upper mediastinal structures is then similar to the sternum-splitting approach (Figure 7).[20]

This technique provides excellent exposure for extensive tumor resection to the T3-4 region. If needed, the clavicle can be used as a stout bone graft for reconstruction. In the original series of 10 patients reported by Sundaresan and DiGiancinto,[20] all achieved complete pain relief and improvement in motor deficits with "minimum" morbidity. The major disadvantage of the approach is the risk of injury of mediastinal structures.

Transaxillary Exposure

A transaxillary approach to the upper thoracic region is occasionally described for exposing the cervicothoracic and upper thoracic vertebrae.[2,20,22] This approach is a high thoracic variant of the transthoracic approach. As an alternative method, transaxillary dissections are most useful for female patients or thin males without pectoral or latissimus dorsi muscle hypertrophy. Levels as high as the C7-T1 interspace are accessible and no major muscle groups require routine sectioning.[21]

Patient positioning is usually in a 60° semilateral position, with the ipsilateral shoulder and arm abducted to expose the axilla. The arm may be fixed in a sling and need not be completely prepped with a stockinet. A transverse incision is made from the border of the pectoral muscle to the border of the latissimus dorsi muscle (Figure 8). Dissection is carried out perpendicular to the plane of the skin to the chest wall using electrocautery. Superficial to the chest wall, a plane is created with blunt finger dissection, working rostrally until the first rib is palpated. The third rib is identified and its periosteum scored with electrocautery. Subperiosteal dissection of the third rib as far ventrally and dorsally as possible is carried out using a Doyen elevator. The rib is then resected with rib cutters or retracted caudally, and dissection is carried through the third rib bed (Figure 9).

The parietal pleura is identified and bluntly swept ventrally and caudally off the dorsal chest wall, thus maintaining an extrapleural plane superficial to the ribs. The costotransverse articulation is identified and the transverse process followed to the vertebral body. A thin, padded retractor facilitates retraction of the lung apex caudally.

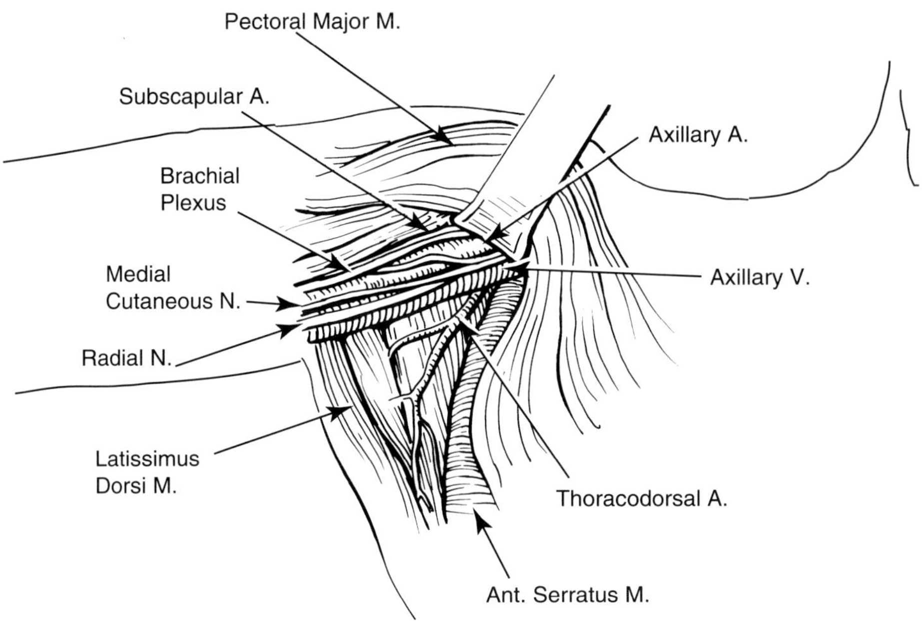

Figure 8. Superficial exposure provided by a right transaxillary approach.

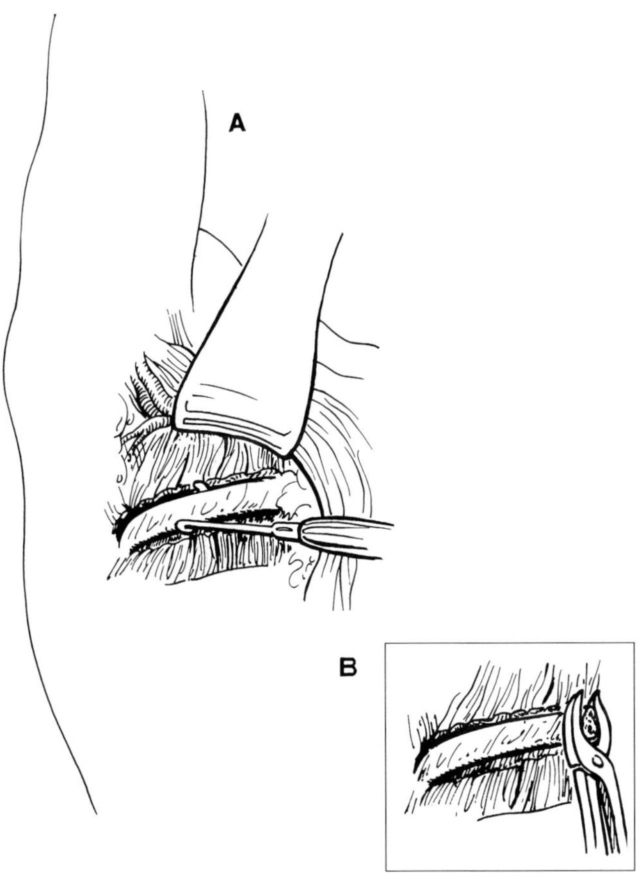

Figure 9. Deep dissection via the transaxillary approach exposes the third rib. This is removed via standard techniques **(A** and **B),** thus gaining access to the extrapleural high thoracic region.

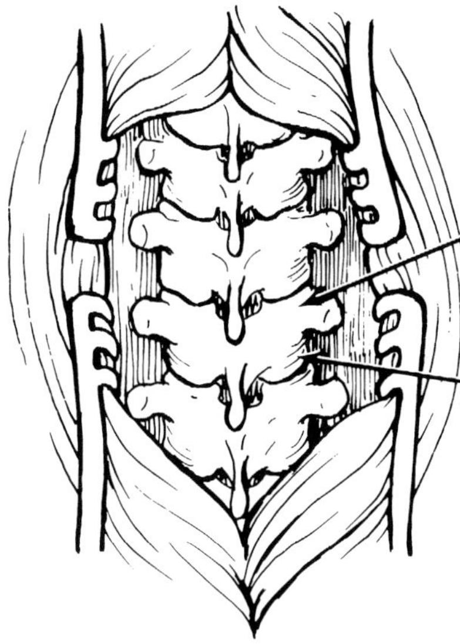

Figure 10. The dorsal exposure of the thoracic spine.

An intrapleural approach is another option. It is helpful in patients with pathology involving the pleura. In this case, the chest is entered through the bed of the third rib, and the upper portion of the lung is retracted caudally. The parietal pleura overlying the bodies of the upper thoracic vertebrae of interest is opened longitudinally and dissected bluntly from the ventrolateral aspect with a Kittner dissector. Intercostal vascular pedicles are identified and ligated as they course around the midportion of the vertebral body. For closure, the parietal pleura may be reapproximated over the vertebral bodies. The lung packing is removed and re-expansion is facilitated by positive pressure ventilation. A chest tube is placed in the midaxillary line, two ribs below the level of the incision.[22]

For closure, the second and fourth ribs are reapproximated with permanent suture, and the axillary soft tissue is reapproximated with absorbable material over a suction drain. Drainage is usually necessary because of trauma to numerous lymphatic channels in the axilla.[21,22]

The major advantage of the transaxillary technique is the preservation of pectoral and shoulder girdle musculature. The approach does require working in a deep, limited space and, if carried intrapleurally, requires chest tube drainage. Complications are similar to those encountered with the transthoracic technique, most commonly pulmonary in nature (atelectasis, hemo/pneumothorax). Additionally, brachial plexus stretch injury, axillary vessel trauma, and intercostobrachial neuralgia have been described after transaxillary dissection.[21]

Dorsal Exposure

The most common route to all levels of the spine is the standard midline dorsal approach. Well known by all spine surgeons, it is used in a large variety of procedures ranging from decompressive laminectomy to fusion, with or without instrumentation. In the cervicothoracic region, dorsal approaches are usually limited to simple decompressions for dorsally situated lesions (e.g., tumor, infection, or other epidural masses) (Figure 10).[11, 17, 20]

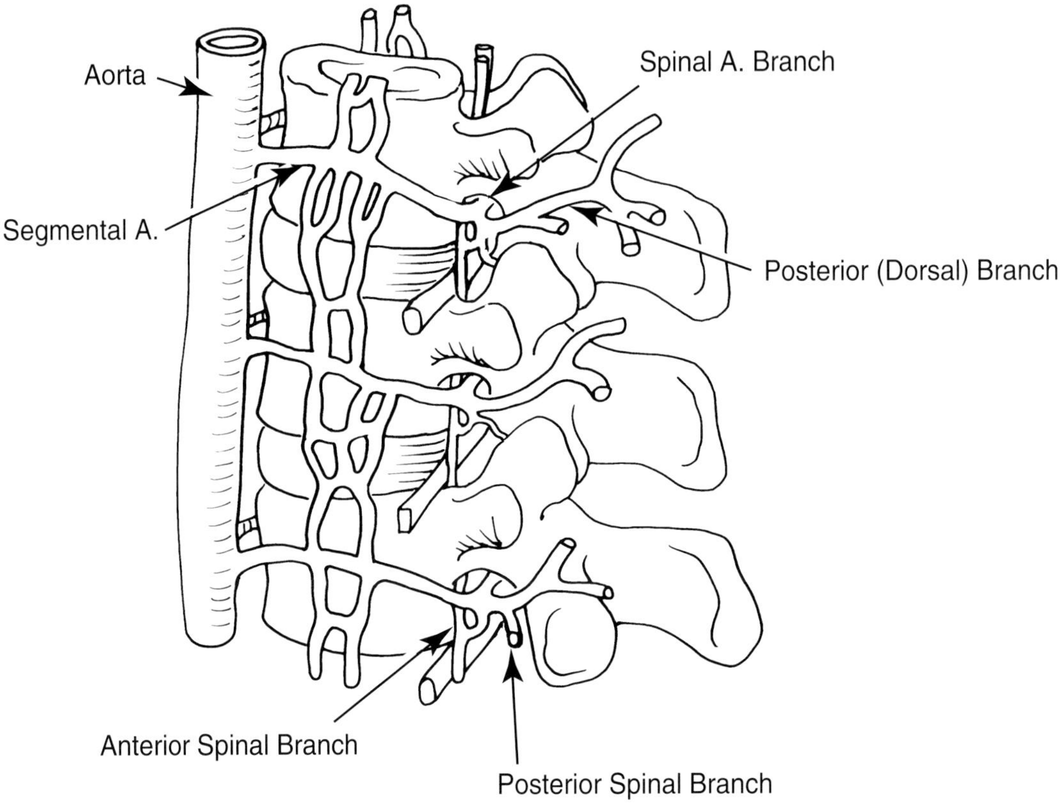

Figure 11. Segmental arteries and their associated collateral plexi are relatively consistent along most of the length of the thoracic and lumbar spine, as depicted.

The patient is positioned prone on a chest frame or on laminectomy rolls. The head is affixed or positioned in a neutral position using either pin fixation or tong traction and a horseshoe headrest. The incision is usually midline, with its position guided by prominent spinous processes. Alternative soft tissue flaps (e.g., curved paramedian) are occasionally necessary, such as in patients requiring future adjuvant radiation or with previous radiation to the area.[20] If a paramedian incision is utilized, the flap is undermined superficial to the thoracodorsal fascia to the midline to allow access to the spinous processes.

In younger patients, a prominent cartilaginous "cap" on the tip of each spinous process can be split sharply and scraped laterally. This maneuver leads to the appropriate plane for subperiosteal dissection along the lateral spinous processes and laminae. Bilateral subperiosteal dissection is continued over the laminae with sharp elevators or electrocautery as far laterally as is required for the particular procedure. Care should be taken to preserve facet capsules in cases not involving fusion.[11] Blood loss may be reduced by progressive packing with sponges and by anticipating the presence of the dorsal branches of the segmental arteries that emerge lateral to the facet joints in the thoracic region and cross dorsally over the pars interarticularis (Figure 11).[1]

Meticulous attention to dissection technique and judicious retraction reduces injury to the erector spinae muscle group, thus minimizing intraoperative blood loss, postoperative swelling, and muscle necrosis. Clo-

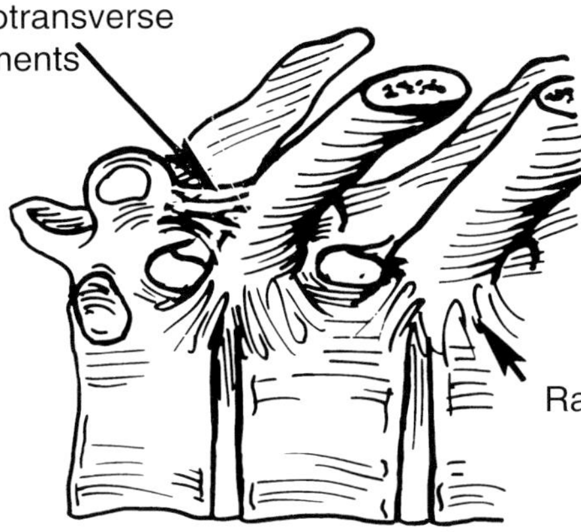

Figure 12. The relationship of the disc interspace to the pedicle in the upper thoracic region. Note that the disc interspace is located just rostral to the rostral margin of the pedicle.

sure simply requires anatomical approximation of the erector spinae muscles and the thoracodorsal fascia over the spinous processes. In the cervicothoracic region, the insertions of the superficial and middle layers of the dorsal musculature become confluent with the thoracodorsal fascia at the midline. Accurate closure of this layer ensures anatomical reconstruction of these stabilizers of the shoulder girdle.

Transpedicular Exposure

A transpedicular approach has been described by Patterson and Arbit[16] as a useful alternative technique for herniated thoracic disc removal and vertebral body biopsy. The procedure can be performed in the cervicothoracic as well as thoracic areas, and is useful for limited exposure to the ventrolateral vertebral body.

The patient is positioned prone in standard fashion on rolls or a spinal frame. A midline incision is made over the region of interest, and paraspinal musculature and soft tissue structures are elevated subperiosteally unilaterally beyond the facet joint of interest. Using a high-speed drill, the entire facet joint and associated pedicle are removed. By drilling deep into the pedicle, the ventral aspect of the vertebral body is accessible. The disc space lies immediately rostral to the rostral margin of the pedicle (Figure 12). Disc decompression may be facilitated by the use of reverse angled curettes.[16] A variation of this approach that spares the pedicle has been described: by removing the facet joint only, the lateral aspect of the disc space is accessible for disc removal without violating the pedicle, which may have a destabilizing effect (CB Stillerman et al, unpublished data).

The transpedicular approach is simple, easy to learn, and safe to perform. It is extremely limited, however, for exposure of ventral structures. Therefore, it is not generally used for extensive tumor resection, multilevel processes, or decompression of medially placed lesions.

Dorsolateral Exposure

Costotransversectomy is a dorsolateral technique that may be used throughout the spine to approach dorsal and dorsolateral structures without violating the pleural cavity.[7,8,11,13] It can be considered an extended transpedicular procedure. Two major variations of costotransversectomy are commonly used, each providing different degrees of access to the ventrolateral aspect of the vertebral body: 1) the midline or medial approach, and 2) the

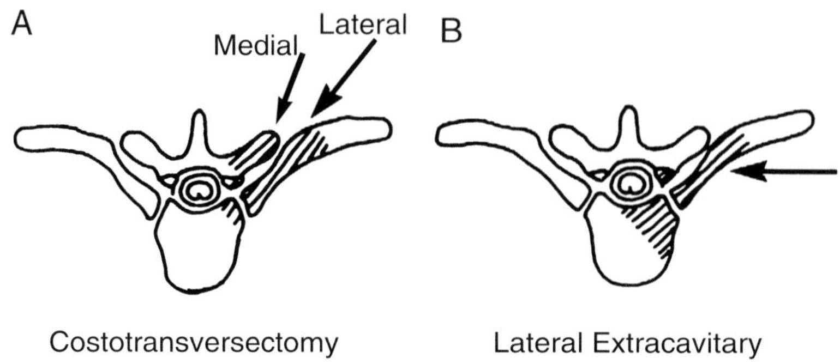

Figure 13. The trajectory of surgery *(arrows)* and the extent of vertebral body that may be accessed via the costotransversectomy **(A)** and the lateral extracavitary **(B)** exposures of the spine.

lateral approach. The lateral extracavitary technique is a specific modification of the lateral costotransversectomy. The principle difference between the medial and lateral techniques is the path each takes to the vertebral body with respect to the erector spinae muscle (Figure 13).

Menard[14] first described the midline costotransversectomy technique for drainage of tuberculous abscesses.[11] This approach uses a straight midline incision, followed by a standard bilateral subperiosteal dissection. The ipsilateral dissection extends beneath the erector spinae muscle laterally to the tips of the transverse processes and proximal ribs. The appropriate rib is incised laterally as far as possible, and its costotransverse and capsular articulations are divided. The rib is then disarticulated. One or several ribs may be removed in this manner. Usually, only two vertebral bodies can be realistically approached by this technique (Figure 14).

The transverse processes and corresponding pedicles are removed using

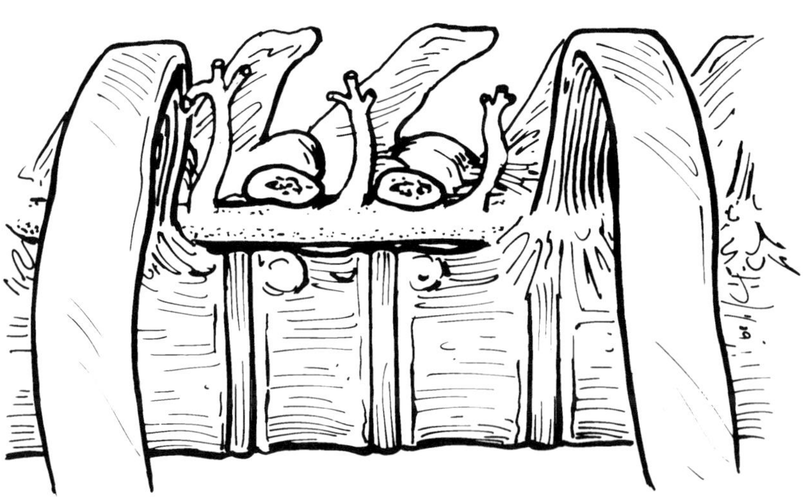

Figure 14. A "skeletonized" view of the exposure gained by the lateral extracavitary approach.

rongeurs, curettes, and/or a high-speed drill, thus exposing the lateral aspect of the thecal sac. Proximal dissection of the intercostal nerve also facilitates identification of the lateral thecal sac, especially in cases of abnormal anatomy (e.g., tumor or trauma). Blunt dissection along the sides of the vertebral bodies improves access to these structures when true ventral decompression is desired. Decompression is limited, however, because of the steep angle of approach achieved with this midline technique.

To improve the working angle to the vertebral body, Capener[3] in 1954 devised a modification of Menard's technique in which the incision is made in a parasagittal location.[13] Dissection is carried through the superficial musculature to the lateral border of the erector spinae muscle group. This structure is elevated in a lateral to medial direction, superficial to the ribs. Alternatively, the erector spinae musculature is divided transversely and reflected. Appropriate ribs are removed to approximately 8 to 10 cm lateral to the midline. The underlying parietal pleura is retracted ventrally, thus exposing the lateral aspect of the vertebral body by a much flatter angle than by using the midline approach.

The improved angle of approach enables access to nearly the entire vertebral body for decompression. Additionally, decompression may be safer because the thecal sac and the compressive lesion are visualized simultaneously from the side.[13] This obviates having to work around neural elements to resect the pathology. Only the contralateral pedicle is not accessible with this technique. Although morbidity is thought to be less than with transthoracic alternatives, the costotransversectomy techniques are technically demanding and can cause considerable blood loss due to epidural vein bleeding after decompression.[11] Complications include neural injury, cerebrospinal fluid leakage, segmental neuralgia, and pleural disruption.

Recently, Larson et al[13] have repopularized Capener's procedure by altering the method of soft tissue approach to allow for dorsal instrumentation. This "lateral extracavitary" approach uses a midline hockey stick incision with an oblique inferior limb. After standard subperiosteal dissection to the transverse processes, a plane is developed on the ipsilateral side beneath the thoracolumbar fascia. A full-thickness myocutaneous flap is retracted laterally, thus exposing the erector spinae muscle group along its lateral edge. A lateral to medial elevation, superficial to the ribs, is carried out in the same manner as the Capener procedure.[13]

The major advantage of the lateral extracavitary technique is that it provides simultaneous access to both dorsal and ventral aspects of the spine. Typically, after ventral decompression of the spinal cord, spinal reduction and dorsal instrumentation can be performed in the same operative setting. A ventral interbody arthrodesis completes the procedure.[13]

Complications are similar to other costotransversectomy techniques and are principally related to the large soft tissue exposure required. This procedure is technically demanding and requires an extended operating time.

Both medial and lateral costotransversectomy methods are appropriate for spinal decompression at all levels. The midline approach is most commonly used in the upper thoracic segments (C7 to T7) and the lateral paraspinal or lateral extracavitary approaches for more caudal levels. Care should be taken to close muscle layers anatomically in order to prevent long-term shoulder girdle dysfunction.

Thoracic and Thoracolumbar Regions

Three procedures are most commonly used for ventral approaches in the thoracic and thoracolumbar spine (Table 1). Dorsal procedures described for the cervicothoracic junction can also be applied at thoracolumbar levels with very little technique modification.

As with other regions of the spine, ventral thoracic exposures afford a direct access to

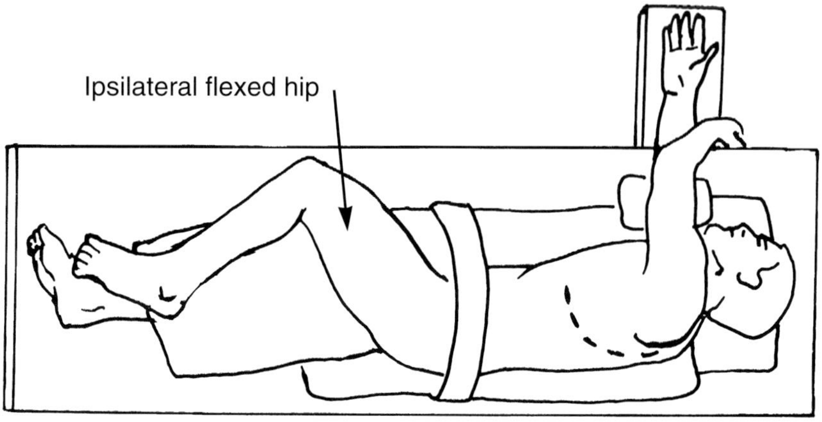

Figure 15. Patient positioning for the transthoracic exposure. Note that the ipsilateral hip is flexed.

ventrally situated pathology.[9,11] Examples of lesions well-suited for this method are vertebral body tumors, osteomyelitis, midline disc herniations, and fixed deformities. The basic technique is that of a transthoracic approach, modified at the thoracolumbar junction to accommodate the unique anatomy of the diaphragm and the transition zone between the pleural and peritoneal cavities.

Transthoracic Exposure

The transthoracic approach is most useful for midthoracic segments between T3 and T11. Advantages include direct access to ventral pathology, extensive decompression, and multilevel exposure.[21] It is the only routinely employed procedure through which ventral spinal instrumentation constructs are installed. Principle disadvantages are the increased morbidity associated with entering the chest cavity, the need for tube thoracostomy, the necessity of decompressing neural structures that lie dorsal to the pathology, and the need for a second procedure in cases requiring dorsal instrumentation.[11]

Patient positioning is either the partial or full lateral decubitus position, using a bean bag apparatus and an arm sling. The side of the approach is usually dictated by the side with the greatest pathological involvement (Figure 15). In midline cases, most surgeons approach mid- and low thoracic levels from the left side because of the greater mobility of the aorta and heart, and a lack of obstruction by the dome of the liver. A slight break in the table positioned beneath the intended incision may facilitate exposure. The ipsilateral hip is flexed to relax the iliopsoas muscle, facilitating its retraction. For midthoracic vertebrae, an incision is made one or two rib levels above the vertebral level of interest. This varies depending upon the downward slope of the rib cage and the degree of exposure required.[21]

A curvilinear incision is made along the line of the chosen rib, extending from the costochondral articulation ventrally to the lateral aspect of the paramedian musculature dorsally. Dissection is carried down to the superficial muscle groups. The latissimus dorsi, the anterior serratus, and the posterior inferior serratus muscles are divided with electrocautery (Figure 16). The periostium of the rib is scored, elevated with a Doyen elevator, and disarticulated from the costochondral junction. The rib is cut dorsally, just medial to the angle. Entry into the chest cavity is through the rib bed periosteum and parietal pleura, and extended the length of the rib bed. The underlying

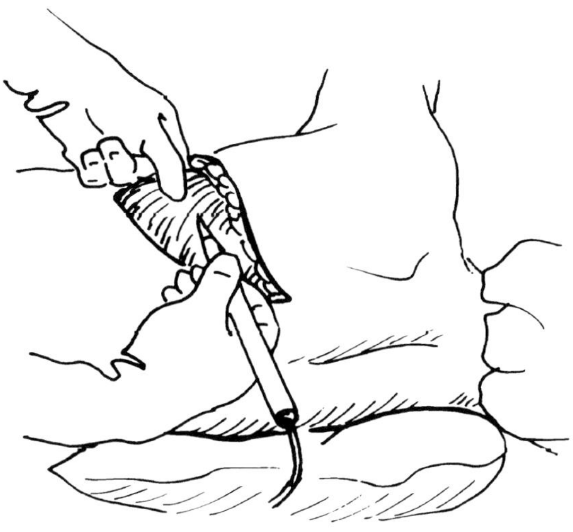

Figure 16. The superficial chest wall muscle groups are incised, thus allowing access to the underlying chest wall.

lung is then manually collapsed. Use of a double-lumen endotracheal tube facilitates collapse and retraction of the lung. A self-retaining padded retractor is useful for retracting the lung ventromedially (Figure 17).[20]

Soft adhesions, if present, are easily broken with a blunt dissecting finger. This exposes the ventrolateral aspect of the vertebral column, which is covered by a thin layer of parietal pleura. Segmental vessels are usually easily visualized, coursing across the midportion of the vertebral bodies. The disc spaces are lighter in color and bulge prominently.[22]

The parietal pleura is incised over the region of interest (Figure 18). The identity of the appropriate vertebral body should then be confirmed by intraoperative radiography.[21] Segmental vessels should be doubly ligated,

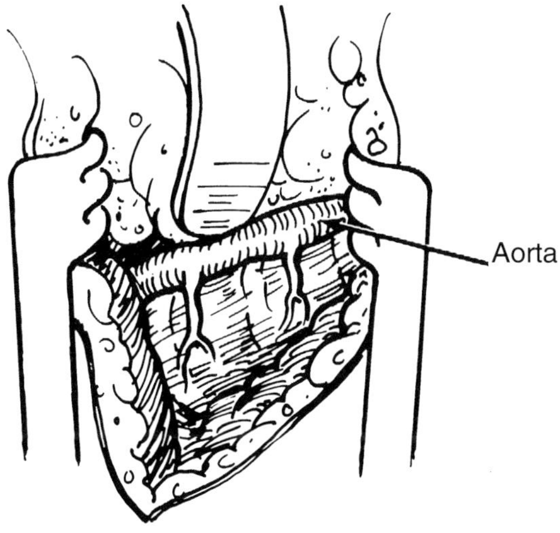

Figure 17. Retraction of the lung provides access to the vertebral bodies, covered by parietal pleura and neural and vascular structures.

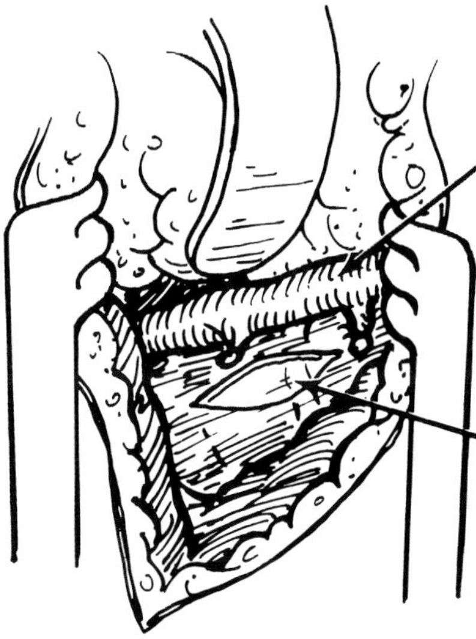

Figure 18. An incision in the parietal pleura and ligation of segmental arteries and veins gains access to the vertebral bodies and disc interspaces.

with care taken to prevent their avulsion from the aorta. Decompression is carried out as required, usually extending between disc spaces. Excessive bleeding should be controlled using liberal packing with bone wax and Gelfoam.

Using this approach, a significant amount of ventral bony material can be resected. The ventrolateral angle of approach also facilitates bone graft impaction for ventral interbody arthrodesis. For closure, the parietal pleura does not necessarily need to be reapproximated over the resection area. The lung is reinflated, and one or two chest tubes are placed two costal levels below the incision. The ribs are compressed and reapproximated with heavy suture. The rib bed is similarly reapproximated securely to reestablish a pleural seal. Superficial muscles are repaired anatomically and soft tissue closure is carried out in the standard fashion.[11]

Postoperative complications of this technique are principally pulmonary. Atelectasis, pneumonia, and pleural effusions should be anticipated.[21] Once drainage abates, the chest tubes can be removed. Infection is uncommon.[11]

Although lower levels of the thoracic spine can be easily reached with the transthoracic approaches, working space is significantly reduced by the dome of the diaphragm. Most surgeons prefer a thoracoabdominal approach for extensive T12 and upper lumbar vertebrae exposure. This requires division of the medial diaphragmatic attachments, thus increasing morbidity. The thoracoabdominal technique provides excellent exposure of the low thoracic vertebrae, but a limited access to the upper lumbar levels. For lesions situated more caudally, the retroperitoneal approach provides a more favorable exposure.

Thoracoabdominal Exposure

Thoracoabdominal approaches to the thoracolumbar junction use rib incisions varying between the T7 and T12 levels. Most commonly, a 10th, 11th, or 12th rib incision is made in a standard transthoracic fashion. The rib is resected and the chest entered. Alternatively, the costal cartilage of the chosen rib is first split longitudinally, and then dissection is carried through the costal rib bed. This maneuver takes advantage of

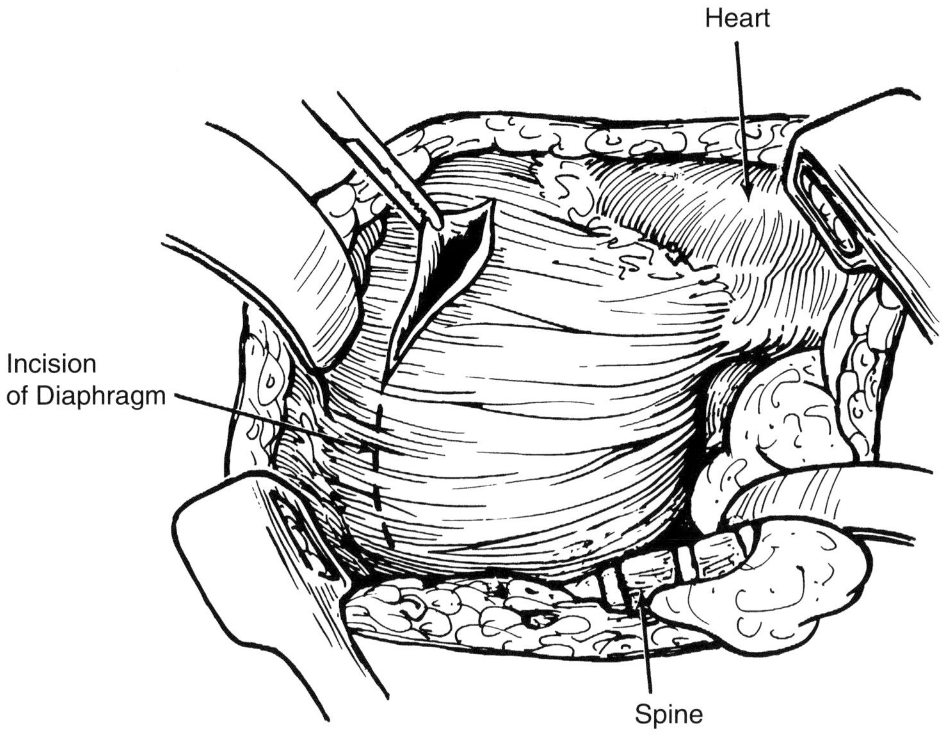

Figure 19. Through the thoracic cavity, the diaphragm is incised. A generous cuff utilizing a peripheral incision allows a margin for suture closure and protection of the innervation of the diaphragm.

the insertion of the diaphragm onto the rostral margin of the costal cartilage and the attachment of the abdominal musculature to the rostral costal cartilage.[22] In this manner, the retroperitoneal space can be entered along the underside of the diaphragm without violating the peritoneal cavity.

An incision is then made through the diaphragm along its peripheral attachment at the costal margin. A generous cuff of muscle is left for later reapproximation (Figure 19). The diaphragm is detached in a lateral to medial direction through the lateral aspect of the lateral arcuate ligament, just above its insertion at the tip of the 12th rib.

The medial arcuate ligament insertion is detached from the L1 transverse process. In this manner, the dorsal aspect of the diaphragm is freed from its medial insertion and retracted. The retroperitoneal plane is then developed beneath the upper pole of the kidney and spleen. Dissection is carried over the quadratus lumborum and psoas muscles to the lateral aspect of the upper lumbar vertebrae, and the left diaphragmatic crus is separated from the ventrolateral margin of L1 and L2 with a sharp elevator. At this point, full ventrolateral exposure of the lower thoracic and upper two lumbar vertebrae has been accomplished. Following decompression and/or stabilization, great care must be taken to repair the diaphragmatic attachments accurately. The

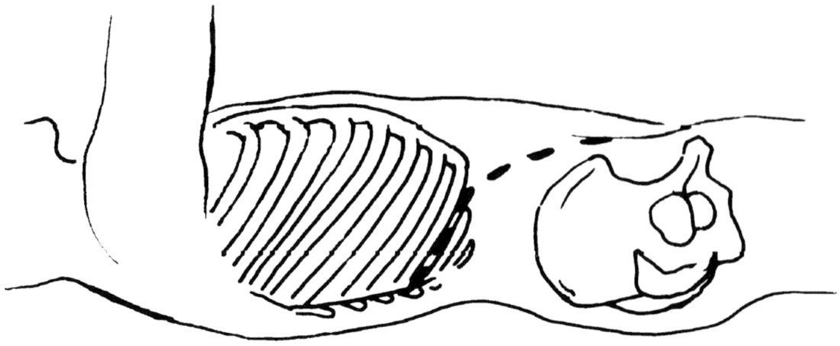

Figure 20. The incision utilized for ventral "thoracolumbar" exposure of the upper and midthoracic spine.

left crus is reattached to the anterior longitudinal ligament, and the peritoneum, if violated, is reapproximated. The medial arcuate ligament is reattached to the transverse process of L1, and the diaphragm is reapproximated to its peripheral muscular cuff. Chest closure is carried out in a standard fashion.

The thoracoabdominal approach violates two major body cavities, thereby producing a significant degree of soft tissue trauma.[11] The most severe complications are related to visceral (spleen, kidney, ureter) injury. As with any transthoracic technique, the patient is at risk for cardiopulmonary complications. This method of extensive exposure of the thoracolumbar area is usually reserved for healthier patients.

Retroperitoneal Exposure

The most caudal approach to the thoracolumbar junction is through the retroperitoneal space, also known as the "ventrolateral flank" approach. It addresses thoracolumbar pathology from the abdominal side of the diaphragm, rather than from the thoracic side. A retroperitoneal dissection does not require disruption of any major body cavity and is consequently a somewhat less morbid procedure.

Like the thoracoabdominal procedure, the incision may vary, depending on the particular lumbar level of interest. The thoracolumbar junction is best approached by an 11th or 12th rib incision, beginning at the lateral aspect of the paraspinous musculature and extending, as needed, obliquely and caudally to the lateral aspect of the rectus abdominis muscle (Figure 20).

The 12th rib is isolated and resected, and the abdominal wall muscles divided or split in the line of the wound. Just deep to the transversus abdominis muscle lies the peritoneum, which is bluntly dissected from the under surface of the diaphragm dorsally and medially toward the dorsal retroperitoneum. At this point, the peritoneum becomes confluent with the transversalis fascia of the abdominal wall and Gerota's fascia behind the renal capsule. The plane is developed bluntly and the peritoneum and its contents are retracted medially with a padded self-retaining retractor (Figure 21). In this fashion, the ventral surfaces of the quadratus lumborum and iliopsoas muscles are exposed. The genitofemoral nerve (on the ventral surface of the iliopsoas muscle) and the sympathetic chain (between the iliopsoas muscle and vertebral column) should be identified and protected, then mobilized and retracted laterally.

This is a relatively quick, uncomplicated exposure of the thoracolumbar and lumbar vertebrae. For simultaneous access to lower thoracic segments, the arcuate ligaments can be detached from their insertions at the tip of the 12th rib and the transverse process of L1 (Figure 22). This mobilizes the medial dorsal aspect of the diaphragm. Careful subpleural dissection provides limited thoracic exposure as high as the T11 level, without violating the pleural space.[12,21] Closure of the wound is straightforward, using simple anatomical

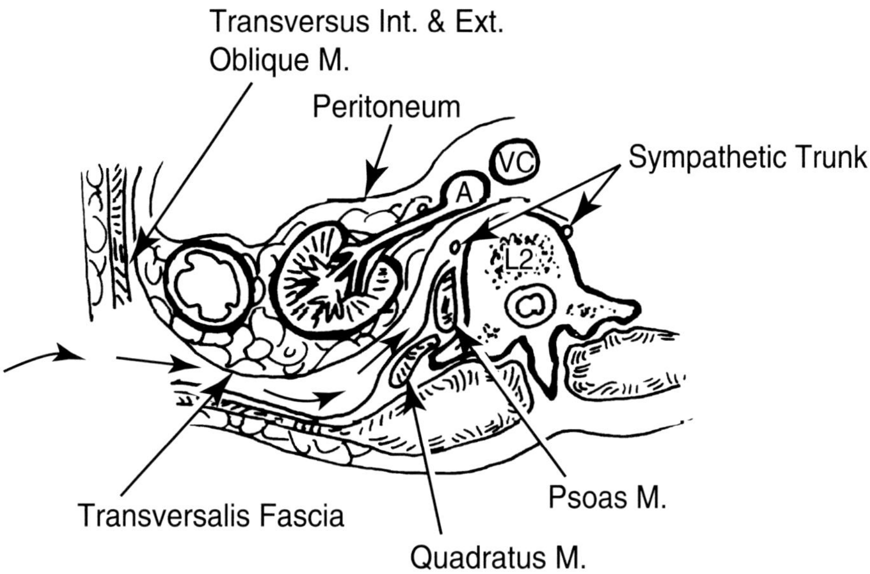

Figure 21. An axial view of the plane of dissection *(arrows)* for the retroperitoneal exposure of the lumbar spine.

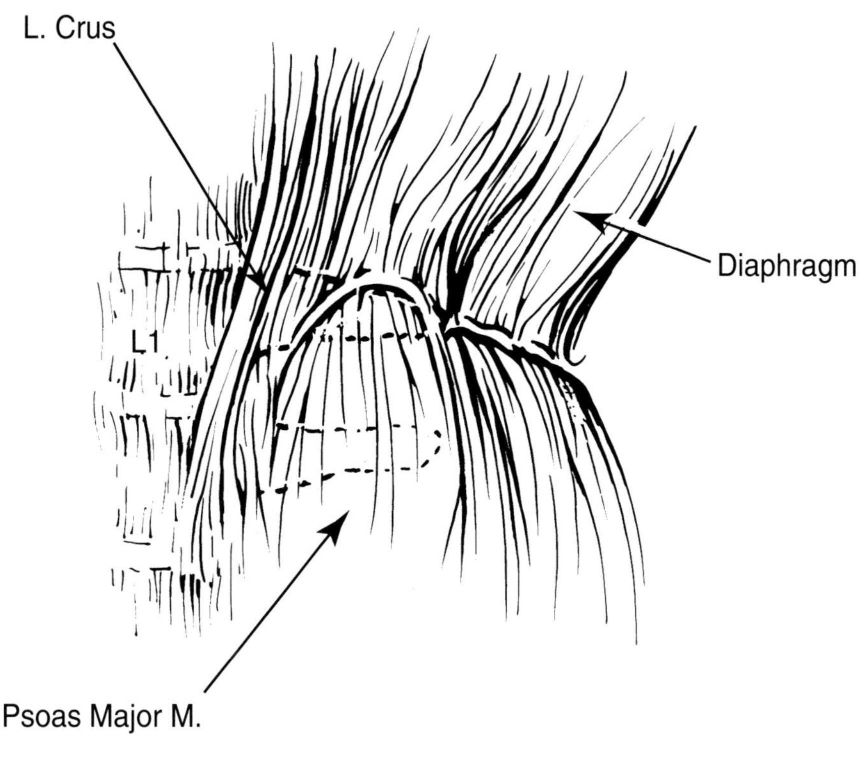

Figure 22. The arcuate ligaments and their attachments to the vertebral body and L1 transverse process (medial arcuate ligament) and the L1 transverse process and the 12th rib (lateral arcuate ligament).

reapproximation of diaphragmatic attachments and abdominal wall layers.

A transient ileus should be anticipated. In addition to wound complications, visceral injury is a potential, but infrequent, problem that is often related to overly vigorous retraction. Dissection and retraction of the sympathetic chain may additionally result in anhidrosis and flushing of the ipsilateral lower extremity.

Lumbar Region

Ventral lumbosacral approaches are generally limited to the retroperitoneal technique described above and the transperitoneal approach to L5-S1 (Table 1).

Retroperitoneal Exposure

Retroperitoneal approaches have become the procedures of choice for many surgeons performing direct ventral decompression, fusion, and instrumentation between the L1 and L4 levels. Advantages include simultaneous access to multiple vertebrae, the ventrolateral angle of approach, and avoidance of the lumbosacral plexus within the substance of the iliopsoas muscle. Because of the constraints of the overlying iliac crest, the lumbosacral lordosis, and the obstructing iliac vessels, the L5 and S1 region is poorly accessed through the retroperitoneum for procedures more extensive than biopsy or simple discectomy.

Transperitoneal Exposure

A direct ventral approach to the lumbosacral junction is afforded by the transperitoneal route. This technique has the advantage of being able to pack the abdominal viscera away from the working area, thus theoretically increasing exposure.

The abdomen is incised in a standard midline fashion, with the dissection being carried between the rectus abdominis muscles. After entering the peritoneal cavity, the bowel is packed rostrally and away from the sacral promontory. A break in the operating table centered under the lumbar lordosis, with slight Trendelenberg positioning of the table, facilitates this maneuver. A table-mounted retractor is useful as well. The bladder may be protected with a "bladder blade" retractor. The dorsal leaf of the peritoneum is then elevated and opened longitudinally over the lower aorta and iliac vessels. This is usually performed from the patient's right side in order to avoid undue trauma to the underlying superior hypogastric sympathetic plexus, which ramifies principally along the left side of the iliac bifurcation.[11,21] Attention should be paid to identify the ureter, as it typically crosses the external branch of the iliac artery. A plane is bluntly developed, working from right to left over the ventral aspect of the L5-S1 interspace for adequate exposure. This usually requires some degree of iliac vessel mobilization and gentle retraction. Electrocautery should be minimized in this area in order to avoid thermal injury to the hypogastric plexus. Great care also should be taken with the iliolumbar veins as they emerge from the iliac vein laterally and distal to the disc space. These structures are generally tightly tethered, and bleeding is difficult to control in the case of inadvertent tearing. Following decompression, fusion, and/or instrumentation procedures, closure involves merely approximating the dorsal peritoneum over the iliac vessels and a standard anatomical abdominal closure.

The main advantage of this approach is full direct ventral access at the L5-S1 junction. Some authors advocate the employment of this technique for extensive L5 vertebrectomy and interbody fusion procedures, when radical resection is indicated.[12] High-grade spondylolisthesis (spondyloptosis) and deficiency of the dorsal elements have been cited as indications for a transperitoneal approach in cases requiring radical resection and reconstruction in the region of the lumbosacral junction.[11,12] The technique suffers, however, from limited exposure (L5-S1 only), intra-abdominal trauma with prolonged ileus, the risk of great vessel injury, and the risk of superior hypogastric plexus injury. The latter may lead to retrograde ejaculation and/or sterility in males and bladder dysfunction in females. However, the reports of this complication with transperitoneal surgery are rare.[11]

Paraspinal Exposure

The standard technique for dorsal exposure of the lumbar spine varies little from that employed for upper spinal levels. With exposure of the transverse processes for dorsolateral fusion, care should be taken to utilize an adequate longitudinal incision. This will decrease the need for overly vigorous paraspinal muscle retraction which, in turn, will minimize muscle injury, swelling, bleeding, and postoperative discomfort. Generous debridement of devitalized paraspinal muscle also facilitates far lateral exposure when required for fusion and/or instrumentation.

The paraspinal approach described by Wiltse et al[23] is a modification of the dorsal approach by minimizing the morbidity of extensive muscle dissection. The technique involves bilateral paramedian incision and a muscle-splitting dissection between the erector spinae and multifidus muscles. This maneuver provides direct access to the intertransverse region and facet joint without access to the dorsal bony elements. The technique has been used for pedicle fixation and intertransverse fusion in cases not requiring a dorsal midline neural decompression.[23]

Dorsolateral Exposure

Lateral extracavitary techniques, as previously described, can be adapted for use in the lower lumbar and lumbosacral areas.[13] Technical points include the lack of a rib plane that guides the dissection in the thoracic spine, and the importance of protecting the distal lumbar nerve roots as they emerge and ramify within the substance of the iliopsoas muscle. This anatomical arrangement limits the lateral exposure of multiple vertebrae by this route and generally precludes most standard techniques of ventral lumbar instrumentation via the lateral extracavitary approach. Similarly, adequate access to the lumbosacral junction can be severely compromised by the overlying iliac crest (which interferes with a true lateral approach), the lordosis of the sacrum, and the difficulty in mobilizing the iliac vessels enough to allow significant dissection in this region. For these reasons, a direct transperitoneal route or a dorsal alternative may be a better choice for exposing this critical region of the spine.

References

1. Amundson G, Garfin SR: Minimizing blood loss during spine surgery, in Garfin SR (ed): **Complications of Spine Surgery.** Baltimore: Williams & Wilkins, 1989, pp 29-52
2. Breslau RC: Transaxillary approach to the upper dorsal spine, in Watkins RG (ed): **Surgical Approaches to the Spine**. New York: Springer-Verlag, 1983, pp 58-63
3. Capener N: The evolution of lateral rhachotomy. **J Bone Joint Surg (Br) 36:**173-179, 1954
4. Cauchoix J, Binet JP: Anterior surgical approaches to the spine. **Ann R Coll Surg Engl 21:** 234-243, 1957
5. Cloward RB: The anterior approach for removal of ruptured cervical disks. **J Neurosurg 15:** 602-617, 1958
6. Cotler HB, Kaldis MG: Anatomy and surgical approaches of the spine, in Cotler JM, Cotler HB (eds): **Spinal Fusion: Science and Technique**. New York: Springer-Verlag, 1990, pp 89-124
7. Cybulski GR: Thoracic disc herniation: surgical management. **Contemp Neurosurg 14(5):**1-4, 1992
8. Garrido E: Modified costotransversectomy: a surgical approach to ventrally placed lesions in the thoracic spinal canal. **Surg Neurol 13:**109-113, 1980
9. Hodgson AR, Stock FE, Fang HSY, et al: Anterior spinal fusion. The operative approach and pathological findings in 412 patients with Pott's disease of the spine. **Br J Surg 48:**172-178, 1960
10. Hodgson AR, Yau ACMC: Anterior surgical approaches to the spinal column, in Apley AG (ed): **Recent Advances in Orthopedics**. Baltimore: Williams & Wilkins, 1969, pp 289-323
11. Johnson RM, Murphy MJ, Southwick WO: Surgical approaches to the spine, in Rothman RH, Simeone FA (eds): **The Spine, ed 3.** Philadelphia: WB Saunders, 1992, pp 1607-1738
12. Kostuik JP: Surgical approaches to the thoracic and thoracolumbar spine, in Frymoyer JW (ed): **The Adult Spine: Principles and Practice**. New York: Raven Press, 1991, pp 1243-1266
13. Larson SJ, Holst RA, Hemmy DC: Lateral extracavitary approach to traumatic lesions of the thoracic and lumbar spine. **J Neurosurg 45:**628-637, 1976
14. Menard V: Causes de la paraplegie dans le mal de Pott. **Rev Orthop 5:**47-64, 1894
15. Nanson EM: The anterior approach to upper dorsal sympathectomy. **Surg Gynecol Obstet 104:** 118-120, 1957
16. Patterson RH Jr, Arbit E: A surgical approach through the pedicle to protruded thoracic discs. **J Neurosurg 48:**768-772, 1978
17. Rengachary SS: Posterior and posterolateral

surgical approaches to the spine, in Sudaresan N, Schmidek HH, Schiller AL, et al (eds): **Tumors of the Spine: Diagnosis and Clinical Management**. Philadelphia: WB Saunders, 1990, pp 488-493

18. Smith GW, Robinson RA: The treatment of certain cervical-spine disorders by anterior removal of the intervertebral disc and interbody fusion. **J Bone Joint Surg (Am) 40:**607-624, 1958

19. Southwick WO, Robinson RA: Surgical approaches to the vertebral bodies in the cervical and lumbar regions. **J Bone Joint Surg (Am) 39:**631-644, 1957

20. Sundaresan N, DiGiancinto GV: Surgical considerations and approaches, in Sudaresan N, Schmidek HH, Schiller AL, et al (eds): **Tumors of the Spine: Diagnosis and Clinical Management**. Philadelphia: WB Saunders, 1990, pp 358-379

21. Watkins RG: Cervical, thoracic, and lumbar complications—anterior approach, in Garfin SR (ed): **Complications of Spine Surgery**. Baltimore: Williams & Wilkins, 1989, pp 29-52

22. Watkins RG: **Surgical Approaches to the Spine**. New York: Springer-Verlag, 1983

23. Wiltse LL, Bateman JG, Hutchinson RH, et al: The paraspinal sacrospinalis-splitting approach to the lumbar spine. **J Bone Joint Surg (Am) 50:** 919-926, 1968

Chapter 13

Anatomically Based Management Strategies

Edward C. Benzel, MD, FACS

The three potential fundamental components of a spine operation are: 1) surgical indications that determine the instability and extent of neural element compression; 2) surgical exposure for neural element decompression and spinal fusion; and 3) spinal stabilization. Each are presented separately in this chapter, and each must, at least, be considered prior to embarking on even the simplest of operations.

In a similar vein, there are two basic indications for spine surgery: spinal instability and persistent neural element compression. They are, however, independent of each other, and are discussed separately herein. Acute and chronic forms of instability are also addressed separately.

Much of the information presented in this chapter has been gleaned from previous works.[2,3] Adaptations have been referenced, when appropriate.

Surgical Indication Determination: Instability

White and Panjabi[16] define clinical stability of the spine as "... the ability of the spine under physiologic loads to limit patterns of displacement so as not to damage or irritate the spinal cord or nerve roots and, in addition, to prevent incapacitating deformity or pain due to structural changes." It is often simpler and more clinically practical to consider the converse of stability, i.e., instability. This may facilitate clinical decision-making. Instability is defined as "the inability to limit excessive spinal displacement."[3] The two fundamental categories of instability are: acute and chronic. These may be subcategorized, as follows:

- Acute instability
  - Overt instability
  - Limited instability
- Chronic instability
  - Glacial instability
  - Dysfunctional segmental motion (mechanical instability)

These categories and subcategories are of significant clinical importance, as depicted in the pages that follow.

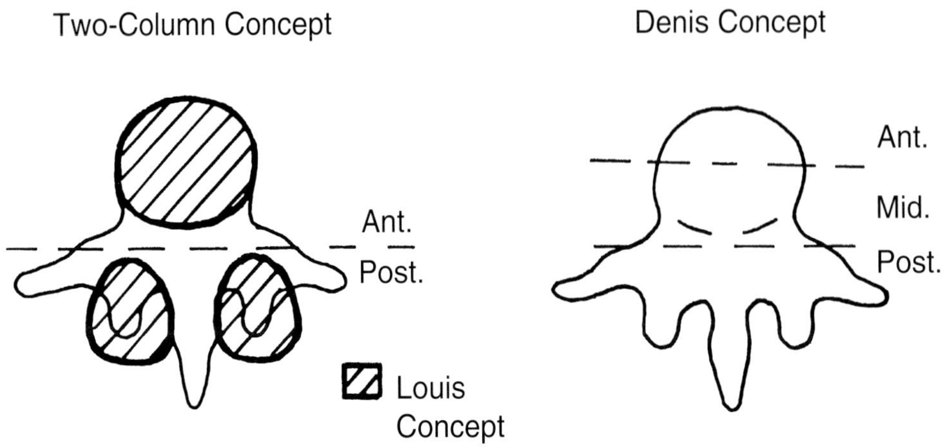

Figure 1. The column concepts of spinal instability. The concept described by Louis[14] **(left)** lends significance to the vertebral body and the facet joint complexes (lateral masses) on either side of the dorsal spine. The three-column concept of Denis[9] **(right)** lends significance to the region of the neutral axis and the integrity of the dorsal vertebral body wall (the middle column). The two-column construct **(left)** relies on anatomically defined structures: the vertebral body (anterior column) and the dorsal elements (posterior column). Louis' three-column concept **(left)** similarly relies on anatomically defined structures.

The Quantitation of Acute Instability

Flexion and extension x-rays may not be useful, or may even be misleading, in diagnosing acute instability.[3,10,11] Instability definition schemes are often based, to one degree or another, on a "column" concept of spinal structural integrity, such as the three-column theory described by Louis;[14] the two-column concept of Bailey,[1] Holdsworth,[12] and Kelly and Whitesides;[13] or the three-column concept proposed by Denis[9] (Figure 1). These schemes are of value on the basis of physician conceptualization assistance only,[2] as they do not truly reflect anatomically or biomechanically relevant information. Nevertheless, the three-column (anterior and two lateral column) theory of Louis is effective in assisting the assessment of bony integrity, because it allows the conceptualization of the bony columns of the spine. It can be quantitated by assessing the extent of collapse or fracture of the vertebral body and the two lateral columns (facet joint complexes or lateral masses).[2]

The two-column concept of Bailey,[1] Holdsworth,[12] and Kelly and Whitesides,[13] and the three-column theory of Denis[9] are more applicable to the clinical situation. They consider both bony and soft tissue integrity (Figure 1). Both of these theories lack anatomical correlation. For example, the middle column of Denis' theory has no anatomical structural analog. However, the anterior column of the two-column theory and the middle column of the three-column theory of Denis encompass the neutral axis (Figure 2) and are thus more clinically relevant in this regard. The use of these schemes, however, may provide insight into clinical situations.

The use of clinically appropriate definitions of instability types is paramount regarding the determination of clinically relevant stability information.

A Point System for Acute Instability Quantitation

A point system that assesses the extent of acute spinal instability is presented in Table 1.[2,3] It is a modification of previous attempts at instability quantitation.[16] It is only useful for acute instability (i.e., overt and limited instability). Five or greater points indicates overt insta-

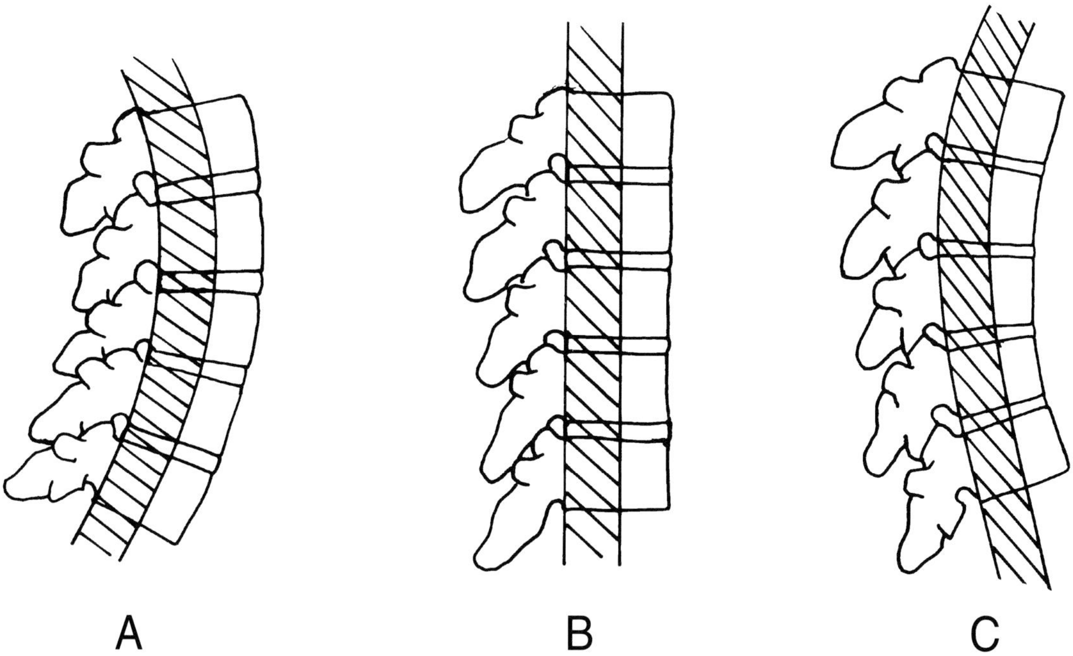

Figure 2. The depiction of the neutral axis *(shaded areas).* The neutral axis is the longitudinal region of the spinal column that bears much of the axial load and about which spinal element distraction or compression does not significantly occur with the assumption of flexed **(A),** neutral **(B),** or extension **(C)** postures.

Table 1. **Quantitation of Acute Instability for Subaxial Cervical, Thoracic, and Lumbar Injuries***

Loss of integrity of anterior (and middle) column+	2
Loss of integrity of posterior column(s)+	2
Acute resting translational deformity†	2
Acute resting angulation deformity†	2
Acute dynamic translational deformity exaggeration§	2
Acute dynamic angulation deformity exaggeration§	2
Neural element injury**	3
Acute disc narrowing at level of suspected pathology	1
Dangerous loading anticipated	1

*Modified from White and Panjabi[16] with care taken to avoid duplication or overlapping of point criteria. Point system: ≥ 5 points implies the presence of overt instability; 2-4 points implies the presence of limited instability.

+By clinical examination, magnetic resonance imaging (MRI), computed tomography (CT), or x-ray. One point only may be allotted if incomplete evidence exists (e.g., only MRI evidence of posterior ligamentous injury, that is, evidence of only interspinous ligament injury on T2-weighted images). Columns are defined as per Bailey,[1] Denis,[9] and Louis.[14]

†From static resting anteroposterior and lateral spine x-rays. Must be the result of an acute clinical process. Tolerance for this criteria is variable with respect to surgeon and clinical circumstances. Guidelines as per White and Panjabi.[16]

§From dynamic (flexion and extension) spine x-rays. Only recommended after other mechanisms of instability assessment have been exhausted and then only by an experienced clinician. Usually only indicated in the cervical region. Must be the result of an acute clinical process. Tolerance for this criteria is variable with respect to the surgeon's opinion and clinical circumstances. Guidelines as per White and Panjabi.[16]

**Neural element: 3 points for cauda equina, 2 points for spinal cord, or 1 point for isolated nerve root neurological deficit. The presence of neural element injury indicates that a significant spinal deformation occurred at the time of impact, implying that structural integrity may have been disrupted.

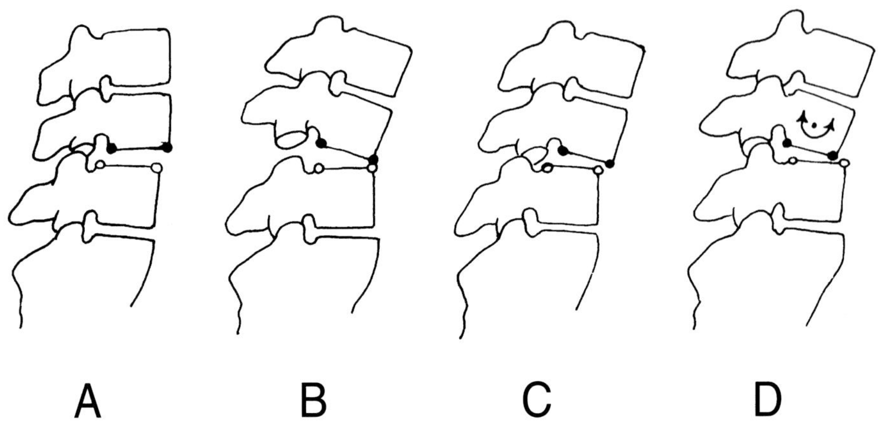

Figure 3. Dysfunctional segmental motion is present if a smooth flexion or extension at the motion segment in question does not occur. This can be assessed by determining the location of the instantaneous axis of rotation. Several types of dysfunctional segmental movement can occur: true translation **(A),** excessive angulation (with flexion or extension) without translation **(B),** translation with angulation **(C),** and pivotal movement about a pathological axis **(D).**

bility, 2-4 points limited instability, and 0-1 point a stable spine. *The spine surgeon must rely upon and liberally utilize common sense, combined with clinical astuteness.* If this or any other scheme is employed without the use of the latter, errors will be common. There is no substitute for common sense.[2,3]

Overt Instability

Overt instability is defined as the inability of the spine to support the torso during normal activity.[2,3] This type of instability may be caused by trauma, surgical intervention, neoplasia, advanced degenerative disease, or infection. With overt instability, the integrity of the spine is insufficient to prevent deformation. In this situation, the loss of integrity of the vertebral body and/or disc interspace is associated with a loss of integrity of dorsal elements (i.e., a circumferential loss of spinal integrity).[2,3]

Dorsal ligamentous disruption may be best assessed by clinical examination and magnetic resonance imaging (MRI).[2,4,15] MRI may, therefore, be useful to assess overt instability. The point system depicted in Table 1 uses MRI for the delineation of soft tissue disruption detection (e.g., the demonstration of posterior column disruption).[2]

Limited Instability

Lesser injuries (compared to overt instability) are often controversial regarding the extent of stability definition and operative indication determination.[2,3] These cases are associated with limited instability. Limited instability is defined as the loss of ventral *or* dorsal spinal integrity, with the preservation of the other. The spine so involved is sufficiently stable to support some normal activity.[2,3]

Overt and limited instability may be confused with each other. The true extent of loss of ventral and dorsal spinal integrity may be underestimated. Furthermore, deformity progression may ensue and, in fact, overt instability may evolve into glacial instability.

MRI is less helpful regarding the definition of extent of injury in the late postinjury situation. This is so because of the absence of acute soft tissue injury changes that were present at the time of the initial injury.

Chronic Instability

Glacial Instability

Glacial instability is a type of spinal instability that is neither acute nor associated with a significant chance for the rapid development or progression of kyphotic, scoliotic, or translational deformities, but, like a glacier, the deformity progresses gradually with time whereas substantial external forces do not cause movement or progression of deformity.[2,3] As previously addressed, since acute soft tissue injury is not a characteristic of chronic forms of instability, MRI is not helpful regarding the determination of the extent of instability. Spine x-rays, however, may demonstrate deformity progression over time.

Dysfunctional Segmental Motion

A dysfunctional motion segment does not involve the overt disruption of spinal integrity nor deformity progression. Most clinical situations involving glacial instability are also associated with dysfunctional segmental motion. All types of glacial instability, however, are associated with deformity progression. Dysfunctional segmental motion is defined as "a type of instability (with or without overtly obvious abnormal segmental motion [Figure 3]) that is related to disc interspace or vertebral body degenerative changes, tumor, or infection that results in the potential for pain of spinal origin."[3] This has also been termed "mechanical instability."[2]

The presence of a characteristic pain pattern (usually worsened by activity and improved by rest and torso positioning in such a manner that spinal stresses are minimized) is suggestive of the diagnosis. This characteristic pain pattern, when associated with degenerative disc interspace changes, tumor, or infection involving the disc interspace, vertebral body, or other vertebral component, suggests the diagnosis of dysfunctional motion segment.[2] The diagnosis may be obvious on the basis of flexion/extension x-rays alone. Often, however, only indirect evidence of its existence is present, including such situations as degenerative disc interspace changes or osteophyte formation. For these radiographic changes to have occurred, excessive stresses or motion must have been placed upon the motion segment(s).

Determining Surgical Indication: Extent of Neural Element Compression

A neurological deficit or symptom that is consistent with the imaging findings may be indication enough for surgery. Exceptions, however, may exist. For example, the presence of a complete myelopathy (no neurological function below the spinal level of the injury) is associated with a minimal, if any, chance for neurological recovery, regardless of whether accompanied by a neural decompression operation.[5,6,8] Therefore, decompression surgery may not be indicated. On the other hand, this patient may benefit from surgery in other ways, namely, the acquisition of spinal stability.

Surgical Exposure, Decompression, and Fusion

Once the decision to operate has been made, it is mandatory to determine the optimal surgical approach to the spine for each of the components of the planned operation. These include: 1) neural element decompression; 2) fusion; and 3) spinal stabilization. If a neural element decompression component of an operation is to be performed, this aspect takes precedence over the others because of: 1) the relative importance of neural element decompression; 2) the fact that stabilization procedures can alter the relationships of compressive lesions with the neural elements in an adverse manner; and 3) the fact that decompression operations often further destabilize the spine.[2]

The orientation of the imaging studies performed can affect the surgeon's interpretation of the pathological anatomy. It, therefore, may be prudent to obtain imaging studies in more than one plane (Figure 4).

The destabilizing effects of a decompres-

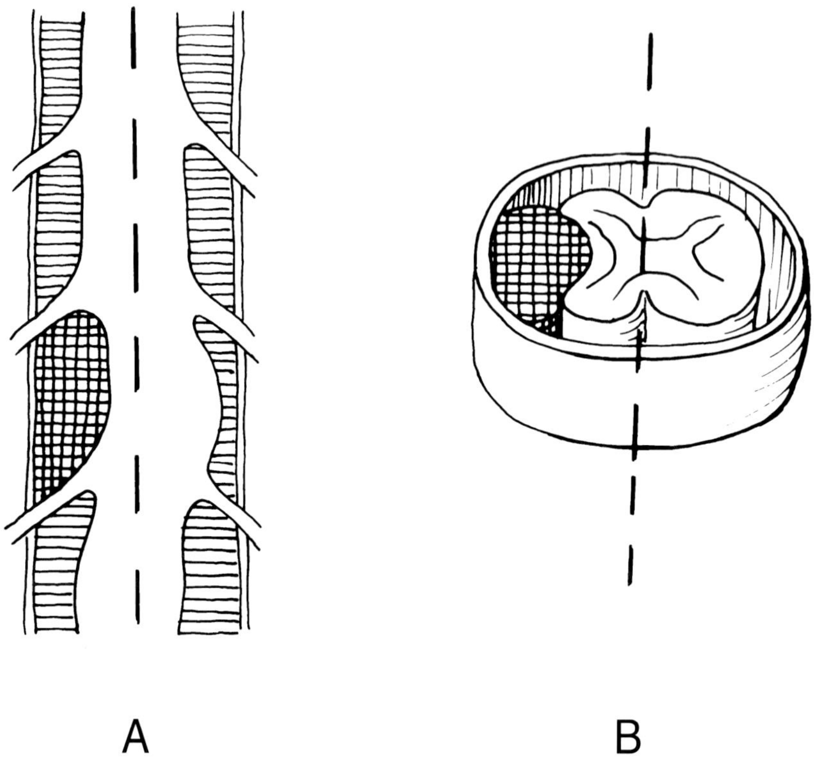

Figure 4. A laterally impinging mass may be missed by sagittal imaging through the *dotted line* of **(A)** and **(B).** Therefore, coronal myelographic or MRI **(A),** or axial CT or MRI **(B)** studies may be critical.

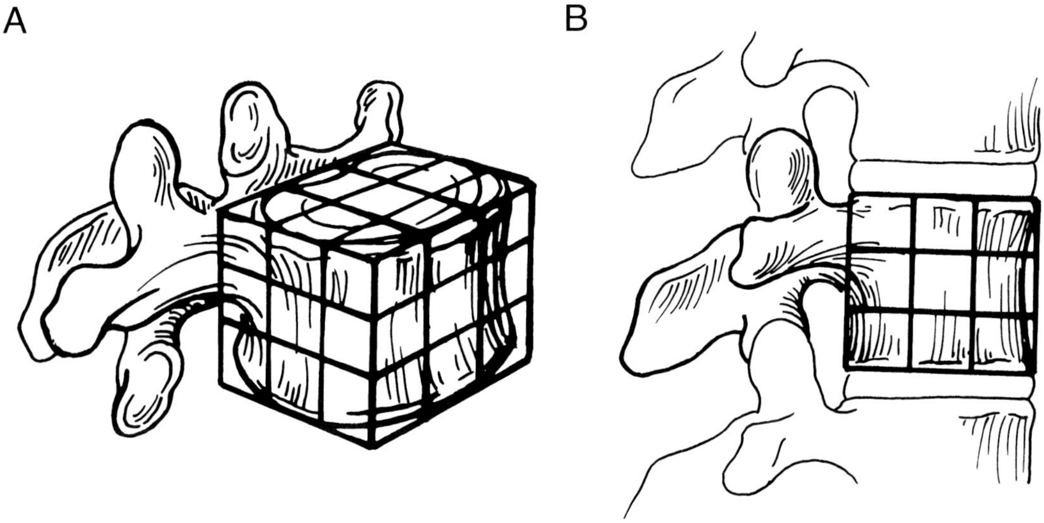

Figure 5A-B. A depiction of a cubical (hypothetical) vertebral body composed of 27 equal, smaller cubes (3 x 3 x 3) in a slightly oblique axial view **(A)** and a lateral view **(B).**

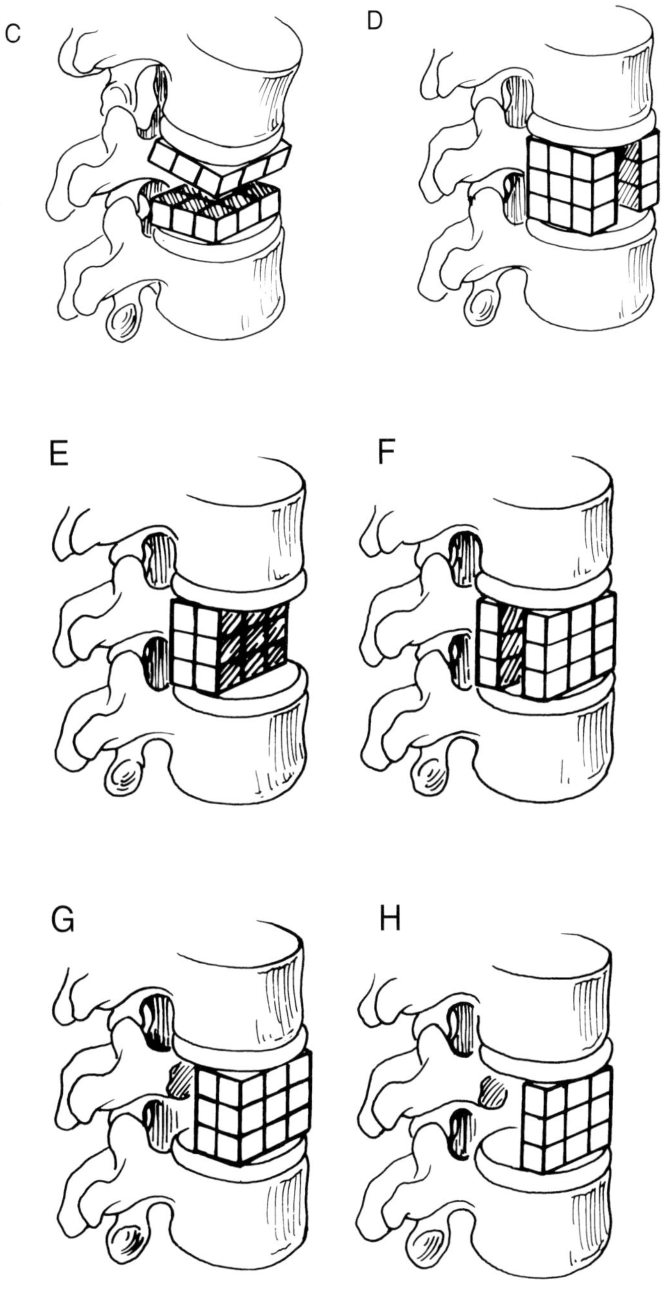

Figure 5C-H. A resection or disruption of the middle axial (horizontal) one-third of the vertebral body, as might occur after trauma, is depicted **(C).** A resection of the middle sagittal (vertical) one-third of the vertebral body is depicted **(D).** Note that the resection depicted in **(C)** destabilizes the spine, whereas the resection depicted in **(D)** does not, despite the fact that both bony resections were of a similar magnitude (similar volume of bone resected). Partial vertebrectomies involving removal of the ventral portion of the vertebral body (in the coronal plane) **(E)** affects stability greater than if the middle **(F)** or dorsal **(G)** portion of the vertebral body (in the coronal plane) were resected. This assumes that an intact posterior column is present. In fact, a resection of the middle and dorsal one-third of the vertebral body (in the presence of an intact posterior column and an intact ventral one-third of the vertebral body) may not significantly disrupt spinal integrity **(H).**

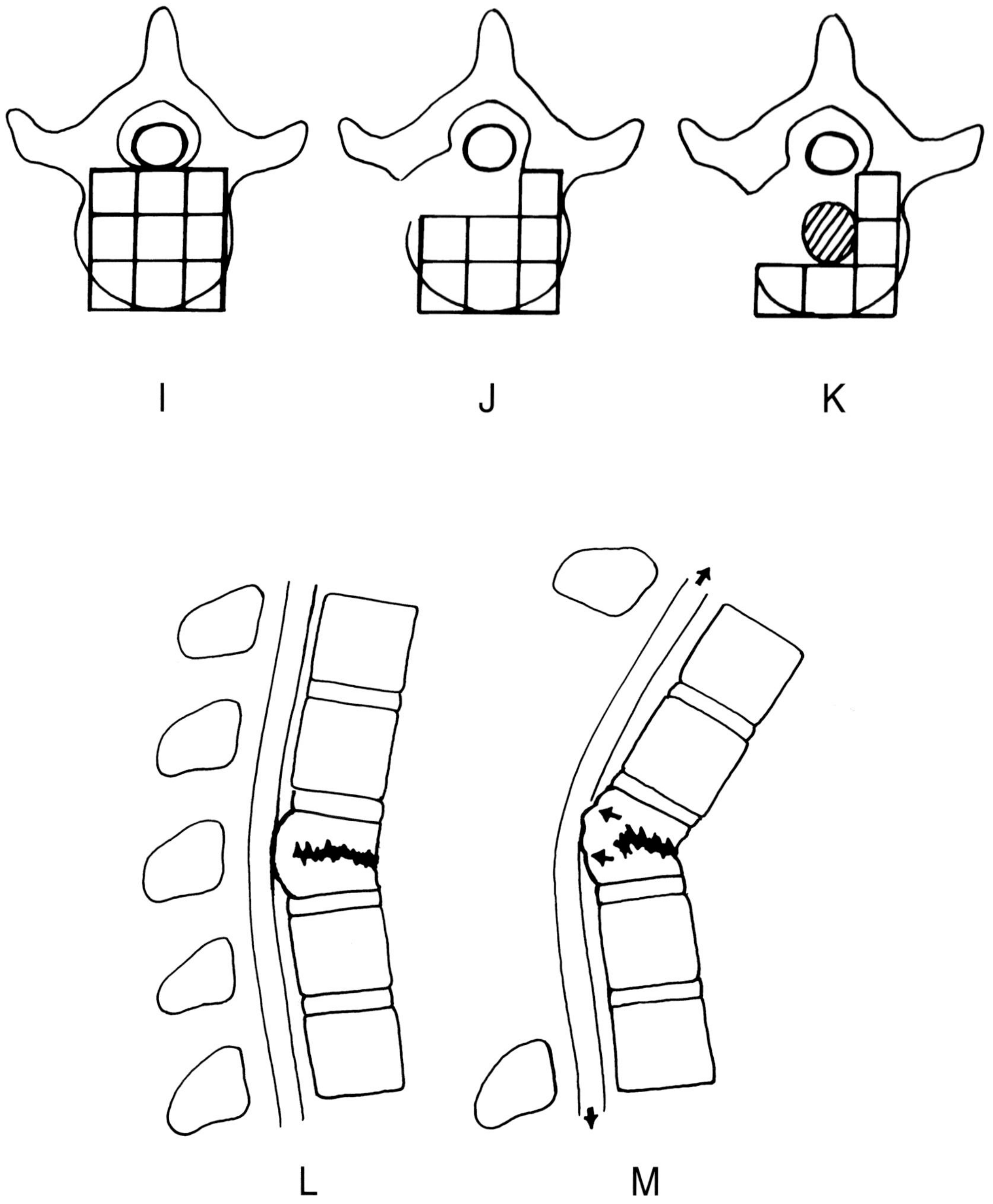

Figure 5I-M. The 27-cube hypothetical cubical vertebral body can be used to depict the bony resection accomplished via a lateral extracavitary decompression of the thoracic or lumbar dural sac. A preoperative view of the spine **(I).** The restriction of bony resection to the most dorsal aspect of the vertebral body allows a substantial amount of preservation of the bony integrity **(J).** Further bony resection is then required for strut graft placement. The final extent of bone removal, with the bone graft in place, is depicted **(K).**

The preoperative **(L)** and postoperative **(M)** sagittal views of a flexion deformity exaggeration after laminectomy are depicted. Note the neural distortion by distraction *(vertical arrows)* and tethering over the ventral compression *(horizontal arrows).*[2,3]

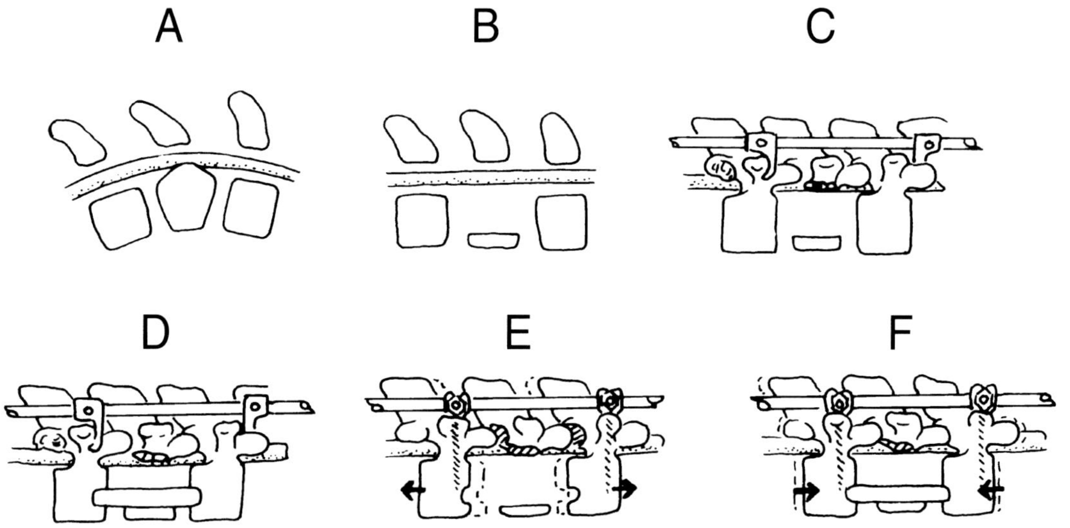

Figure 6. For most ventral interbody bone-grafting situations, the appropriate order of procedural components is to: 1) perform a neural element decompression and accomplish spinal alignment (**A** and **B**); 2) perform a spinal stabilization procedure **(C);** and 3) place the bone graft **(D).** An obvious exception is a situation where it is mandatory to place the bone graft before the instrumentation construct placement. In the case depicted, the bone graft is placed prior to the instrumentation construct. This, in fact, may be used to an advantage in a situation where the dynamics of the reconstruction of the pathology may be augmented by the application of bone healing-enhancing forces intraoperatively. In this situation, the decompression may be accomplished first **(B).** Then, the pathological segments may be distracted by the implant (in this case via pedicle fixation) *(arrows)* **(E)** and the bone graft inserted. Finally, the construct may be compressed *(arrows)* **(F)**, thus allowing for the accomplishment of load-sharing between the ventral interbody bony structures and the dorsal instrumentation construct.[2,3]

sion operation should be carefully scrutinized before, during, and following the operation. This destabilizing effect most certainly alters instrumentation or decompression plans (Figure 5).

Surgical Exposure

The orientation of the approach for the surgical exposure is primarily dictated by the orientation of the planned neural decompression operation. Particularly with ventral decompression operations, the decompression and fusion are usually performed through the same surgical exposure.

In general, for most combined ventral decompression, fusion, and instrumentation procedures, the order in which the operations should be performed is: 1) neural decompression; 2) placement and attainment of spinal implant, with the simultaneous attainment of spinal stability; and 3) the placement of the fusion (Figure 6).[7] Obviously, situations may exist that alter this sequence; for example, plate interference with fusion placement during ventral cervical fusion and plating operations.

Often, the best method of depicting what is achieved via a particular surgical exposure is by thinking in terms of axial "views." These are depicted for the thoracic and lumbar spine in Figure 7.[2]

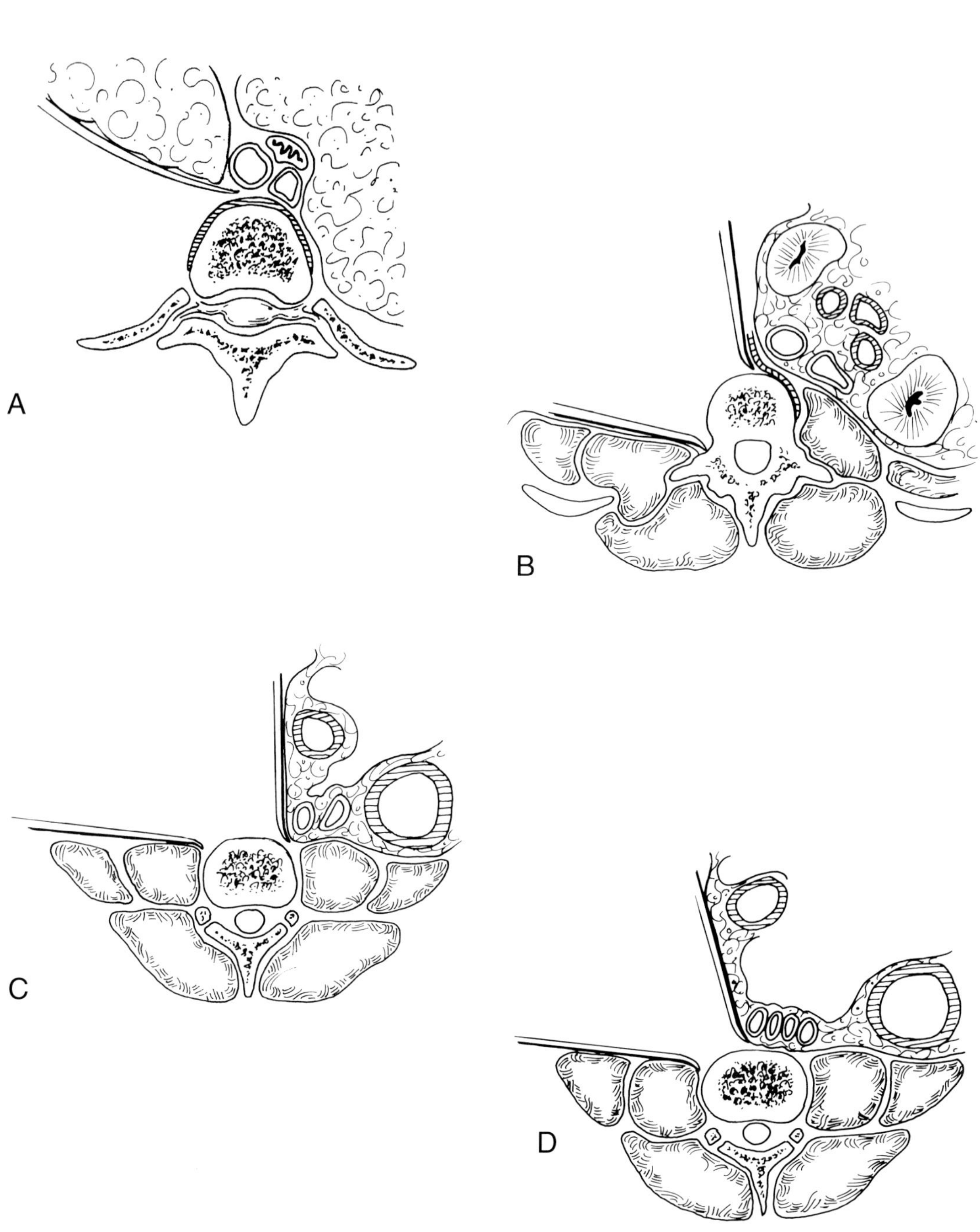

Figure 7A-D. Axial depictions of various approaches to the thoracic and lumbar spine. **A)** The ventrolateral transthoracic approach to the spine. **B)** The transdiaphragmatic approach to the thoracolumbar spine. Note the significant soft tissue violation required for this approach. **C)** The ventrolateral extraperitoneal approach to the lumbar spine. **D)** The pelvic brim extraperitoneal approach to the low lumbar spine. Note that the vertebral body exposure is less than that achieved with more routine approaches due to the confinements related to the iliac vessels.

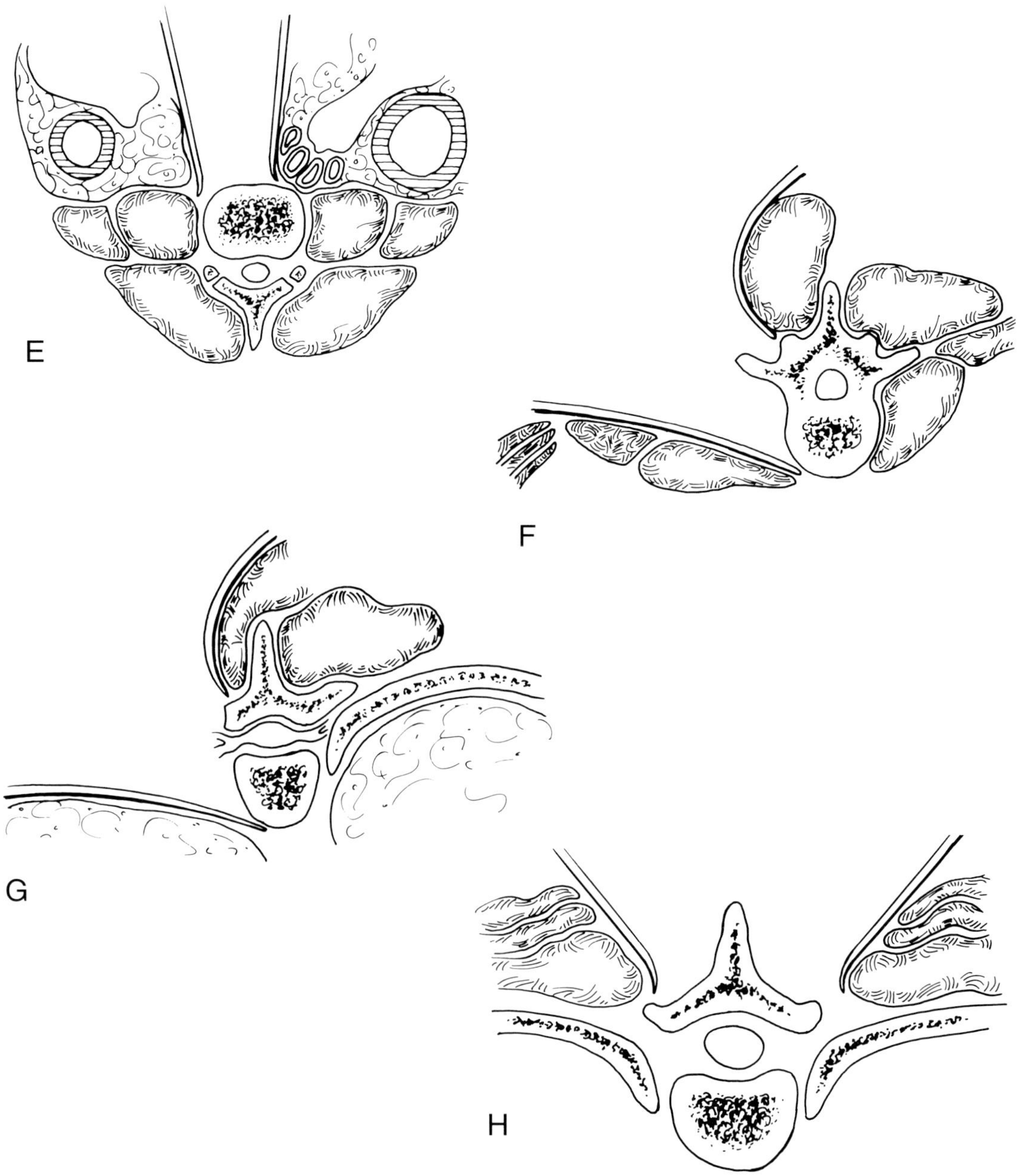

Figure 7E-H. E) The transperitoneal approach to the low lumbar and lumbosacral spine. **F)** The lateral extracavitary approach to the lumbar spine. **G)** The lateral transcavitary approach to the thoracic spine. **H)**The dorsal approach to the subaxial spine.[2,3]

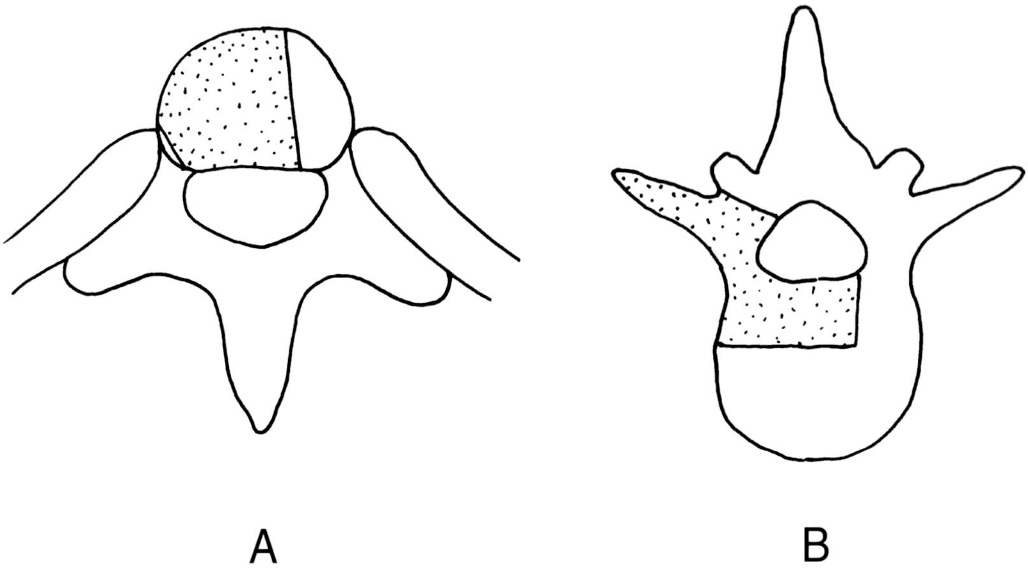

Figure 8. Axial depictions of the ventral and lateral operative exposures of the dural sac. **A)** Ventrolateral transthoracic, transdiaphragmatic thoracolumbar, ventrolateral extraperitoneal lumbar spine, extraperitoneal low lumbar spine, pelvic brim extraperitoneal low lumbar spine, and transperitoneal low lumbar spine. **B)** Lateral extracavitary and lateral transcavitary thoracic and lumbar spine.[2,3]

Neural Element Decompression

In general, compressive lesions located ventral to the dural sac should be decompressed from a ventral exposure and dorsal lesions should be decompressed dorsally. It is emphasized that it is the decompression aspect of the operation that ultimately dictates the approaches used for the fusion and implant placement components. In this vein, it may be beneficial to consider the extent of decompression achievable via the variety of surgical exposures available to the surgeon. Ventral dural sac decompression, via a variety of surgical exposures, is depicted in Figures 8 and 9.

Although ventral surgical exposures decompress the dural sac via direct vision, they provide inadequate surgical exposure for dorsal spinal implant placement.

Ventral surgical exposures may be associated with an unexpected element of risk. The visualization of the dural sac is not achieved until the vertebrectomy is complete. Furthermore, ventral surgical exposures are usually performed through deep wounds. Both may aggravate the surgeon's ability to appropriately protect the dural sac during decompression and, thus, to perform an adequate and safe operation. On the other hand, the lateral and dorsal approaches provide the opportunity to visualize the dural sac prior to its decompression.

The lateral and dorsal operations provide a variable extent of ventral dural sac decompression (Figure 8). A wide variation of surgical angles of view are achieved. Of significance is that the costotransversectomy and lateral extracavitary surgical exposures approach the spine from medial and lateral sides of the erector spinae muscle mass, respectively. An additional 20° in the ventral dural sac surgical viewing angle is attained

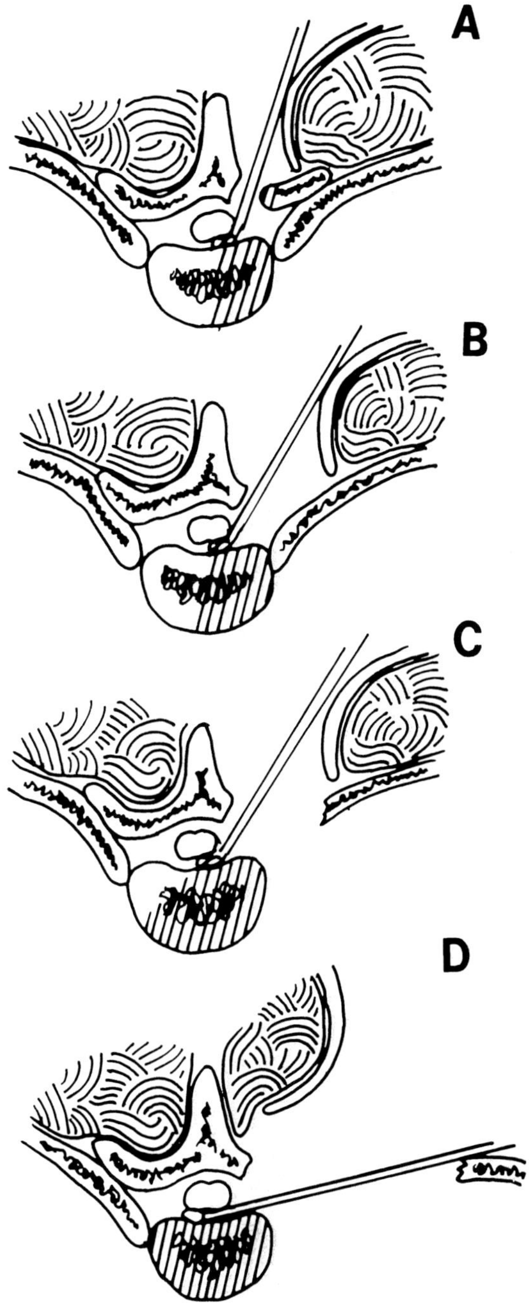

Figure 9. Axial depictions of the potential ventral dural sac decompression achieved via a reverse-angled curette through the variety of dorsal surgical exposures: **A)** laminectomy; **B)** transpedicle approach; **C)** costotransversectomy approach; and **D)** lateral extracavitary approach. Note that the differentiation between the costotransversectomy approach and the lateral extracavitary approach is predominantly via the direction of the retraction of the erector spinae muscle (medial for the lateral extracavitary and lateral for the costotransversectomy approach). Also note that an approximately 20° to 40° angle of view advantage for ventral dural sac decompression is realized with the lateral extracavitary approach vs. the costotransversectomy approach. Resection of the erector spinae muscle eliminates much of this difference.[2,3]

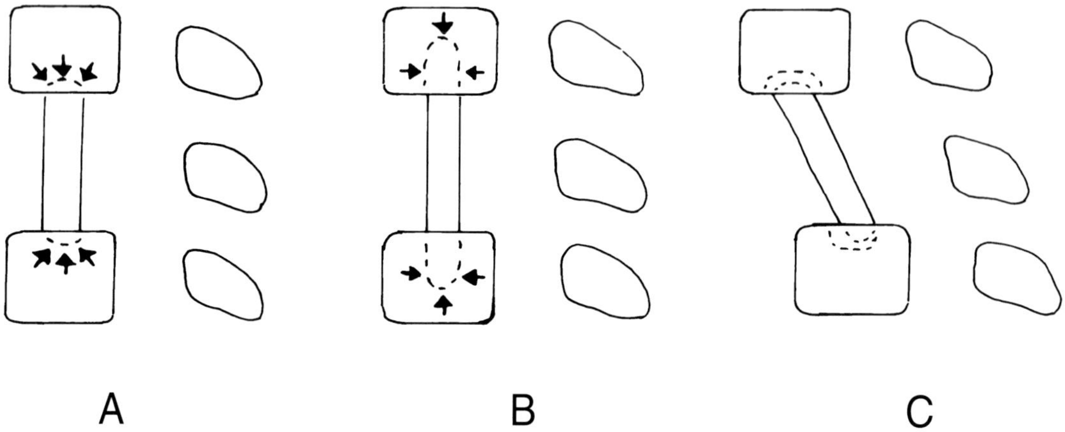

Figure 10. If the only stresses resisted by an interbody bone graft are axial, the bone graft itself only functions in a distraction or axial load-resisting mode **(A).** The creation of a deep mortise in the vertebral bodies can provide some translation resistance if the integrity of the vertebral body and the bone graft are adequate, the mortise is deep enough, and the bone graft and the mortise are fashioned meticulously **(B).** If the mortise is not so constructed and is exposed to shear stress (and circumferential instability [overt instability] is present), the construct may fail via a "pole-vaulting" mechanism **(C).**[2,3]

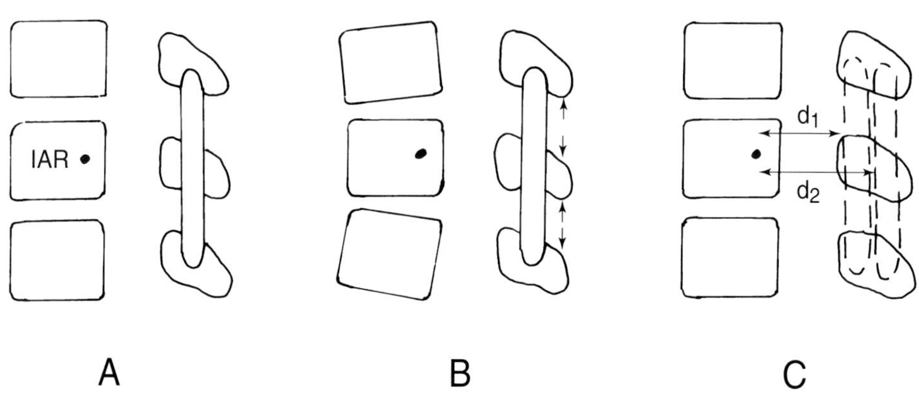

Figure 11. Acutely, a dorsal bone graft does not resist axial loads well **(A).** Flexion causes distraction of all points dorsal to the instantaneous axis of rotation (IAR, the axis about which a vertebral segment rotates). This causes a dorsal bone graft to be exposed to bone-healing-inhibiting (distracting) forces *(arrows)* **(B).** Upon maturation of a dorsal fusion, the graft itself can resist significant flexion deformation, if adequate axial load-resisting abilities are present. This is accomplished by applying a flexion-resisting moment arm. The longer the moment arm, the greater the flexion deformation prevention ability. d_1 and d_2 depict a short- and long-moment arm, respectively **(C).**[2,3]

by viewing the spine from under this muscle mass (i.e., via the lateral extracavitary surgical exposure).[2]

Spinal Fusion

Situations exist where a fusion and decompression are not optimally achieved through the same exposure. Multiple additional considerations also may be present, depending on the clinical situation, including the availability of autogenous bone, the ability of the patient to withstand the surgical scheme planned, biomechanical considerations, and the armamentarium of the surgeon. In a situation where decompression and fusion are not optimally achieved through the same exposure, alternative exposures for each component or the utilization of an accompanying instrumentation construct to augment both stability and the fusion rate may be appropriate.

Finally, the location of bone graft plays a role regarding both acute (Figure 10) and long-term (Figure 11) stability. Acutely, interbody grafts provide stability to one degree or another (Figure 10), whereas dorsal grafts do not (Figure 11). After maturation of a dorsal fusion, however, translation and flexion-extension deformation resistance (but not significant axial load-induced deformation resistance) are provided by dorsal fusions (Figure 11).[2]

References

1. Bailey RW: Fractures and dislocations of the cervical spine. Orthopedic and neurosurgical aspects. **Postgrad Med 35:**588-599, 1964
2. Benzel EC: The anatomic basis of spinal instability. **Clin Neurosurg 41:**224-241, 1993
3. Benzel EC: **Biomechanics of Spinal Stabilization: Principles and Clinical Practice.** New York: McGraw-Hill, 1995
4. Benzel EC, Hart BL, Ball PA, et al: The definition by MR imaging of soft-tissue injury associated with acute cervical spine trauma. **J Neurosurg 78:**355A, 1993 (Abstract)
5. Benzel EC, Larson SJ: Operative stabilization of the posttraumatic thoracic and lumbar spine: a comparative analysis of the Harrington distraction rod and the modified Weiss spring. **Neurosurgery 19:**378-385, 1986
6. Benzel EC, Larson SJ: Functional recovery after decompressive operation for thoracic and lumbar spine fractures. **Neurosurgery 19:**772-778, 1986
7. Benzel EC, Larson SJ: Recovery of nerve root function after complete quadriplegia from cervical spine fractures. **Neurosurgery 19:**809-812, 1986
8. Benzel EC, Larson SJ: Functional recovery after decompressive spine operation for cervical spine fractures. **Neurosurgery 20:**742-746, 1987
9. Denis F: The three column spine and its significance in the classification of acute thoracolumbar spine injuries. **Spine 8:**817-831, 1983
10. Dvorak J, Panjabi MM, Chang DG, et al: Functional radiographic diagnosis of the lumbar spine. Flexion-extension and lateral bending. **Spine 16:**562-571, 1991
11. Dvorak J, Panjabi MM, Novotny JE, et al: Clinical validation of functional flexion-extension roentgenograms of the lumbar spine. **Spine 16:**943-950, 1991
12. Holdsworth FW: Fractures, dislocations and fracture-dislocations of the spine. **J Bone Joint Surg (Br) 45:**6-20, 1963
13. Kelly RP, Whitesides TE Jr: Treatment of lumbodorsal fracture-dislocations. **Ann Surg 167:**705-717, 1968
14. Louis R: Spinal stability as defined by the three-column spine concept. **Anat Clin 7:**33-42, 1985
15. Orrison WW, Hart BL, Benzel EC, et al: MRI, CT and plain film comparison in acute cervical spine trauma. **Neurosurgery** (In press)
16. White AA, Panjabi MM: **Clinical Biomechanics of the Spine, ed 2.** Philadelphia: JB Lippincott, 1990, pp 30-342

Index

Page numbers for figures and tables are followed by *f* and *t*, respectively.

A

B

C

D

E

F

H

I

L

M

N

O

P

R

S

T

U

V